Patient-Centered Primary Care

Alexander Blount

Patient-Centered Primary Care

Getting From Good to Great

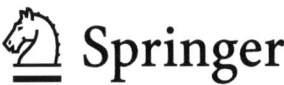 Springer

Alexander Blount, EdD
Department of Clinical Psychology
Antioch University New England
Keene, NH, USA

ISBN 978-3-030-17644-0   ISBN 978-3-030-17645-7   (eBook)
https://doi.org/10.1007/978-3-030-17645-7

This Springer imprint is published by the registered company Springer Nature Switzerland AG.
The registered company address is: Gewerbestrasse 11, 6330 Cham, Switzerland

For Francesca

Foreword

For those of us laboring for the betterment of primary care, this modest volume by Sandy Blount is of outsized, even monumental, importance. Our efforts at advancing the field, and thereby improving primary care, have been stultified along the way by a number of complications and difficulties. This book – exquisitely turned, perfectly timed – explains how we got here, dissects the elements of primary care that stubbornly resist improvement, and describes a way forward that is entirely within our capacities.

Let me call out a few markers along this path to better care. Fifty years ago, we catalogued the problems that primary care patients presented with and understood those problems as the content of primary care. We soon discovered the staggering prevalence and clinical importance of chronic diseases in our practices and, in tackling the rudiments of chronic disease management, realized that *how* we practice is as important as the clinical content we had so carefully documented. We adopted registries, care managers, team-based care, and other components of chronic disease management programs. It quickly became evident that multimorbidity, the norm for most of our patients, does not yield to a disease-by-disease approach, and we began formulating *personal* care plans, rather than disease care plans, that give primacy to the patient's individuality. Early on, some advocated for incorporating the mental, emotional, and behavioral elements of care into the fabric of all personal care plans; in fact, behavioral scientists and clinicians were a feature of many first-generation patient-centered medical homes, but their role in this expanded version of a primary care team has always been somewhat ambiguous – or at least variable. Along the way, Barbara Starfield et al. elucidated the elements of primary care that confer value, and in 1994, the IOM enshrined these essential features of primary care into a definition that has held fast to this day. These elements – access, personal relationship, comprehensiveness, coordinated care, continuity, and practicing in the context of family and community – are highly variable in their ease of implementation.

Meanwhile, technological "advances" and changes in our nation's healthcare system – the EHR and the unfulfilled promise of access to useful clinical and practice information, the availability of patients to online information that is highly variable in quality and accuracy, the compelling incentives toward productivity over quality, and the advancing hegemony of the pharmaceutical and hospital system industries – continually knock us off course and require adjustments just to avoid losing ground.

Despite these headwinds, we're making progress – primary care is getting better. We should not overlook how variable this progress is across our nation's practices and clinics and should remember that each practice will have its own particular problems to solve, but taken as a whole, primary care is getting better – even though progress just seems to be harder and take longer than it should and always seems to come at a cost that also needs to be recovered. Advanced practices have accomplished, at great cost, relatively dramatic changes in their practice operations, with demonstrably better quality of care for, say, chronic diseases, but so far, the translation of these quality improvements into actual health improvements has been disappointing.

Dr. Blount comes in at this point and explains how the structural, practice-level changes we've made so far are necessary but not sufficient for the improvements in health that we hope for. He makes the case that up to this point, our rhetoric about patient centeredness has far outstripped our actual practice, and our next great push needs to be the creation of substantive, meaningful partnerships with patients – making them fully vested members of their own care team. We've heard this before, and there have been noteworthy efforts to this end – facts that Dr. Blount fully credits and describes. Chapter 4, entitled Getting from "Delivering Care to Patients" to "Partnership with Patients," is one of the most radical in the book. Here, Dr. Blount describes the elements of true patient partnership, how previous efforts at this have been helpful and partially successful but ultimately incomplete, and how a comprehensive approach, *using material that is already available to us*, can effect a fundamental transformation in the relationship between the patient, her family, and the healthcare team. This and nothing less than this radical transformation is essential in realizing our full potential as primary care clinicians.

Dr. Blount is under no illusion that this will be easy or painless. In one of this book's more brilliant devices, he shows how this plays out for that large and important group of primary care patients we call complex or challenging or difficult – multiply-disadvantaged, he calls them – and spends the remaining two-thirds of his pages showing how to braid together the threads of the existing patient-centered care efforts to create, for even these patients, a true partnership that can serve their best interests and preferences, that can make best use of their strengths and resources, and that can withstand the sometimes countervailing pressure of our healthcare system.

The steps in this transition will be familiar to students of patient centeredness, but they have never been put together to such good effect before. Dr. Blount weaves together the elements of health literacy, motivational interviewing, appreciative inquiry, shared decision-making, minimally disruptive care, trauma-centered care, enfranchisement coaching, relationship-centered care, and family-informed care into a clinical approach that works within the constraints of primary care practice.

As if that weren't enough, he then devotes a chapter on how to sustain this expert team in the face of the inevitable changes in team composition.

Dr. Blount in this book recognizes where we are in our quest for more effective, more advanced primary care, recognizes what we have accomplished, marks where our work has been disappointing or difficult, and describes the good work we have done in pressing through to better partnerships with patients. And then he takes us through a step-by-step process, awake to the nuances, the variation written into this by our patients, our own temperaments, our readiness to change, and the problems our practices are facing – in the face of all this, he lays out a process by which we can actually move into partnership with our patients, calling out from their problems hidden assets, linking arms and borrowing strength from each other, and finding in their voices not just complaint and despair but also sustenance and solution and song.

This volume is a perfect and perfectly timed gift to the field, a gift made of gifts, of what others have learned and bequeathed to the field, and of Sandy's imagination and good thinking and formidable hard work. I for one am deeply grateful for this book and have already begun using it to help patients be healthier.

Aurora, CO, USA   Frank deGruy, MD, MSFM

Preface

This book is the product of a 40-year career in healthcare, about evenly divided between mental health settings and primary care medical settings. The actions, approaches, and interventions described in the book are based on evidence. The synthesis of these into a method is based on my experience as well as on innovations from other programmatic attempts to deliver team-based patient-centered care. In general, the older the programmatic attempt to deliver transformed care, the more likely it has received formal implementation and evaluation. This is the first articulation of the T.E.A.M. Way. It is my hope that formal implementation and evaluation will follow in the future. I believe that in the meantime, there will be interventions and ideas that will make it useful to the readers from a broad array of disciplines and roles, including the role of the patient.

A book about how to improve primary care written by a psychologist rather than a physician could be suspect to some of the readers I hope to reach. For that reason, it seems reasonable to go into more detail about my experience in primary care than I would otherwise offer. At least, the reader will have a context for making their own judgment about the credibility of the work.

In 1996, after a 20-year career as a psychologist working as clinician, administrator, and trainer in outpatient mental health, I came to the Department of Family Medicine and Community Health at the University of Massachusetts Medical School as the director of Behavioral Science. I already had the bug for integrated primary care, a term that I created in 1994 (Blount and Bayona 1994). My job in the Department was to oversee the training of the resident physicians in family medicine in the psychosocial aspects of primary care and to provide behavioral health services in one of the residency practices. The psychosocial aspects of primary care include the many elements of the doctor-patient relationship, plus mental health, substance abuse, and health behavioral change that primary care physicians need to be able to address. Most of the actual training in these aspects, as was true of the biomedical aspects of primary care, were delivered by experienced family physician faculty members who precepted (oversaw and taught) the residents. My job was to add elements that the physician faculty members could not provide and to design training methods that assured that each resident met the minimum levels of competency in "behavioral science."

The conceptualization of behavioral science at the time was as a set of skills, distinct from generalist medical skills. I was expected to be the specialist in those skills, just as specialists in other areas of practice, such as cardiology, OB/GYN, and infectious diseases, taught the finer points of their specialties to the residents, while the family medicine faculty taught and precepted the delivery of the generalist care the residents were providing. The problem with this idea, as I learned from observing the residents as they saw their patients, was that behavioral health needs were present and behavioral science skills were needed in virtually every visit. The idea many residents had that there were patient visits with "no behavioral science issues" was a product of the way it was defined in the curriculum and the field, not a perception drawn from the experience providing care. Several of my family medicine faculty colleagues shared my observation that it would be helpful to broaden the definition of behavioral science and the residents' perception of behavioral health factors in primary care.

In my earlier career as a trainer in family therapy in mental health settings, I had learned the power of working with the one-way mirror as a clinical and training approach. I had seen how the observation of clinical interactions by supervisors using the one-way mirror provided a myriad of opportunities for immediate supportive training and clinical interventions that were not available through simply discussing cases or observing on closed circuit TV. I knew how the conversation of the team behind the mirror could make possible more targeted suggestions to the trainee in front of the mirror, suggestions that took into account the learning style of the trainee as well as the needs of the patients. I also wanted to create a training venue in which medical and behavioral training became as inseparable as were the medical and behavioral problems that patients brought to primary care. With Ronald Adler[1] as my physician faculty partner, we initiated the weekly training process we called "team precepting." Over the course of a year, the process was expanded to all three residency practices. The "team" was composed of a medical faulty member and a behavioral science faculty member in an observation room behind the one-way mirror, working with a resident who saw their scheduled patients for the morning in a regular exam room with the mirror in one wall. Patients were asked for their permission for the observation, and they rarely withheld it. When they learned that senior faculty members were observing and consulting to their doctor about their care, they were willing to allow this extra training element to be part of their visit. At times, when an examination might involve exposure of the patient, a shade was drawn across the mirror for their privacy.

The person in the room who was likely to feel most exposed was the resident physician. We worked to counter their feelings of vulnerability by, as much as possible, catching them in the act of doing things well. We augmented our strength-based feedback with a limited number of suggestions for improving the care they

---

[1] Over the course of many years, most of the training and clinical projects that I was able to initiate were made more effective and credible by the expertise, consultation, and support of Dr. Adler.

provided. Over time, most residents came to look forward to their sessions of team precepting as a rich and supportive learning experience.

For me, team precepting was an experience afforded to very few psychologists. I observed between 10 and 15 patient visits a week, discussing the details of each visit with a physician colleague behind the mirror while the resident conducted the visit. These were not patients who were, in some way, identified as needing psychological care. They were the people who happened to be on the resident's schedule that morning. In the discussion between behavioral science faculty and medical faculty, the details of the way the medical and behavioral issues interacted in a patient's life could be made clearer. The perceptions of all team members were sharpened. I was afforded a multi-year training in the routines of primary care practice and the problems and challenges faced by physicians.

During my years of team precepting, I gradually learned to adapt interventions that were developed in the mental health arena so they could be used to improve the engagement, support, and influence that physicians could offer patients, particularly their patients presenting the most complex mixes of medical and behavioral health problems. I learned to help residents add these interventions by framing suggestions within their understanding of their work rather than by asking them to learn a new vocabulary of therapy or behavioral healthcare. Suggestions had to be familiar and to be easily understandable to be something a resident could use again when I was not around. The fact that so many alumni of the residency later talked about having "Sandy on my shoulder" as they conducted their daily practice testified to the effectiveness of our team precepting training approach.

Over the years, I began to look for a time when I could organize the many clinical and training interventions we developed into a clear method, based on an articulation of the principles that were common to these interventions from the beginning. These principles can be useful in understanding some of the developments and challenges of primary care as a field, as well as providing the underpinning for a method that can allow primary care practices to be more reliably successful with the "complex" patients that often fail to benefit from many of the transformation efforts underway in healthcare today.

Keene, NH, USA   Alexander Blount, EdD

Reference

Blount A, Bayona J. Toward a system of integrated primary care. *Fam Syst Med.* 1994;12:172–80.

Acknowledgments

The two most important mentors and teachers in my career have been Don Bloch and Carlos Sluzki, who gave me the jobs and the intellectual leadership that allowed me to build the foundation of experience and understanding on which this work is based.

For the existence of this book, I should begin by thanking Jose Bayona, my coauthor on the original article that coined the term "integrated primary care" (Blount and Bayona 1994), who read and commented on each chapter as it was drafted. His judgment about what was truly patient-centered care was my North Star in this endeavor. At that time, he had created an integrated, team-based, patient-centered medical home in his solo primary care practice in Rochester, NY, before any of those concepts were in circulation. His practice staffing and routines of care, which he sought to make a catalyst for healing in the community as a whole, grew out of his determination to meet the needs of his patients and his fundamental belief in partnership with the health professionals, who were his colleagues, and with his patients. He believed in the healing power of relationships, particularly within families, assumed his patients would have a role in designing their care, and saw each patient as a potential resource, not only for themselves but for other patients in the practice. In addition, he made his practice a source of new connections between his patients and a creator of connections for his patients with the larger community.

I owe my experience in primary care to the Department of Family Medicine and Community Health of the University of Massachusetts Medical School and to the faculty, residents, psychology trainees, and, most especially, patients in the practices of the Department. The commitment to whole person care, especially for underserved and vulnerable populations, was a core value of the faculty, led by Daniel Lasser, the chair of the Department during my tenure. His support of my work was unwavering, even when I gave him cause to waver. I especially appreciate Drs. Ronald Adler, Gerald Gleich, Peter McConarty, Jeremy Golding, Michael Ennis, Frank Domino, Mark Quirk, Lucy Candib, Sara Shields, Tina Runyan, Daniel Mullin, Samuel Pickins, and Steven Earls for the inspiration, the support, and the challenges they offered me.

Dr. Michael Fine, a family doctor, leader in healthcare in Rhode Island, medical visionary, and self-proclaimed warrior for radical transformation in healthcare in the USA, has been a friend, mentor, and coconspirator for healthcare change for many years.

Though they appear rarely or not at all in the text, this work would not have been possible without the friendship, support, and intellectual influence of C.J. Peek, Frank deGruy, Susan McDaniel, Macaran Baird, Larry Mauksch, Parinda Khatri, Rodger Kessler, Ben Miller, and my fellow members of the National Integration Academy Council, the Society of Teachers of Family Medicine, and the Collaborative Family Healthcare Association.

In addition to Jose Bayona, I owe an important debt to David Artzerounian and Lora Council for their close reading of drafts and for providing a crucial physician perspective on the work and Dave deBronkhardt (EPatient Dave) for providing equally important feedback from the patients' perspective.

I am very grateful to Sari Chait, Lora Council, Kirsten Meisinger, Jackie Ross, Bertha Safford, Andrew Schutzbank, and Amy Valeras, each of whom offered me a substantial and very useful conversation about the practices in their settings.

About the Book

This book is designed to be a handbook for patient-centered care for the present and the future of healthcare. It is targeted at the care of adults in primary care settings, but there is little in it that would not be relevant to ambulatory specialty settings and, in fact, to most other healthcare settings. The special issues in pediatrics were more than I could address this time, even though pediatricians see the multiply-disadvantaged patients described here both as children and as parents. The work contains an attempt to assemble and organize evidence on the latest patient-centered approaches to care and then to add a method to take patient-centered care further in being able to engage complex patients. It is intended for every member of the primary care health team (e.g., physicians, nurse practitioners, physician assistants, medical assistants, nurses, psychologists, social workers, care managers, community health workers, health coaches, translators), plus practice transformation facilitators, administrators, health policy professionals, regulators, and clinical educators who train the members of any healthcare team. It is my hope that it also will be seen as useful to the many people supporting "participatory medicine" from the patients' perspective.

The book outlines the challenges of true patient-centered and team-based care. It attempts to be realistic about the pressures, stresses, and alienation faced by physicians and other members of the healthcare team. It tries to clarify the characteristics of a group of patients that are the most challenging to the team, for whom current patient-centered approaches are commonly unsuccessful and who currently receive less effective healthcare. It outlines a method with four component principles to transform practice in ways that improve engagement and health behaviors for patients and that lower stress and burnout for health team members. The four principles of the method are transparency, empowerment, activation, and mutuality. These form the mnemonic T.E.A.M. and together are called "the T.E.A.M. Way" in the text. These components actually are much more general and concerned with more aspects of patient-centered practice than just team process. The excuse for using a mnemonic that doesn't quite match the focus of its elements is that a mnemonic that is impossible to forget may be worth the occasional need to remind the reader that we are working at a more general level than the team alone.

Abbreviations

AAP	American Academy of Pediatrics
ACA	Affordable Care Act
ACE	Adverse Childhood Event
AHRQ	Agency for Healthcare Research and Quality
AMA	American Medical Association
BH	Behavioral health
BHC	Behavioral Health Clinician (or Consultant)
CCM	Collaborative Care Model
CM	Care manager
CYA	Cover your acts
DIGMA	Drop-in group medical appointment
ED	Emergency department (same as ER – emergency room)
EHR	Electronic Health Record
FIC	Family-informed care
HCA	Healthcare assistant (British category similar to a community health worker)
HI/SI	Homicidal ideation/suicidal ideation
HP	Health professional
IOM	Institute of Medicine
IPC	Integrated primary care
MA	Medical assistant
MDM	Minimally disruptive medicine
MI	Motivational interviewing
NDP	National Demonstration Project, PCMH implementation
NHPCBHWI	New Hampshire Primary Care Behavioral Health Workforce Initiative
PAC	Patient Advisory Committee
PAM	Patient Activation Measure
PCAM	Patient-Centered Assessment Method
PCCP	Patient-Centered Care Plan
PCMH	Patient-Centered Medical Home

PCOF	Patient-Centered Observation Form
PCP	Primary care provider (physicians, nurse practitioners, physician assistants)
PDSA	Plan, do, study, act
PFEC	Patient and family engaged care
PPDSA	Partnering, plan, do, study, act
PTSD	Post-traumatic stress disorder
QI	Quality improvement
RCC	Relationship-centered care
SA	Substance abuse
SCP	Shared care plan
SDM	Shared decision-making
SES	Socioeconomic status
SFI	Solution-focused interviewing
SMHC	Specialty mental health clinician
T.E.A.M. Way	Transparent, empowering, activating, and mutual way to providing patient-centered care
TIC	Trauma-informed care
UPOC	Urgent plan of care
USFHC	Union Square Family Health Center
WHO	World Health Organization

Contents

About the Author

Alexander Blount, EdD, has been a licensed psychologist since 1977. In the first 20 years of his career, he worked as a clinician and trainer in a private mental health center, a director of clinical services in a public mental health center, a faculty member at the Ackerman Institute for the Family in New York, and the director of an outpatient psychiatry service in a regional medical center. In 1996, he was appointed director of Behavioral Science in the Department of Family Medicine and Community Health at the University of Massachusetts Medical School in Worcester, MA, where he worked until 2015. Currently, he is a professor emeritus in the Department and continues to consult to the Center for Integrated Primary Care, which he founded at the Medical School, teaches clinical psychology at Antioch University New England graduate school, and offers consultation and training in behavioral health integration, patient-centered care, and workforce development around the USA and overseas. In addition, he is a member of the National Integration Academy Council; a past editor of *Families, Systems, and Health*; and a past president of the Collaborative Family Healthcare Association. He lives in Amherst, MA, with his wife, Francesca Maltese, and spends his spare time with his three grown daughters and their families.

Chapter 1
Getting to Patient-Centered Care

1.1 Primary Care Is Powerful

Primary care is the most important service setting in any comprehensive health system on a number of dimensions. It is where the majority of the population receives the majority of its care. It is the setting with which people are likely to engage over longer periods of time, the setting where they can be known personally and in the context of their families. It is where people can bring any problem to get help in understanding what sort of problem it is and where in the system it can best be addressed. It is the setting that focuses on keeping people healthy, in addition to returning them to health. Primary care is the place where advances in research and policy can be implemented on a population basis. If done well, it is the leverage point for improving the health of the population while reducing the overall cost of care.

Some of the most influential research on the importance of primary care in a health system has been done by Barbara Starfield and her colleagues. Before her death in 2011, she led a team at the Johns Hopkins Medical School studying the impact of primary care services on health and on the healthcare system as a whole. Perhaps more than anyone else, her work provides the evidence about what is right with primary care. Starfield defined primary care as "the provision of integrated, accessible healthcare services by clinicians who are accountable for addressing a large majority of personal healthcare needs, developing a sustained partnership with patients, and practicing in the context of family and community" (Starfield [1], p. 19).

Over the course of many studies, the evidence produced by Starfield and her teams made unassailable the importance of primary care for the improvement and maintenance of health [2]. They showed that people in areas with more primary care physicians are healthier, that people who get their care from primary care physicians instead of solely from specialists are healthier, and that people who receive the elements of care provided in primary care, no matter where they get them, are healthier.

© Springer Nature Switzerland AG 2019
A. Blount, *Patient-Centered Primary Care*,
https://doi.org/10.1007/978-3-030-17645-7_1

The studies of the workforce of primary care physicians (PCPs) (family medicine and general internists, who, along with general pediatricians, nurse practitioners, and physician assistants, comprise the primary care workforce), measured in generalists per 10,000 population in each state, showed that for adults, increasing the ratio of PCPs to population correlated with significantly better outcomes and lower mortality from all causes. This relationship was specifically seen in lower mortality from heart disease, cancer, and stroke; lower infant mortality and infants born with low birth weight; and better self-perceived overall health.

To see if this might be related to some difference in the demographic characteristics of populations in different states, Starfield's team analyzed the data controlling for age, gender, ethnicity, race, income, education, health insurance coverage, urban or rural living, reported physical health, and health behaviors such as smoking. The significant correlation held up, especially for the ratio of family doctors to the population. Interestingly, the correlation was in the opposite direction for the size of the specialty physician workforce, a higher ratio of specialists to the population correlated with higher mortality rates [2].

Not only did Starfield's research show that a higher ratio of PCPs to the population correlates with higher-quality care and lower death rates, it also documented the correlation of more PCPs with lower overall cost of medical care. In the case of acute illnesses, such as pneumonia, and chronic illnesses, such as diabetes, care is less costly when it is provided by a generalist than when provided by a specialist, and the outcomes are the same [2, 3].

Why is primary care so powerful in improving the health and the cost of care for the population? Starfield suggested that there may be several mechanisms behind its effect on improving health and reducing cost, among them: (1) better access to health services, (2) improved quality of care, (3) emphasis on prevention, (4) identification and early management of conditions, and (5) reduction of unnecessary specialist care [2]. These are current fundamentals of a high-functioning primary care system.

There is an additional aspect of primary care that needs to be taken into account: primary care as a relationship. In a study of "connectedness" of patients and doctors,[1] people who had continuous relationships with one primary care doctor, and whose doctor thought of them as "my patient," as opposed to care by various doctors in the same practice, showed better quality of care as measured by the completeness of the preventive care patients received. The study also showed better health outcomes as measured by the successful management of chronic illnesses [4]. The effect seems to be due to a mutual identification of the unique physician-patient relationship and is not impacted by likeness or unlikeness in the race or ethnicity of the physician and patient.

Perhaps at the most general level, the impact of "connectedness" that is a feature of primary care more than specialty care is for two reasons: (1) the continuity over

---

[1] I use the word "doctor" to designate physicians, nurse practitioners, and physician assistants. It saves a lot of extra words, and it is what most patients call the person in the role of primary care provider anyway. I use "physician" when that is the only discipline indicated.

time of the relationships in primary care makes it the medical setting most likely to be able to influence people's behavior, and (2) the majority of the determinants of people's health, especially their longevity, are impacted by their own behavior. The most common contributors to premature death in the USA are tobacco use, diet and activity patterns, alcohol abuse, microbial agents, toxic agents, firearms, sexual behavior, motor vehicles, and illicit drug use [5]. Of these premature deaths, 86% are the result of a person's behavior. If you add all the deaths that aren't demonstrably "premature" but that would not have come as early as they did if there had been better preventive care, the case is even stronger. The health behavior of patients, how well they take care of themselves including getting preventive care from the health system, has by far the largest impact on the cost of their care, on their functioning, and on their health and longevity.

It is clear that primary care should be the jewel in the crown of the USA or any other healthcare system. But at the same time that Starfield and her colleagues were documenting the importance of primary care in the overall healthcare system, other experts were taking that same healthcare system to task for its inefficiency, second-rate health outcomes when compared to other countries, organization to fit the preferences of professionals rather than those of patients, and poor record on patient safety.

1.2   The Call for Patient-Centered Care

In 2001, the Institute of Medicine (IOM), now the National Academy of Medicine, published its watershed report, *Crossing the Quality Chasm: A New Health System for the 21st Century*. The report has profoundly influenced subsequent efforts to save the US healthcare system from a future of economy-breaking costs and relatively poor quality. The plan for a new health system had a reconceptualized and revitalized primary care service at its center.

The Quality Chasm report was the follow-up to a previous IOM report called "The Urgent Need to Improve HealthCare Quality" [6]. The problems of quality were summarized as overuse, underuse, and misuse of care. "Staggering" levels of harm and unnecessary cost were attributed to these problems. Primary care was seen as the possible laboratory for developing solutions. At the time of the "Urgent Need" report, the authors called for a reorganized primary care that would improve access and make the routines and processes of care more understandable to patients, more evidence based, more efficient, and better coordinated [7].

As medical leaders described the pathway toward a reorganization of primary care, the role of the doctor in relation to the patient gradually became more of a focus for change. When the "Quality Chasm" report appeared in 2001, the vision of the way healthcare should change was different from the one expressed by the "Urgent Need" report [6]. Donald Berwick [7], one of the authors of both reports, describes a contentious conversation that went on in the committee as the Quality Chasm report was being prepared. He reports that the disagreement was over the question of how much patients should have control of their own care. He suggests the disagreement can be framed as a struggle between those advocating an approach he calls "consumerism" and those advocating an approach he terms "professionalism." Consumerism is based on an understanding of a healthcare interaction between a doctor and a patient as a consumer purchasing a service. The consumer should be able to determine what service they want based on information about the service from the service provider. Professionalism is based on the idea that the group that has the most scientific knowledge and expertise will do better than the patient in making decisions about what care is best and how to deliver it. They will also do best at holding themselves to high standards of professional behavior. "Patient-centered care" and "the patient as the source of control" were compromise concepts that came out of this discussion [7].

The "Quality Chasm" report put forward rules for improving healthcare that were radical for the time.

The IOM's ten rules for improving healthcare:

1. "Care based on continuous healing relationships." This indicates both continuous in the sense of longitudinal, and continuous in the sense of available any time.
2. "Customization of care based on patient needs and values." The system should be able to respond to individual patient choices and values.
3. "The patient as the source of control." Patients should be given adequate information to actively participate in decisions about their care, based on their values, using approaches such as shared decision-making.
4. "Shared knowledge and free flow of information." Patients should have "unfettered" access to their own medical information and to clinical knowledge relevant to their health.
5. "Evidence-based decision making." Care should be based on the latest scientific knowledge with minimum variation between clinicians and settings that is not based on patient populations.
6. "Safety as a system property." Patients should not be at risk from harm caused by their healthcare system.
7. "The need for transparency." Their health system should make all information available that is relevant to patients making informed decisions including possible alternative treatments. This should also include information about stakeholders, effectiveness, and costs of the health system and its components.
8. "Anticipation of needs." The health system should anticipate patients' needs in addition to responding to needs they bring to the system.
9. "Continuous decrease in waste." The health system should work to decrease waste of resources, including wasting patients' time.
10. "Cooperation among clinicians." Clinicians and organizations should actively collaborate and exchange information for coordination of care (IOM [8], pp. 8–9).

The rules on system change for quality improvement, safety, and reduction of waste (1, 5, 6, 8, 9, 10) might have been expected in response to the report outlining the need to improve quality. These could be called the "systems change" rules, the ones that depend on the health system to reorganize itself. Rule 1 is in this group because it indicates expanded time access for patients.

It was the strategy of enfranchising the patient, both to improve patient experience and to add a new judgment to the discussion of quality that was the most significant new direction for healthcare to come out of the report (1, 2, 3, 4, 7). These could be called the "relationship change" rules. Rule 1 is in this group as well in that it indicates continuity of relationship for patients with their chosen doctor or team.

The latter group of rules proposed a changed relationship between the health system and the patient. Under these rules, the patient would be treated very differently than was then (or currently) the case in most health settings. Patients would be given access to all the information about themselves that the professionals had. They could expect to be consulted on choices involved in determining a care plan. They would be able to make choices based on knowledge about the cost and effectiveness of their care elements, including having the ability to choose to let the professionals make the decisions. They could expect to see their chosen team of people with whom they had long-term relationships. Care would be more egalitarian and more accountable. Care would be "patient-centered" in that the patient would be central to determining its direction, not just because the professionals would direct their efforts in the patient's best interest.

The IOM rules became the guiding vision for a number of efforts to transform the patient experience, the quality of care, and the cost of US healthcare [9]. When the Affordable Care Act was designed, many of these elements became part of the transformation of health delivery mandated in the law and in the regulatory and funding authority that the law gave to various government agencies.

The discussion among the members of the IOM committee working on the Quality Chasm report could be said to embody the challenge of the patient-centered care movement: "How can we have a health system in which the people who are receiving the care, and directly or indirectly paying the cost, don't have primary control of what care they receive and how they receive it? The patient has to have control." vs. "How can we have a health system in which decisions about care are made by people who are not scientifically and professionally trained to make those decisions? The professionals have to hold the reins." Listening to the conversation in a vacuum, most professionals (and most patients) would lean toward the side advocating that decisions be made by those professionally and scientifically trained to make them.

In practice the choice is more complicated. The patient can be remarkably influential in determining the success of their own care. In the hospital, the setting in which the greatest acute need is addressed in the shortest possible time; "the professionals should guide care" point of view would seem particularly crucial. Yet making patients, even elderly patients, more central players on their care teams can significantly improve some outcomes. A major source of expense and an indication of unnecessarily poor patient experiences is the phenomenon of patients being readmitted to the hospital shortly after discharge, especially for the same illness that took them there in the first place. Eric Coleman [10] developed a brief intervention in which elderly patients who are transitioning out of the hospital are coached so that they can promote communication between the hospital and the setting to which they are returning. They are helped to take a more active role in their care by asserting their preferences. In a randomized controlled trial of the intervention, the elders who were coached to be assertive were readmitted significantly less than controls who got usual care. The coached patients came back 30% less at 30 days from all causes. They came back 46% less at 90 days from the cause that took them to the hospital originally. On average their total cost of hospitalizations was 19% less [10].

A moment's thought about how relationships of care work in the real world is enough to recast the argument between the professional deciding and patient control. Over the long term, control of what care is received and what plans are adhered to belongs to the patient. People go to their doctor when they decide to. If they don't choose to go, the doctor in most primary care practices has no impact. When they are in the doctor's office, the majority are polite and accepting of their doctor's recommendations; however what they do with those recommendations in their lives is often another matter. What they understand of their diagnosis and treatment plan and how likely they are to follow the plan are commonly very different from the way they present themselves in the doctor's office. The patient, or the patient's life circumstances, ultimately makes the decision about what medicines of those prescribed she obtains and takes, what exercise she gets, and on and on. In the primary care relationship, the professionally and scientifically trained one makes a few decisions about what treatments will be available, but the patient decides what treatments will occur. Only in a mutually influential relationship between the doctor or team and the patient can a synthesis between professional guidance and patient control be forged.

The current movement to implement the patient-centered medical home (PCMH) is cast as the successor to the movement started by the Quality Chasm report. It developed over several years, driven first by pediatrics and later by the other primary care disciplines, family medicine, and general internal medicine. It can be seen as a way of implementing a somewhat evolved version of the rules in the IOM report. Under the influence of the Affordable Care Act (ACA) and other regulatory and disciplinary efforts, the Patient-Centered Medical Home has become a model for practices that would carry out the spirit of the IOM report, designed to put primary care back on its feet as the leading edge of a new, higher-quality, and more efficient health system. In a number of regions, primary care practices that become accredited as PCMHs are eligible for increased recognition and improved payments for their services. Accrediting bodies such as the National Committee for Quality Assurance have had a profound effect on primary care practice by their requirements for PCMH designation.

While the PCMH is presented as one model, it can be useful to keep an eye on the different elements that combine under that title. Berwick distinguishes "medical home" from "patient-centered care." He defines the medical home as "a practice team that coordinates a person's care across episodes and specialties" (Berwick [7], w555). Patient-centered care is defined in the following way by the Institute for

Healthcare Improvement, the organization that Berwick founded: "Care that is truly patient-centered considers patients' cultural traditions, their personal preferences and values, their family situations, and their lifestyles. It makes the patient and their loved ones an integral part of the care team who collaborate with healthcare professionals in making clinical decisions. Patient-centered care puts responsibility for important aspects of self-care and monitoring in patients' hands—along with the tools and support they need to carry out that responsibility" (IHI [11]).

We may loosely assign the five "practice design" rules plus Rule 1 of the IOM report to "the medical home" and the five "relationship rules" to "patient-centered care." The efforts have been combined in the Patient-Centered Medical Home, but the distinction will be useful as we look at the development of this model.

When the PCMH was first implemented broadly, the focus of the regulations was to a large extent on the "systems change" elements of the organization and information management of the practice (e.g., [12]), the "medical home." The driving belief was that if a primary care practice couldn't produce data about its patients, their needs, their care, and their outcomes, it could not improve itself. This required a number of changes in most practices in their approaches to administration and care so that they were more predictable and reportable. These changes were so taxing on practices that commonly when a practice started its transformation to being a PCMH, patient satisfaction with the experience of care in the practice went down [13]. Becoming a medical home negatively impacted patient-centered care. The doctors usually found the changes burdensome as well.

Crabtree and his team of colleagues report on a large-scale implementation of the Patient-Centered Medical Home through the transformation of existing primary care practices, either by their own efforts or with the help of practice transformation facilitators [13]. In their study of the National Demonstration Project (NDP), they found that the transformation of a primary care practice to the PCMH takes a lot of uncompensated time, a lot of effort, and therefore a lot of motivation. The study highlighted the fact that the change in the design of the practice to being a medical home was one on which the transformation team of the practice could focus effectively, especially if a practice coach or facilitator was made available. On the other hand, the NDP report highlighted that the relationship change elements are particularly challenging for physicians and their teams. It is a major challenge for physicians, people who are trained to be responsible for every element of care on the team, to be facilitative in their relationship with patients' health behavior, and to give up expecting to be the leader of the healthcare team in all situations. The study found that to truly make the transformation to being patient-centered requires shifts in roles and in the "mental models of care" and therefore a shift in professional (and self) identity, by doctors and staff.

What the National Demonstration Project of the PCMH accomplished was to move practices in the direction of achieving the model components of care that the health system thought should be provided or improved to achieve the goals of the Quality Chasm report. Access improved, which the NDP designers thought would improve health and satisfaction of patients. In the course of the project, however, health status, satisfaction with the service relationship, patient empowerment, comprehensiveness of care, coordination of care, consistency of the patient relationship with one provider and team over time, and patients' global experience with their primary care practice did not improve. In general, it seems clear that the system change elements are not enough to significantly impact the relationship change elements.

Changing practice to develop what the health system has assumed patients want and need does not seem to be the best plan for impacting patients' reports of receiving what they think they want and need. The systems change elements are hard but can be done with time and support. The relationship change elements are harder and not possible for every practice, even with time and support. The NDP evaluators did not find that the coaching or facilitation that was provided to the health professionals succeeded in helping practices make the shifts involved in changing the "roles and mental models of care."

In a more recent and broader survey of the research on the implementations of the PCMH, Jabbarpour and her colleagues [14] summarized all of the evidence that was made available, in journals or in credible professional reports, in the previous year. They found that, while there is no "manual" emerging for implementing the PCMH, team-based interventions, including case management, and having a usual source of care have a reliably positive impact on patient experience. Patient experience is a core measure of successful transformation. The longer a practice has transformed to the PCMH model, the more significant the positive effect of the transformation. It takes several years for the medical home changes to begin to be integrated so that the patient-centered care changes are manifested. There does not appear to be a shortcut, at least within the PCMH transformation process, to get to patient-centered care without the medical home changes. All of the practices that showed positive impacts of transformation met quality metrics of the medical home model. Finally, the patients who present the highest risk, in terms of most comorbid conditions, show the greatest impact of transformation, especially in terms of cost savings.

1.3   Change in Payment Models

If primary care is to make the changes mandated in the Quality Chasm report, a change in how care is paid for has been assumed to be necessary. If a payment system that pays for each element of care tends to generate more care, what would be possible if we changed to a system that pays for better health for the patient? In concept, this is clear and sounds like a good idea. In practice, working toward this simple goal has often been a nightmare. A "carrot and stick" strategy that incents the adoption of the IOM recommendations was contained in the implementation steps of the Affordable Care Act. These transformations were aimed at paying more for better health outcomes and imposing financial penalties for poor outcomes or excess costs. As they have been implemented, a great deal of the transformed payments have been for compliance with the elements of the PCMH, not for patient health [15]. When payments are based on patient health metrics, the targeting of the measurable often impacts care of some patients negatively. A reward for lowering the average measure of blood sugar in a population of patients with diabetes can be good for the population, but this may foster a more rigid protocol that keeps a practice from engaging some if its more complex patients, patients who need an individualized approach to determine the best place to start addressing their needs. Rewarding the achievement of targeted readings like blood pressure is counter to another desired benefit of payment transformation that whatever the payment model, the practice would be incentivize to be as active as patients need to engage them. Freeing the practice from using the "doctor visit" as the main way of communicating with and supporting patients should allow numerous opportunities for contact with and support of a patient by team members other than the doctor. This creates an opportunity to use multiple different staff roles to reach out to patients, supporting them in maintaining and improving their own health.

If practices are paid for the health of their patients and not for delivering service, the calculation involved in what counts as a quality clinical interaction may change dramatically. Under the "professionalism" approach to care, the responsibility of primary care, and of the health system in general, has been thought to stop at prescribing treatments and giving patients information about what is best for their own health and longevity. The autonomy of the patient, in this way of thinking, includes the right to make their own decisions about their health behavior, once they had been supplied the latest evidence about what that behavior might mean for their future. While that approach has long since been deemed inadequate by healthcare leaders involved in policy and payment, it is still the understanding of a great many healthcare providers.

In the old system, a note in a patient's chart after a visit for asthma (for example) that said "counseled about smoking cessation" reflected an interaction that met the standard of care at the time. The counseling increased the complexity of the service offered in the patient visit, and the payment was correspondingly higher. This was true even though telling someone to quit smoking, by itself, is unlikely to have the desired effect. The patient is likely to go on smoking and needing more care, more emergency room visits, and more in-patient stays and to die earlier. Under payment transformation, these outcomes will impact the measures of effectiveness of the primary care practice and therefore the payment the practice receives. The practice has to move on from giving good advice (evidence-based practice) to finding a way to influence patients to follow it (patient-centered care). As the details of payment transformation are codified and simplified, especially if the doctor is part of a health system that is at risk for the total cost of a given patient's healthcare, the line of what is effective will be much more the arbiter of payment. This increases the pressure on doctors to foster longer term patient engagement and adherence over short term measures like blood pressure for the most complex and most costly patients.

Though primary care has been shown to be the foundation of an effective healthcare system, and though the model of the medical home, when contrasted to the way care was previously organized, has been shown to improve outcomes and to lower cost [16], there remains the challenge of the transformation of the role of the patient, including their values, preferences, culture, and beliefs, in guiding their care. To achieve this requires a change in "mental models of care" [13] on the part of doctors and other members of the team. Changing one's mental models is not something most people can simply decide to do. Changing mental models of care occurs through actions in the practice (quality improvement) rather than through changing beliefs (classes). These changes coevolve; models of care evolve as the roles in delivering care evolve and as the clinical routines in care delivery evolve [17].

1.4   Doctors Under Pressure

Doctors, patients, policy-makers, health plans, and payers such as employers, Medicare, and Medicaid have known for some time that primary care is under intense pressure. Because of its central position in the health system, primary care bears the burden of expectations from many larger elements of the health system and the society. Is there a new screening procedure that can save lives? Primary care sees the largest slice of the population and so primary care should implement it. Are the emergency services overused? Primary care should reach out to engage overutilizing patients before they get to the ER. Has depression been discovered to be the common comorbidity for patients with chronic illnesses that are the most costly to treat? Primary care should integrate evidence-based depression treatments. Did health coverage expand to a large number of previously uncovered people? Primary care should absorb them and help them catch up on preventive care. Is there an opioid crisis in the state? Primary care is the best place to engage potential users and over-users to address the terrible increase in overdose deaths. Primary care practices should add the new treatments for opioid addiction.

The evidence about the inevitable role of primary care in the treatment of mental health and substance use disorders creates a substantial new mandate. The majority of mental health and substance use disorders are presented in primary care and other medical care settings, but not in a mental health or substance abuse treatment setting. Most people coping with these disorders will not go to a mental health facility even if referred by their primary care doctor. So primary care has become the de facto mental health system in the USA [18].

Each new mandate adds another challenge to the job of the primary care doctor, a job with a large list of challenges already. Studies of the time needed to meet each mandate have shown that a physician in adult primary care would need 18 hours per day, every day, to meet all the mandates (as of 2005) for a panel of 2500 patients. It would take 7.4 hours to deliver all the recommended preventive care [19] and 10.6 hours to deliver all the recommended chronic care services [20]. This is before they see the first visit based on a patient complaint. This means that primary care physicians are always making compromises between what is recommended and what is possible. It is a constant stress for a group of professionals who want to "get it right." They did not go to medical school and pick primary care for their careers in order to provide care "as right as time allows."

One would think that the evidence of the importance of primary care would have led to higher financial reward for primary care physicians, especially if the whole system clearly benefits from a robust and stable workforce in this crucial role. In the USA, general internal medicine, family medicine, and general pediatrics are three of the four lowest paid medical disciplines. Specialist physicians average 46% higher income than primary care physicians [21]. While there is some effort to change this at the national level, such efforts proceed very slowly and are often not welcomed by specialists. A "relative value scale" is used by Medicare to attach dollar values to medical actions and procedures. The Relative Value Scale Update Committee (RUC) that recommends to Medicare how the scale should be weighted is overwhelmingly comprised of specialists. The method of picking membership on the RUC honors specialties with comparatively small numbers of members and patients (e.g., otolaryngology and thoracic surgery) with the same representation as primary care specialties (e.g., family medicine and pediatrics) each of which has much larger membership and number of patients [22]. The result is that Medicare pays disproportionally higher rates for procedures as opposed to the core elements of primary care: diagnosis, patient teaching, and prevention. Medicare pays for "doing" over "talking." State Medicaid plans and most private health plans take their lead from Medicare in matters of payment. Talking is the central action that is required as primary care doctors are compiling their sterling record for controlling cost and keeping people healthy, and it is less rewarded in money or in time allotted.

If primary care physicians chose their specialty on considerations of income alone, the situation in the workforce would be much worse than it is. In family medicine, for example, it appears that medical students choose the field because they have a societal orientation (want to focus on patients in their communities, value long-term relationships with patients, feel a social commitment, and want to promote health) and because they are interested in addressing a variety of conditions and problems during the course of a workday [23]. Over time, the issues of income, the challenges of complex patient needs, the struggle with each new electronic health record (EHR), increasing productivity targets, the connection of payments to changing outcome metrics, and the lack of resources to meet the range of needs brought to primary care practices every day can make for a surprising level of alienation in the primary care workforce. Physicians currently have the highest rate of suicide of any profession in the USA [24], and their degree of alienation is steadily growing [25].

Though they tolerate more frustrations than they are paid for, primary care doctors are still leaving the profession in droves, and they are not being adequately replaced. By 2020, the American Association of Medical Colleges predicts the USA will have a shortage of 45,000 primary care physicians [26]. A similar situation is developing in Europe with the aging of the physician workforce and an imbalance of primary care and specialists. The undersupply of primary care doctors puts pressure on the remaining workforce, making the time for the doctor to spend with each patient shorter and the relationship that both parties want harder to establish and maintain. Primary care physicians are feeling the pressure. Family physicians have the highest burn out rate of any specialty [25]. This statistic should be of concern to everyone, because doctor burnout is associated with a twofold increase in unsafe care, unprofessional behaviors, and low patient satisfaction [27].

And what prevents burn out? According to a Rand Corporation study commissioned by the AMA, it is reducing the administrative complexity that gets between the doctor and the patient (e.g., the EHR) and enabling the doctor to feel that he or she is providing high-quality care to their patients [28]. These apply to the impacts of the multiple levels of systems in which physicians practice: the US healthcare system, the health system in which they are employed, the practice in which they see patients, and the team of colleagues who work with them in delivering care [29]. To increase the enjoyment that physicians have in their work also requires a better balance than most have between their work lives and their personal lives.

If we describe the routines of practice that might bring doctors greater job satisfaction and lower the chance of their burning out, we begin to envision interactions that look remarkably similar to those that were shown to be most correlated the patient satisfaction. Doctors would work on teams that took over much of the administrative work that a person does not need to go to medical school to do. The team would add new expertise and types of services, such as behavioral health and case management, that would mean the patients of the team received high-quality care, and the doctor would see patients consistently over time to see the impact of high-quality care on improving their lives and their health.

So here is what we know:

The most achievable changes of those recommended by the IOM are in the practice routines and information infrastructure, the medical home elements, of primary care.

Making the medical home changes, at least in the first few years of the transformation, makes little difference in bringing about patient-centered care. It generally increases stress on health professionals, particularly physicians, and hurts the patient experience of care.

The changes that make a difference to the experience of patients include receiving team-based care, seeing the same team members consistently, and having access to case management.

No program in the studied PCMH implementations that showed improvement in patients' experience of care failed to show improvement in the quality metrics prescribed for the medical home.

The more complex the health burden of the patient, the more likely that successful practice transformation, medical home, and patient-centered care will correlate with saving costs.

The longer the period of time a practice has to integrate the transformations required by the medical home model, the more likely it is to have made progress on the patient-centered care it provides.

The more effective physicians and other health professionals are in the care they provide, the less likely they are as a group to burn out or to seek to find ways other than patient care to make a living.

Any approach to reorganizing or reconceptualizing primary care that is to have a chance for success will allow non-physician team members to take on functions that free physicians from tasks that can be done by others and at the same time will increase the range of expertise and of services provided by the team, especially behavioral health and case management services. This increases the effectiveness and engagement of physicians and the whole team with the patients who present the most complex health needs.

The rest of this volume is an attempt to describe such an approach.

References

1. Starfield B. Primary care: balancing health needs, services and technology. New York: Oxford University Press; 1998.
2. Starfield B, Shi L, Macinko J. Contribution of primary care to health systems and health. Milbank Q. 2005;83:457–502.
3. Greenfield S, Rogers W, Mangotich M, Carney MF, Tarlov AR. Outcomes of patients with hypertension and non-insulin dependent diabetes mellitus treated by different systems and specialties. Results from the medical outcomes study. JAMA. 1995;274:1436–44.
4. Atlas SJ, Grant RW, Ferris TG, Chang Y, Barry MJ. Patient-physician connectedness and quality of primary care. Ann Intern Med. 2009;150:325–35.
5. McGinnis JM, Foege WH. Actual causes of death in the United States. JAMA. 1993;270:2207–12.
6. Chassin MR, Galvin RW, the National Roundtable on Health Care Quality. The urgent need to improve health care quality: Institute of Medicine National Roundtable on Health Care Quality. JAMA. 1998;280:1000–5.
7. Berwick D. What 'patient-centered' should mean: confessions of an extremist. Health Aff. 2009;28:w555–65.
8. Institute of Medicine. Crossing the quality chasm: a new health system for the 21st century. Washington, DC: National Academy Press; 2001.
9. Barry M, Edgman-Levitan S. Shared decision making — the pinnacle of patient-centered care. N Engl J Med. 2012;366:780–1.
10. Coleman EA, Parry C, Chalmers S, Min S. The care transitions intervention: results of a randomized controlled trial. Arch Intern Med. 2006;166:1822–8.
11. Institute for Healthcare Improvement (IHI). http://www.ihi.org/resources/Pages/Changes/PatientCenteredCare.aspx. Downloaded 2 Sept 2017.

12. Shaller D. Patient-centered care: what does it take. Commonwealth Fund. 2007. http://www.commonwealthfund.org/publications/fund-reports/2007/oct/patient-centered-care%2D%2Dwhat-does-it-take

13. Crabtree B, Nutting P, Miller W, Stange K, Stewart E, Jae'n C. Summary of the National Demonstration Project and recommendation for the patient-centered medical home. Ann Fam Med. 2010;8(Supplement 1):S80–90.

14. Jabbarpour Y, DeMarchis E, Bazemore A, Grundy P. The impact of primary care practice transformation on cost, quality, and utilization: a systematic review of research published in 2016. Patient-Centered Primary Care Collaborative and Robert Graham Center. 2017. https://www.pcpcc.org/resource/impact-primary-care-practice-transformation-cost-quality-and-utilization

15. Porter ME, Teisberg EO. Redefining health care. Boston: Harvard Business School Press; 2006.

16. Nielson M, Gibson A, Buelt L, Grundy P, Grumbach K. The patient-centered medical home's impact on cost and quality. Patient Centered Primary Care Collaborative. 2015. PCPCC.org. Accessed 23 Sept 2017.

17. Blount A, Bayona J. Toward a system of integrated primary care. Fam Syst Med. 1994;12:171–82.

18. Regier DA, Narrow WE, Rae DS, Manderscheid RW, Locke BZ, Goodwin FK. The de facto US mental and addictive disorders service system. Arch Gen Psychiatry. 1993;50:85–94.

19. Yarnall KS, Pollak KI, Ostbye T, Krause KM, Michener J. Primary care: is there time enough for prevention? Am J Public Health. 2003;93:635–41.

20. Ostbye T, Yarnall KS, Krause KM, Pollak KI, Gradison M, Michener JL. Is there time for management of patients with chronic diseases in primary care? Ann Fam Med. 2005;3:209–14.

21. Medscape Physician Compensation Report. 2017. http://www.medscape.com/slideshow/compensation-2017-overview-6008547. Accessed 5 Sept 2017.

22. American Medical Association (AMA). Composition of the RVS update committee. 2018. https://www.ama-assn.org/about/rvs-update-committee-ruc/composition-rvs-update-committee-ruc

23. Wright B, Scott I, Woloschuk W, Brenneis F. Career choice of new medical students at three Canadian universities: family medicine versus specialty medicine. JAMC. 2004;170:1920–4.

24. Shaffer,J.Physicianandmedicalstudentdepressionandsuicide.Non-ProfitQuarterly.July28,2016. https://nonprofitquarterly.org/2016/07/28/physician-medical-student-depression-suicide/

25. Shanafelt TD, Hasan O, Dyrbe L, Sinsky C, Satele D, Sloan J, West CP. Changes in burnout and satisfaction with work-life balance in physicians and the general US working population between 2011 and 2014. Mayo Clin Proc. 2015;90:1600–13.

26. Brown KD. Precarious future for primary care. Boston Globe. June 23, 2015. https://www.bostonglobe.com/metro/2015/06/22/the-thinning-ranks-medicine-front-line/GdG27Z26BD1i5u4Fh6aM6H/story.html. Downloaded 5 Sept 2017.

27. Panagioti M, Geraghty K, Johnson J, et al. Association between physician burnout and patient safety, professionalism, and patient satisfaction: a systematic review and meta-analysis. JAMA Intern Med. 2018;178:1317–30.

28. Friedberg MW, Chen PG, Van Busum KR, et al. Factors affecting physician professional satisfaction and their implications for patient care, health systems, and health policy. Rand Health Q. 2014;3(4):1–122.

29. American Academy of Family Physicians (AAFP). Family physician burn out, well-being, and professional satisfaction. 2018. https://www.aafp.org/about/policies/all/physician-burnout.html

Resources

Patient Centered Care

What is Patient-Centered Care? New England Journal of Medicine Catalyst, January 2017. https://catalyst.nejm.org/what-is-patient-centered-care/

Physician Depression and Suicide

Why Physicians Kill Themselves: https://www.tedmed.com/talks/show?id=528918

Chapter 2
From a Squad to a Team: Creating Team-Based Care

2.1 Understanding the Change

The changes represented by the implementation of the PCMH model that make a positive difference for the experience of patients include receiving team-based care, seeing the same team members consistently, and having access to case management [1]. Certainly, a commitment to patient-centered care would require an understanding and implementation of team-based care.

"Team-based care" is a concept that is applied broadly within and across healthcare settings. A "high-functioning team" could describe care in an inpatient setting, in which case it would describe an improvement in the sequential care given by different shifts of clinicians and staff. Another use of "team" might represent clinicians and staff that a patient would encounter across different healthcare settings who work to achieve continuity of care plans and to share information. For our purposes, "team-based care" represents care from a group of people who work together in real time to serve a shared panel of patients in a primary care setting.

In an Institute of Medicine discussion paper on the principles and values of team-based care [2], the principles of successful team-based care are identified as shared goals, clear roles, mutual trust, effective communication, and effective process and outcomes. These represent a good list for assessing the functioning of a care team in primary care. They also represent a challenge. Creating a team that exhibits these qualities requires a substantial process of evolution for most practices, one that can be stressful on clinicians, staff, and patients.

In Chap. 1 we discussed the fact that the practice change elements of the patient-centered medical home have been studied extensively, whereas the fundamental change in the relationship of the doctor to the patient and how to create that change have been much less well outlined. Looking at the guidance for developing a PCMH, one could assume that a better organized practice that is easier on the doctor and that delivers better care more smoothly will create the core change in the doctor-patient relationship such as the IOM calls for in the "rules" for patient-centered care. The

© Springer Nature Switzerland AG 2019
A. Blount, *Patient-Centered Primary Care*,
https://doi.org/10.1007/978-3-030-17645-7_2

evaluators of the National Demonstration Project *did not* find that to be the case. The change in the doctor's role, from being the creator of a treatment plan which the patient should follow to being a facilitative guide to better health who offers whatever type of leadership is needed by each patient, constitutes a challenge, in skills and in identity, for many doctors.

A similar situation exists in the realm of team-based care. Ways of getting to the routines of interaction that characterize high-functioning teams have been described at some length. How to do a huddle and how to develop workflows that involve other members of the team more substantively in the care process and that take pressure off the doctor have been described in detail [3]. There are good examples of tools for making this transition on the web. One particularly well-worked-out example is the Steps Forward program offered by the American Medical Association (www.Stepsforward.org). The change in the role of the doctor in relation to the rest of the team, from the creator of the treatment with a supporting cast to a facilitative leader enabling the self-organizing energy of the same group, has been much less extensively described. For many doctors that change is the most challenging aspect of the transition. The ways to effect this change need to be outlined in much better detail.

Reorganizing the practice, in itself, does not bring about the wanted change in doctor-patient relationship, and reorganizing the team, in itself, does not bring about the wanted change in doctor-team relationships. It was the assumption at the start of the National Demonstration Project that if the whole team, physicians, and support staff met regularly, communicated more intensively, and worked together to improve the quality of the care based on meaningful data, the transition in roles and in the experience of team members would happen. The authors of the NDP evaluation did not find this to be true [4]. They reported a finding that was unexpected, the necessity for new "mental models of care" that go along with a team-based practice organization as well as those that are needed for patient-centered care. Specifically referring to the relationship of the people and their roles on the practice team, they offer an account of the difficulties that were discovered.

> Nevertheless, as the NDP unfolded, it was observed that the effect of integrating NDP model components required roles of practice participants to transition in ways that met unexpected resistance. Becoming a PCMH requires more than just implementing sophisticated office systems: it involves adopting substantially different approaches to patient care that require moving away from a physician-centered approach and toward a team approach shared with prepared office staff. (Crabtree et al. [4], p. 586)

This move to team-based care changes the roles of staff and physicians, with the most immediately noticeable change demanded of the physician who previously had been the only leader.

Some people who were part of the practices in the National Demonstration Project expressed concerns about the possibility that the patients' experience of the team members' enhanced roles would be a loss of the focal relationship with the physician. The centrality of the physician-patient relationship was asserted in the initial definitions promulgated by the primary care physician guild organizations for the PCMH model which required a "physician-led team." Crabtree and his colleagues on the NDP evaluation project, two thirds of whom were physicians, felt this definition of the physician-led team could be a disservice to physicians, staff, and, in the long run, patients.

> Perhaps from the patient's perspective there will need to be a physician-led team, but from the practice's perspective, this concept needs to transform into one wherein the physician is part of a team, and not even necessarily the team leader. (Crabtree et al. [4], p. S86)

They recognized that this is a challenge for most physicians. It is a "change in their professional identity, and the ways in which they have been trained to deliver primary care. Training programs are not set up for future practice models as they are currently envisioned" (Crabtree et al. [4], p. S86).

The basics of teamwork or leadership are rarely topics in coursework in the training of medical students [4]. When leadership is mentioned, it is with an emphasis on the physician being responsible for what happens in the practice and on the team. For a doctor trained in this way, the sort of "change of identity" described by the NDP evaluators is often experienced as making them vulnerable. "My license is at risk here," and similar statements have been heard numerous times as practices attempt to make the transition to team-based care. Having one more thing to feel stressed about would seem to make this sort of transition an non-starter for many physicians.

These are not trivial concerns, yet for many sites, they are not taken as concerns that stop the development of teams.

> The issue of team leadership has sometimes been contentious, especially when approached in the political or legal arenas, where questions about team leadership often become entangled in professional "scope of practice" issues. In particular, arguments have arisen around "independent practice" versus team-based care and, where care is team-based, whether all team functions must be "physician-led," and what this would imply for other health professionals with regard to care management decision-making… . While the teams we interviewed acknowledged that physicians are clinically and often legally accountable for many team actions, the physicians on the teams we interviewed were not micromanagers; instead, they were collaborators who did not seek or exercise authority to override decisions best made by other team members with particular expertise, whether in social work, chaplaincy, or care coordination, etc. (Mitchel et al. [2], pp. 11–12)

Being realistic about the challenges is important in a developing a successful team. Team size can be an issue with 4–8 seeming ideal and over 12 being too big to work [3]. Using a process in which everyone's input is needed on every decision likely takes too much time and is unrealistic in areas in which the expertise of the physician or nurse needs to prevail. Finally, in fee-for-service payment systems, there are some functions that are compensated when performed or adequately overseen by a physician or nurse, but not when performed independently by another team member. Keep in mind, however, that in many practices there are divisions of labor based on understandings of payment regulations that are out of date. These have been used as reasons not to expand the roles of team members based on unrealistic fears of risk and consequences. The development of a team requires efforts on the part of administration to seek and exploit flexibility in regulations in addition to the work to seek and exploit flexibility in care routines on the part of clinical staff.

2.2   From a Squad to a Team

One way of understanding the difference in leadership styles that the IOM [2] and the NDP evaluation team [4] describe between poorly functioning and well-functioning teams may be thought of as the difference between a squad and a team. A squad is a small group of people with a clear leader and a shared purpose, often associated with the military. The leader does not change because of the context or the task. Leadership is permanently designated by the hierarchy of rank.

A team is different. "A team is a group with a specific task, the accomplishment of which requires the *interdependent* and *collaborative* efforts of its members" (Wise et al. [5], quoted in Bodenheimer [3], emphasis added). A team may have a clear leader, but the implication of the inflexible hierarchy of a squad is gone. Teams can have situational leaders. Each member of the team can be the eyes and ears of the whole team. Each can make discoveries that will influence everyone's functioning with a given patient. Each can make suggestions about improvements in clinical routines, suggestions that may become the usual practice of the whole team after a team discussion.

The transition from a squad to a team is a reorientation for all members. The expectation in a squad is that each member knows their job and carries it out under the continual direction of the squad leader. In specialty medical settings, this is sometimes possible. The array of situations that are presented to the practice may be reasonably narrow and fairly predictable. Each member's job, therefore, can be predictable. Roles and routines can meet the definition of a squad and still be very functional. In an acute setting such as the operating room or intensive care unit, a squad organization is necessary. In most primary care practices, a squad organization is not optimal. The array of problems and situations presented to the practice team is extremely broad. When you consider the complexity of diagnoses, complaints, and demands patients present as they are receiving preventive care, chronic care, and urgent care, it is necessary that team members display more flexibility of approach. Though primary care can be informed by protocols, a protocol that was developed for "patients like this one" (e.g., patients with type 2 diabetes) is often not a fit for "this patient" (patient with type 2 diabetes, congestive heart failure, anxiety, and substance use disorder) [6]. A team in which each member is trained and enfranchised to adapt their approach based on the needs of an individual patient and that maintains adequate communication in the flow of care to include a helpful adaptation or a new piece of information into the work of all its members will do better for most of its patients.

The evidence related to high-functioning teams reveals the benefits to everyone on the team when physicians take the facilitative rather than the directing approach. Rachael Willard-Grace and her colleagues [7] looked at the relationship of team structure and culture to burnout or emotional exhaustion for both primary care clinicians and support staff. "Team structure" in their study indicated the consistency with which the same primary care clinicians and support staff worked together. They called a small group that worked together on a regular basis a "teamlet." They used the term "team culture" to describe what might be called the cohesion of the team built on elements such as communication, participation, effort, social support, respect, and shared objectives (essentially the IOM list of the elements of a good team). The study was done in 16 primary care practices, ten serving primarily low-income or uninsured patients, and six serving more commercially insured and Medicare patients, in total encompassing 264,000 visits in the year before the study. They found that a strong team culture seemed to protect against emotional exhaustion for both clinicians and support staff. Tight team structure, consistency of working as a team, helped to promote team culture particularly for the clinicians. Where there was a lack of team culture, consistency of working together did not help to lower burnout.

One way to help doctors make the transition to a different sort of leadership and to a team vs. squad organization is to make it possible for them to practice with the same group of support staff and other clinicians regularly. Consistency of working as a team also helps the support staff members to keep from getting the message that they are interchangeable, as can happen when they work with different doctors on different days without a pattern that relates to their particular preference or skills. People who know they are going to be regularly working together tend to invest more attention to getting to know each other personally, to working together smoothly, and to solving problems amicably. They are more likely to attend to elements that Willard-Grace and her colleagues called team culture.

At first glance, organizing a practice in consistent teams is not the most convenient or efficient way for administrators. Some people want to work part-time. That complicates scheduling. Sometimes people are out for one reason or another. If a doctor is at a conference, does the rest of the team stay home? These are not trivial questions to people who are trying to keep the practice organized and who are watching the budget. When the longer-term effects of promoting teams that are cohesive are considered, the equation changes. Consistent team structure contributes to better team culture for doctors, who contribute to a team culture for everyone, culture that reduces emotional exhaustion or "burnout." Burnout of clinicians or staff is associated with higher errors, poorer communication with patients, and lower patient satisfaction. Lower patient satisfaction is associated with poorer patient adherence to care plans and poorer health outcomes [7].

Job satisfaction, when studied as an aggregate measure of the whole team, correlates with higher-quality metrics [8]. One knowledgeable interpretation of this data attributes the finding to the "flattening of the current knowledge-based hierarchy" and "more efficient matches between individual team member knowledge and skills and the actual work that they do" (Kimberly [9], p. 8). A team that can promote the importance and involvement of support staff in the core services of the patient visit also promotes higher-quality care, better patient satisfaction, stronger team culture, better job satisfaction, and lower burnout for clinicians and staff.

It might help to think of the change in the leadership role of the physician and the change from squad leader to team leader, from directive to facilitative, and from setting the tasks to developing the mission and the culture, as being a version of the same change that is called for by the IOM relationship rules for the doctor-patient relationship. The change is isomorphic (of the same form) as the change in the clinician-patient relationship identified as true patient-centered care. The transition of the squad to a team is preparing the doctor for a second transition, the transition from "delivering care to" patients to "partnering with" patients to achieve better health. This allows the challenge of team-based care to be seen in a new light. Attending to a different form of leadership for the doctors is an intervention in quality and sustainability of the practice as a whole by developing the skills for patient-centered care.

Getting to a new approach to leadership can go wrong. Team leaders sometimes make an effort to enfranchise other team members to participate by exerting less leadership, allowing things to rock along hoping that the leadership vacuum will be filled by other team members. It is a strategy that aims to be egalitarian, but that usually fails. In an undefined situation, historical patterns of hierarchy based on job title, race, gender, and socioeconomic and educational status are likely to exert unbidden influence on team members expectation about leadership. People, who are supposed to feel enfranchised or empowered by this approach, instead can feel anxious when they are unclear about what they are supposed to do. It makes people feel vulnerable if the person, whom they expect to be providing leadership and who will have an impact on their evaluation, retention, and promotion decisions, denies his or her own role in guiding of the team process. It tends to make people more likely to work from a "CYA" mindset as they go through the day.

2.3   Communication in the Team[1]

Successful transition to a highly functioning team is based on a significantly richer exchange of information both at regular meetings and through brief exchanges of information to keep each other up to date in the flow of care. It is a fair generalization that primary care practices, and medical services in general, commonly try to have as little time in meetings as possible. This often leads to a practice having barely enough communication to keep things moving and not nearly enough communication to effect any meaningful changes. Lack of adequate communication means a lack of coordination of action and to team members feeling unsupported and alone, even with colleagues all around. In this situation team members are more likely to feel overwhelmed.

---

[1] Some of the ideas in this section appeared previously in a chapter: Blount, A. (2018). Building your team. In Gold, S. & Green, L. (Eds.) *Your Patients are Waiting: Integrating Behavioral Health for the Primary Care Physician*. Springer, New York.

The idea that more communication is needed to plan changes in workflows, to evaluate the results, to do brief targeted training, or to talk about mission or values and that the investment in more communication could leave everyone less stressed and help the practice provide better care more efficiently can be very hard for administrators to translate into quantitative value. It is also true that time spent in meetings which is not productive in the experience of team members, or in conversations that don't relate to the jobs the team has accomplish will lead to meetings losing the engagement of team members.

There are a number of approaches possible to address the need for more communication in the team. One health system that has done an exemplary job in building primary care teams, including behavioral health clinicians and multiple "health coaches" supporting each doctor, expects that teams will meet for a 45-minute huddle at the beginning of each day and use an additional 3 hours per week for team meetings and training [10]. This health system considers team functioning in the architecture of practice facilities. Team members work stations are designed so that they can't help seeing each other. The unscheduled exchange of information that is facilitated improves group cohesion and patient care.

For regular meetings, some practices have one meeting a week to address a range of matters. Other practices have more than one kind of meeting and address different sorts of issues at different times. Some have longer meetings to get it all done, while some have briefer meetings because those are more efficient for them. It is very hard to say what schedule and organization works for a practice.

Examples of topics for regularly occurring meetings:

1. One or two patients that team members feel the team could engage or manage better, e.g., nonadherent patients, scary patients, dissatisfied patients, patients who aren't getting better, and patients with complex lives or family situations that need to be understood better.
2. How can we improve? The team looks at data, something that is being counted and sees where the numbers look good and where there might be a place to try something different. They remember together one or two specific instances when things didn't go smoothly and think about how those specific situations could be handled better in the future. Before spending too much time looking for a fix, it is important to spend some time looking for instances when that same process or task went well. They see what various team members did in those instances that made things work. Whatever the sequence, the work in the successful case is something they already know how to do and could be the basis for making that success more frequent.
3. Highlight excellence. The team takes a moment to let team members recite things that other members did that were noticeably helpful or insightful or caring or courageous. They make sure they describe very specifically what their teammate did that they appreciated.

Some have a weekly meeting time with rotating topics so that the time is always interesting and useful.

Perhaps the most useful regular meeting, in terms of value per minute spent, is the huddle before each session of patient care. A huddle is commonly a 10- to 15-minute meeting in which all of the people who will be providing or assisting in patient care during the session exchange information that will help everyone work in a coordinated and efficient way. When the decision is made to hold huddles, there will likely be pushback. "We could use this time better to each get ready for our individual roles." The clinical and administrative leadership in the practice is wise not to give in. Once team members see how much better the half-day goes, how much less stressed everyone is, and how much less follow-up work there is, they will come around.

2.4   Team Roles

In the medical group that we have been calling a squad, roles and the functions that go with each role are often determined by discipline. The person who can give injections, the person who can take vital signs, the person who can instruct the patient to temporarily increase or discontinue a medication, or the person who can assess the acuity of a patient's complaint and dispense medical advice over the phone, each of these tends to be determined by the discipline and training level of the squad member. In the move from squad to team, team members are likely to take on additional functions that are not identified with a particular discipline. A team member who is helping a patient articulate their health goals, who is teaching sleep hygiene, or who is scoring a depression screen might be from any of a number of disciplines or have any of a number of different levels of training. This team member might be in a role with any of a number of different names.

Bodenheimer [11] summarizes a study of 15 sites with teams that exhibited some or many aspects of what could be called "high functioning" in a paper called "lessons learned." It is a product of 112 interviews with team members representing the variety of the team roles. The study found that a number of functions that physicians had been performing could be distributed to other team members, especially in the care of chronic illnesses, using protocols, standing orders, oversight, and training. When the "care enhancers" (my term for the different roles and job descriptions that are part of the care team but not licensed clinicians) were used more broadly in chronic illness care, the quality of the practices' care of chronic illnesses improved, especially in the areas of monitoring and patient teaching. Attention to team cohesion and shared decision-making led to team input on defining and refining the roles of team members which led to improved care metrics and more efficient use of the time of the most expensive team members, physicians, and RNs.

Using the structure of the usual primary care interaction, pre-visit, visit, post-visit, and between visits [3] can be helpful in delineating functions that should be added or that can be passed to different team members. The structure helps in developing protocols for various chronic illnesses or common presentations. Pre-visit care can be done by team members who have been taught specific routines for preparation or for handling aspects of care that can be checked by the doctor in the visit.

In the visit there can be clinical support roles and, more recently, the role of scribe, a person who creates the documentation of the visit and who accesses information and resources during the visit under the direction of the doctor. In some models this scribe is a person who accompanies the patient through all of the stages of the visit [3].

Post-visit can be a time for clarifying or extending information offered in the visit and for setting up monitoring or other contacts in the between visit periods. This period can encompass programs of chronic illness teaching, monitoring, or care. It can include visits with subgroups of the team or outreach by team members. It can include time spent connecting the practice and the patient with resources for the individual patient or for a population. A good deal of the creativity being shown by high-functioning teams in enfranchising team members to providing excellent care without using the direct contact time of the doctor is occurring in this space.

In designing the roles, teams try to make a balance between adding functions for "care enhancers" and limiting the number to handoffs in the process. Though roles are evolving over time, at any one point all of the team members ought to be able to describe the roles of each member involved in a patient's care to the patient. These descriptions should allow the patient to know why the person is participating in their care and what they are contributing to the treatment. It helps when these explanations are made to the patient as part of the introduction of a team member, either by the team member themselves or by another team member. When one team member introduces another in terms of their role in the care, the skill set they bring, and the contribution they are making to the treatment plan, and when this introduction is followed by an introduction of the patient to the team member in terms of the reason for their visit today and the efforts they have made to promote their own health, the relationship of the first team member with the patient is partially passed to the second. This is especially true when the introducing team member is the doctor, the person with the clearest reason for relating to the patient. When patients have the experience of working with the same team members repeatedly, this introduction can be modified, but there could be reasons to go back to introductions of a sort depending on the reason for the visit on a given day.

Team-based care is often part of a larger reorganization of primary care practices that is going forward around the country. In some settings the goal of the reorganization is to better serve patients with complex health needs who tend to require a great deal of medical services from a healthcare system while failing to obtain the benefit the services are designed to provide (see the Union Square model below). In these instances, the team increases the intensity and variety of services the doctor can offer. This is designed to promote, in the long run, better health and lower cost. In other settings, the reason for creating team-based care is to increase doctors' work satisfaction and lower their burnout rate (the APEX model). In primary care, attending to the problem of physician burnout is important for the quality of patient care as well as for maintaining the workforce. In Chap. 1 we saw that physician burnout is associated with twofold increased odds for unsafe care, unprofessional behaviors, and low patient satisfaction [12]. If we consider the RAND finding that the way to counter burnout is to reduce the administrative complexity that gets between the doctor and the patient (e.g., the EHR) and to enable the doctor to feel that he or she is providing high-quality care to their patients [13], both of the approaches to reorganization below are likely to serve both the goals of improved patient care and lowered burnout. They differ in the degree to which they are designed to support or change the physician-led team approach.

2.5   The APEX Model

A model of team-based care specifically designed to lower physician burnout and improve their experience of providing healthcare is called the APEX model (standing for "ambulatory process excellence" or "awesome patient experience") [14] which was piloted first in the University of Colorado health system. Building on the "team-let" as the central unit of care [3], the APEX model is designed to reduce burnout by adding substantial support for doctors in each patient visit. This is done by greatly expanding the role of the medical assistant (MA) and more than doubling the number of MAs supporting each doctor, from <1:1 to 2.5:1. In addition managing the flow of patients into and out of exam rooms and taking vital measurements, the MAs' role in the visit is expanded to spend added time before each visit to do the following:

- Elicit a comprehensive patient agenda.
- Collect or update elements of the patient's past medical, surgical, social and family history in the EHR.
- Conduct detailed medication reconciliation …
- Use templates to document the history of the illness or complaint that was the reason for the visit (History of Present Illness) and ask standard questions covering other aspects of the patient's health (Review of Systems).
- Using protocols, initiate certain clinical tasks such as rapid strep or urinalysis.
- Review preventive care gaps such as screenings or immunizations and either arrange for them or mark the gaps for the physician's review. (Paraphrased from Lyon et al. [14], pp. 7–8)

The MA remains in the visit when the doctor comes in. They provide "documentation support," writing in the EHR, thereby freeing the doctor from the having to look at a computer screen rather than the patient during the visit. The doctor reviews the information gathered by the MA, finalizes the agenda for the visit, conducts the conversation, performs any examinations, makes diagnoses, and makes the recommendations needed for ongoing treatment. When the visit is over, the MA remains with the patient, to reinforce the patient's understanding of the information and advice offered in the visit, to add additional protocol-based teaching, to carry out any orders from the visit such as lab draws or immunizations, and to arrange follow-up. Finally, the MA escorts the patient back to the waiting room.

Early outcomes have been very promising. The expanded participation by the MA has allowed attention to preventive health elements that might not have been able to be addressed in the physician visit. Colon cancer screening, hypertension control, and diabetes care such as foot exams and retinal exams increased modestly, and breast cancer screening increased by almost 50%. The largest measured improvement has been in the work life of the doctors. Measurements of burnout symptoms decreased by half. Doctors willingness to take on additional clinical hours increased. Doctors spending extra time logged into the EHR after hours dropped. Scores improved in all measured domains, including overall doctors' satisfaction, efficiency, documentation, and actions defined as patient-centered or as improving patient engagement. Perhaps the most telling outcome for administrators has been the greatly improved success in recruiting new doctors.

Patients' experience improved in the areas of better communication with their health professionals on the team, particularly in the area of feeling their concerns were listened to. Their willingness to recommend the practice to others went up as well.

In its impact on provider stress and potential burnout, the APEX model seems to be having the results seen in other implementations of team-based care. Because it was explicitly designed and studied as an intervention on provider burnout, the results of its effect on burnout may be somewhat more robust than other studies. An unintended result of the program is its usefulness as an example of a transition from a squad to a team organization. Lyon, English, and Smith have done us a favor by including brief descriptions of the organizational challenges that accompanied the APEX implementation.

The increased involvement of MAs and the extra support of doctors set off a cascade of other organizational changes, changes that probably should be expected as part of a plan to move from a squad to a team organization. There were challenges in the health system and in the relationships in the team itself. The increasing importance of the MA's role to the success of the model required increased organizational attention to their training and their needs. They needed ongoing training and support equal to about 40 hours of additional classroom training as well as time to observe doctors' visits with patients and do simulated practice in their new roles with the physicians. Several meetings about the purpose of the change were held with all concerned, and ultimately a transition facilitator was hired to help in the process. With the increased responsibility and increased training came an expectation from MAs for increased salaries, which had to be met before the recruiting of the additional MAs could be successful and the existing workforce could be stable. If there was any belief that MAs would be happy with receiving just the "professional development" the program offered, especially in a medical setting where the difference in levels of payment between doctors and staff can be so stark, that proved to be wishful thinking. The changes in roles and salaries in the pilot practice encountered the sort of pushback within its large health system that is common when exceptions to usual job descriptions and pay levels are requested. To keep the program going, budgetary and human resources administrators had to be brought on board by the support of top administrators.

The evolution of roles within the team was a challenge. In the previous organization as a squad, the role of the MA was much narrower and better defined. In the expanded role, no matter how clear the protocols that were developed, the increased complexity of the role created the need for increased use of judgment by the MAs and gave opportunities for increased variance between their actions and doctors' expectations. For their part, MAs needed to understand and to participate in developing the overall vision and mission of the program. Doctors found they needed to treat MAs more as team members who required personal support for their learning and participation in planning. The "squad" approach of offering gentle corrections if an MA made a mistake was not workable, because they felt more vulnerable when doing tasks that were new to them. The "flattening" of the leadership structure of the teams occurred to some degree even though it does not appear to have been a goal of the program.

Both before and after the transition to the APEX model, behavioral health clinicians were part of the practice. Their contribution was more as specialty services available within the practice space than as members of the "teamlet." Both the report on the APEX model and on the "Union Square" model assume the presence and importance of behavioral health services. They are not the focus in the transformations that are reported.

2.6 The "Union Square" Model

This model was developed at Union Square Family Health Center (USFHC) in Somerville, Massachusetts. It was designed to provide effective care to a particularly challenging patient population, to serve the complex health needs of low-income immigrant families in an urban setting. The model involves segmenting the patients of a large health center into smaller practices within the clinic called "pods." Each pod has 4000–5000 patients, 2–4 primary care physicians, 1.5 physician assistants (PAs), 1.5 nurses, 1 receptionist, and 3–4 MAs. Patients are assigned to pods without regard to their diagnoses or risk profiles. Every attempt is made to have continuity between patients and providers within the pod. For the PAs, the continuity is about 90%. The continuity with the pod is almost 100%.

In their reorganization of the roles in the multidisciplinary team, USFHC has gone farther away from the physician-led team and has distributed functions more broadly than simply enhancing the MA's role. Here is how they describe the roles they developed:

- Medical receptionist: Frontline staff represents the local community and serve as cultural ambassadors for the clinic, helping bridge language barriers. Receptionists are familiar with each team's patients and can schedule immunizations and appointment for the whole family. They help ensure consistent follow-up, leveraging mobile technology like secure texting to contact patients.
- Medical assistant (MA): Considering the "boss" during clinic sessions, MAs manage clinic flow and guide patients through blood pressure checks, immunization and other activities. Before a clinic session, the MA coordinates with the physician around care needs for patients visiting that day. The MA also has a panel of patients to outreach for screening and prevention.

- Registered nurse: Nurses facilitate chronic disease management, developing relationship with patient through longitudinal educational visits. They also undertake outreach to complex patients and manage transitions of care, following patients after discharge from the hospital.
- Physician: Because other team members handle many of the screening, prevention, education, and administrative efforts that often consume physician time in primary care practices, physicians at Union Square focus on the work of diagnosing, treating, and developing relationships with patients.
- Physician assistant: Physician assistants share a panel of patients with physicians. Patients can choose the kind of provider they want to see, and many receive care solely from PAs. For example, Haitian patients on one physician's team may opt to see a PA who is fluent in Haitian-Creole (Jain et al. [15]).

"The multi-disciplinary team employed innovative workflows to be able to address many different types of needs with different intensities of contact at the same time. In a three-hour period, the team of one physician, one nurse practitioner, two medical assistants and one nurse would have contact with 30 patients. All would huddle at the beginning of the session. Two patients with complex needs could get visits with increased physician time. Patients with acute needs could be seen quickly by the NP, both physician and NP supported by an MA. In addition, the nurse could do 2 hours of care management outreach calls, the physician did a half hour of e-visits and phone visits and half hour of coordination with specialists and hospitalists.

The physician, NP and nurse could meet, and the medical assistants had significant time for panel management or patient health coaching (see Jain et al. [15]). Over the course of 3 years of implementation, the average number of visits per year was cut in half, reducing wait times. This does not mean that the average number of contacts with patients by the practice fell. These increased."

In addition to the pod organization, USFHC tracks 20 chronic conditions using registries. Each registry has a group of staff that meets weekly to discuss the patients they are tracking. There is a team especially set up to provide care management for complex patients, and behavioral health clinicians are available to work with any team and any patient. Communication about patients is enhanced by placing the workspace of all providers in a common area. This facilitates unscheduled exchange of information in real time rather than asynchronous communication using the EHR. The success of the model is continually monitored by 20 measures used by the health system, Cambridge Health Alliance, of which USFHC is a part. In 2016, USFHC met or exceeded 15 out of those measures.

Lora Council [16], Senior Medical Director for Primary Care of Cambridge Health Alliance, makes the point the additional members of the primary care team are not just relieving doctors and nurses of some tasks so that their jobs will be more managed. There is a new dimension to the care introduced because of the way these other members relate to patients. It is important to consider the idea that the care enhancers do not just take on task but they may take on aspects of the therapeutic relationship. The patient benefits from having a relationship with someone who may more directly support them rather than instruct them. In a heterogenous large patient panel, the doctor or the nurse may not be the best people to serve the therapeutic relationship needs of every patient. It is both threatening to professional identity and immensely relieving simultaneously if a care enhancer on the team is the primary "owner" of some of the emotional relationships of the 2500 patient panel.

The examples detailed here are but two of many reorganizations to team-based care that are happening around the nation. Whatever the emphasis or goal of these reorganizations, all involve increasing the involvement in and responsibility for important aspects of patient care by non-physician team members. With these changes come increased need for training, additional exchange of information among team members, flexibility in the types of services offered, and increased involvement, support, and flexibility on the part of administration to keep the transformation from stalling.

2.7   Team Training

The training a team will need to create or to find will depend on the approach it takes to adding functions for its members. Faster transitions call for more extensive training, usually from an outside sources, though the results are less reliable (see Chap. 11). More evolutionary changes may be achieved with training developed by the team itself. Many of the functions done by the doctor or a nurse could be done by someone with lesser training if the team member who has the skills can take the time to develop a training experience for other team members. This will include time given to overseeing the development of the team member in using the new skill.

One way that mutual skill improvement can be done is to have a regular routine of mutual observation and feedback on the team. It takes some planning to schedule mutual observation in a way that does not take too much of the team's time. Some teams do mutual observation during the visit of the first patient of the day. In this approach each team member joins the team member who works with the patient before or after themselves, observing the work of that member. This is done with the permission of the patient, who usually is happy to be part of the self-improvement that this represents for the team. Each member notices specific behaviors that the team member whom they observe does well in addition to noticing opportunities for improvement. As each team member completes their role in the care of the first patient, they return to their usual routines. The team shares observations when they get together for a planned lunch meeting at the end of the morning patient care. Substitutions in who observes whom can be made based on trainer or mentor and trainee relationships on the team (see Chap. 11).

2.8   Conclusion

The benefits of high-functioning teams are many. A high-functioning team allows tasks that do not need a doctor's level of training to be performed by other members of the team. The evidence indicates that working in a high-functioning team increases job satisfaction and reduces burnout for doctors and staff. Team-based care increases patient satisfaction. Having participation by team members in monitoring care and addressing problems allows for patients to feel more constant support and for the team to care for a patient's needs without needing to have the patient come for a visit each time.

Sustaining team-based care is hard in a fee-for-service payment environment. Union Square calculated that its model lost money in fee-for-service because of the many types of service it offered for which there was no payment code. When the center had 63% of its patients covered by capitation, the model showed financial gains [15]. Some very innovative team-based care has been developed by for-profit health systems who only work with patients covered by capitated payments, such as in the Medicare Advantage program [10]. On one hand, payment transformation allows this flexibility for team-based care, and on the other, it appears that having a high-functioning team in a practice makes moving to an alternate payment approach a safer bet for payers.

The dedication of additional time to regular meetings, meetings in the flow of care each day or by the week or month, does not in itself lead to the change from a squad to a team. It is perfectly possible for these meetings to become opportunities for the squad leader to give more detailed directions to the squad members without creating any new ways of relating. The transition comes when the patterns of exchange of information are transformed. Some accounts suggest that additional meetings could lead to increased coordination and effectiveness of care and that could lead to better satisfaction and esprit de corps for team members. Yet, at the point that a practice decides to take on this transition, what does the current squad leader say or do to create successful team process? It is unreasonable to expect that doctors or other team members will create a method that fosters the transformation on their own. Having a method that can be used to build engagement with patients and with fellow team members, such as the T.E.A.M. Way, can make the entire transformation easier (see Chap. 11). Finally, adding a team member with expertise in group processes and in mental and behavioral health can be a way to help all team members to be more successful in their additional levels of responsibility for overall patient care. However it is achieved, team-based care, when it includes the changes in relationship and communication patterns described here, and when it is supported by data on its performance with its particular panel of patients, seems to be a necessary foundation block for patient-centered care.

References

1. Jabbarpour Y, DeMarchis E, Bazemore A, Grundy P. The impact of primary care practice transformation on cost, quality, and utilization: a systematic review of research published in 2016. Patient-centered primary care collaborative and Robert Graham Center. 2017. https://www.pcpcc.org/resource/impact-primary-care-practice-transformation-cost-quality-and-utilization

2. Mitchell P, Wynia M, Golden R, McNellis B, Okun S, Webb CE, Rohrbach V, Von Kohorn I. Core principles & values of effective team-based health care: a discussion paper. Washington, DC: Institute of Medicine; 2012.
3. Bodenheimer T. Building teams in primary care: lessons learned. San Francisco: California Healthcare Foundation; 2007.
4. Crabtree B, Nutting P, Miller W, Stange K, Stewart E, Jaén C. Summary of the National Demonstration Project and recommendation for the patient-centered medical home. Ann Fam Med. 2010;8(Supplement 1):S80–90.
5. Wise H, Beckhard R, Rubing I, Kyte AL. Making health teams work. Cambridge: Ballinger Publishing; 1974.
6. Montori V. Why we revolt. Rochester: The Patient Revolution; 2017.
7. Willard-Grace R, Hessler D, Rogers E, Dube' K, Bodenheimer T, Grumbach K. Team structure and culture are associated with lower burnout in primary care. J Am Board Fam Med. 2014;27:229–38.
8. Mohr DC, Young GJ, Meterko M, Stolzmann KL, White B. Job satisfaction of primary care team members and quality of care. Am J Med Qual. 2011;26:18–25.
9. Kimberly JR. The relationship between job satisfaction of primary care team members and quality of care: a comment on Mohr et al. Am J Med Qual. 2011;26:8–9.
10. Schutzbank A. V.P. of Iora Health. Personal communication, 9/29/18. 2018.
11. Bodenheimer T. Building teams in primary care: 15 case studies. San Francisco: California Healthcare Foundation; 2007.
12. Panagioti M, Geraghty K, Johnson J, et al. Association between physician burnout and patient safety, professionalism, and patient satisfaction: a systematic review and meta-analysis. JAMA Intern Med. 2018;178:1317–30.
13. Friedberg MW, Chen PG, Van Busum KR, et al. Factors affecting physician professional satisfaction and their implications for patient care, health systems, and health policy. Rand Health Q. 2014;3(4):1–122.
14. Lyon C, English AF, Smith PC. A team-based care model that improves job satisfaction. Fam Pract Manag. 2018;25(2):6–11.
15. Jain N, Okanlawon T, Meisinger K, Feeley TW. Leveraging IPU principles in primary care. NEJM Catalyst. June 27, 2018.
16. Council L. Personal communication. 2018.

Resources

Getting to team-based care: https://www.stepsforward.org/modules/team-based-care

Chapter 3
Behavioral Health and Care Enhancement: Building a Team to Do the Whole Job

3.1 New Expertise for Better Patient Care

Truly patient-centered primary care attempts to address the entire array of needs and problems that patients bring to their doctor. These needs and problems tend to be as challenging and complex as patients' lives. Since the beginning of the development of the patient-centered medical home, it has become clearer and clearer that when the "squad" that was providing medical care transforms into the team providing patient-centered care, the collective expertise represented by the team members needs to match the complexity of the most common problems presented by patients in primary care. A great many of those needs are mental health, substance use, or health behavior change, the three elements of what we term "behavioral health needs." In addition, there are numerous needs that wouldn't be called behavioral health but are nevertheless behavioral in nature such as difficulty in understanding one's disease or its treatment; fear of bad news that keeps a person away from care, anxiety, or defensiveness in responding to a doctor's suggestions; and many more. Behavioral expertise in all of these situations can increase the effectiveness of the team in engaging and caring for patients.

In Chap. 2 we discussed the importance of the team-based care to patients and to doctors and some of the possibilities for organizing team-based care that are emerging around the country. For patients, a consistent relationship with a small group of people who work together delivering coordinated aspects of care is key to their positive experience of their care [1]. This positive experience and the trust that it builds in turn correlate with improved self-management of their chronic health conditions by patients with complex health needs [2]. For doctors, the key to low burnout and greater satisfaction in their work seems to be spending less time on administrative tasks and more time delivering what they experience as high-quality care [3]. If the care is better at meeting the needs of their patients, doctors are likely to be more satisfied, even if they are not the team members delivering that care. [4] found that doctors' burnout rate was lower when they perceived their

© Springer Nature Switzerland AG 2019
A. Blount, *Patient-Centered Primary Care*,
https://doi.org/10.1007/978-3-030-17645-7_3

clinic had greater capacity to meet the social needs of their most vulnerable patients by having a social worker, behavioral specialist, psychiatrist, or pharmacist on staff.

It is commonly believed that biopsychosocial (BPS) care characterizes the best primary care [5]. Particularly for "complex" patients whose health needs are easily identifiable as biological, psychological, and social, the lack of any one of the elements of biopsychosocial care is likely to limit the effectiveness of other elements of care that are offered. Consider the patient whose diabetes would be under control and whose depression would be improving if he had housing and could get to appointments, or the patient with new housing whose diabetes would likely be better if he weren't so depressed that he keeps losing his sobriety. For the healthcare team to be effective for patients with complex health needs requires that they are able to deliver biological, psychological, and social types of interventions.

In this chapter we will go into detail about the addition of health team members who represent the introduction of new expertise and new service capability in behavioral health and the social elements of care.

The array of problems brought by a patient in primary care may be quite common without being simple. A 35-year-old woman with diabetes and a history of trauma, who is struggling with depression and a number of somatic symptoms for which no cause can be found, whose housing is tenuous and whose employment is only as reliable as her child care and her sobriety, is a person presenting an array of problems whom many primary care doctors will recognize as common in their practice. She is also a patient whose needs can severely challenge the services in most primary care practices.

When this patient (whom we will call Mary) comes to her doctor's office, and she comes often, she presents what she considers "medical" symptoms to her doctor (whom we will call Dr. Kelsey). She is tired all the time. She can't concentrate on things. She worries about the headaches she has been having and wonders if she has a brain tumor. On one particular visit, for example, she is back with somatic complaints. The medicine that Dr. Kelsey prescribed for her diabetes at her last visit didn't make her feel any better, so she stopped taking it. She is hesitant to admit this to Dr. Kelsey, lest her doctor become impatient with her and stop seeing her. She knows people who have been "fired" by their doctors for "non-compliance," and she appreciates the way Dr. Kelsey listens to her, even if she doesn't always follow her advice.

Entering the exam room, Dr. Kelsey is very concerned about the findings of the laboratory tests Mary had since her last visit. Her hemoglobin A1c (a measure of the level of sugar in her blood over the previous 3 months) is at 10 (above 7 is concerning). Mary has gained more weight since her last visit when they had discussed her starting on a diet and getting a bit of exercise regularly. If Mary senses some frustration behind Dr. Kelsey's always-professional demeanor, it is not because she is angry at Mary, but because she is feeling pessimistic about the prospect of making a difference for her patient during the visit. She is imagining trying to address the concerns that brought Mary in today, concerns for which she may find no medical cause, in a way that will engage Mary more actively in care while still having time to influence her toward adherence to her diabetes medication, her diet, her exercise regimen, and her continued sobriety, all in the 15 minutes allotted for the visit.

Dr. Kelsey's pessimism about influencing Mary toward changing her health behavior to manage her diabetes is reasonable. Mary does not share her doctor's level of concern about her disease. Dr. Kelsey has seen the havoc in people's lives that uncontrolled diabetes can cause: loss of vision, severe neuropathic pain, loss of limbs, and early heart attacks. She can describe vividly and with urgency what a dangerous disease it is. When Mary heard this list as part of the patient education that is routine when someone is first diagnosed with diabetes, she thought these warnings sounded overstated. She assumed that Dr. Kelsey was benevolently trying to scare her into following her diet in the same way that she (Mary) sometimes tries to use scare tactics to keep her kids from doing dangerous things. And besides, when she tried to change her diet a bit, to cut out sugary drinks and eat more fruits and vegetables, she got nothing but complaints from her family. It was not worth the increased expense for the fruits and vegetables.

In a moment of candor, Dr. Kelsey might tell a peer that when she considers how she spends most of her time with patients, she often feels that they are talking about the topics that are least important for improving her patients' lives. In the case of Mary, as a prime example, Dr. Kelsey often thinks that if she (Dr. K.) were expert at treating depression or alcohol misuse or symptoms of PTSD, her skills would be a better fit for her patient's needs. If she could find a way to relieve some of Mary's stress by making her childcare more reliable, teaching her ways to manage her children's behavior more comfortably, teaching her how to improve her relationship with her children's school, influencing her to make a better choice of a love partner, meeting with her and her partner to elicit his support for her diet, or helping her repair the cutoff between herself and her family of origin and the support they could provide, Dr. Kelsey is confident that helping her manage her diabetes and control her weight would be easy by comparison. The keys to beginning to help her patient escape the net of problems in which she seems caught are not what Dr. Kelsey thinks of as "medical." In the terms of the biopsychosocial model that was discussed in her residency training, she sees herself presented with problems framed as biological that she perceives to be predominantly psychological and social at their root.

It is not that Dr. Kelsey has been shirking her responsibility to the array of her patients' needs. She regularly has offered treatment in the form of antidepressant medication to her patients who seem down and depressed. She has gone to continuing medical education classes to improve her skills at prescribing for the cases of depression and anxiety that she identifies in her patients. She is familiar with the first-line medications for depression and anxiety, but does not feel confident in her skills when the first or second medication that she prescribes does not seem to make a noticeable difference. She knows that primary care doctors tend to prescribe antidepressant medication in accordance with the latest evidence only about half the time, but because she doesn't feel competent with mental health disorders at a specialty level, she still finds herself uneasy about using diagnoses such as "major depressive disorder" or with prescribing the levels of medication that were recommended in the classes she took.

Dr. Kelsey knows that many of the symptoms of depression are physical symptoms such as rapid changes in weight, difficulty sleeping, and difficulty concentrating and that other symptoms, not formally on the list of depression symptoms, are common for people with depression. Symptoms such as pains for which there are no medical findings seem to be a part of the presentation of many of her patients whom she is treating for depression. Still she is hesitant to suggest the idea of depression to people presenting these symptoms who are not overtly sad or suicidal. For most people she tends to follow each physical symptom, evaluating for a list of possible medical diagnoses before suggesting a diagnosis of depression that she suspects the patient will not like or accept.

Dr. Kelsey has learned that making a diagnosis of a mental health or substance use disorder can be the beginning of more headaches for her. When she offers such a diagnosis, the question of what sort of treatment to pursue becomes a challenge. She was trained that for a condition that she is not fully trained to manage, a referral to a specialist, in this case a mental health service, is the logical next step. When she suggests such a referral, her patients, like patients in primary care generally, are likely to agree to accept her referral when they are in the visit with her, but, also like many patients in primary care, the number who follow-up and start treatment is a small minority. Some get lost in the complexity of the world of mental health intake, giving up after facing the insurance issues and long waiting lists that they encounter when they call a mental health or substance use facility. The majority, however, simply don't make the call. They agreed to the referral because they didn't want to argue with their doctor, but they still wondered if they had a physical ailment the doctor was missing. Many felt stigmatized or rejected by her when she suggested the referral to mental health services and never intended to pursue the new treatment. For this reason, Dr. Kelsey tries to treat some patients herself and saves her energy for the referral of only the most urgent cases. Dr. Kelsey is enacting a pattern that is true in the health system as a whole: for the vast majority of people with mental health and substance use needs, unless there is treatment for those needs in primary care, there will be no treatment at all [6].

The service Dr. Kelsey would use most often in her current role as the only clinician providing behavioral health treatment to her panel of patients is the service she has given up trying to access: referring a patient to a psychiatrist to obtain a specialist's expertise in prescribing for them. Many of the psychiatrists in her area no longer take the insurance that her patients carry. The demand for their services is so great that most can keep a practice busy while treating only people who can pay cash for treatment. That saves the psychiatrist the headaches of the lower payment rates and oversight regulations that are enforced by behavioral health-managed care companies. For the minority of psychiatrists who work in the public mental health service system, new openings in their patient schedules are rare. Many of the mental health centers in which they work will not allow them to see patients as consults to other physicians or to treat patients who are not also seeing therapists who work in the center.

When she has succeeded in referring a patient who did begin treatment at the mental health center, her only source of information about the patient's treatment and any medication that may have been prescribed has been the patient himself. Many mental health centers are very reluctant to share information with patients' primary care doctors or any other clinicians outside of the mental health center staff. Primary care doctors often jokingly use the term "black hole" when referring to the mental health system. Like the gravitational pull of a black hole that keeps any light from escaping, the practices of the mental health system can appear to take patients in and prevent information of any kind about their progress or treatment from "escaping" to other doctors. Because patients can be such unreliable sources of information about medication, this creates risk for the primary care doctor who must prescribe for her patients' "medical" illnesses without being sure what other medication they are taking.

The descriptions of Mary's situation and of Dr. Kelsey's practice are not meant to be stereotypes of patients, of doctors, or of the way all primary care works. Far from it, they are meant to be examples that primary care doctors and others in the field will recognize as common. The story of Dr. Kelsey and Mary, as composite examples of many others in each role, was created with respect and empathy for both patient and doctor. Finally, they are meant to make more experiential the many statistics that are used to document the importance of integrating behavioral health clinicians into primary care as part of the primary care health team [7, 8] and to underline the reasons for the urgent efforts of state and national medical authorities to address the fragmented health system in the USA.

3.2 Adding a Behavioral Health Clinician

Consider how the situation would change if Dr. Kelsey or her practice decided to involve a behavioral health clinician in Mary's care, a clinician who is part of the practice staff. One of the first impacts will be, in all likelihood, a change in Mary's reaction to the suggestion that she receive behavioral healthcare. Mary generally perceives her complaints as medical in origin, and having a behavioral health team member in her doctor's practice allows her to perceive her treatment for the symptoms of depression as part of her medical care. People who hesitate to be involved in care that is defined as for mental health problems are often perfectly comfortably accepting care that is defined as helping them cope with the stresses that they are experiencing or as directed at teaching them new skills for managing their pain, insomnia, fatigue, or chronic illness. The fit of behavioral healthcare to the needs of primary care patients is one phenomenon behind the fact that one of the first outcomes of adding a behavioral health clinician in primary care is the doctors' satisfaction with the addition and their improved satisfaction with providing primary care generally [9]. Doctors get to focus on the areas in which they feel most competent and to be able to involve a behavioral health clinician where they feel they need help.

The decision to add a behavioral health clinician to the primary care health team in Dr. Kelsey's practice would make the practice part of a movement to integrate behavioral health into primary care that is national in scope. The resulting enhanced primary care service is called integrated primary care (IPC) [10] or behavioral health integration (BHI). It is an effort that currently is being pursued in numerous countries around the globe. In the USA, the movement is led by government health agencies (the Center for Medicare and Medicaid Services (CMS), the Health Resources and Services Administration (HRSA), the Agency for Healthcare Research and Quality (AHRQ), the health systems of all of the branches of the military, the Veterans Administration (VA), and the Substance Abuse and Mental Health Services Administration (SAMHSA)). The impetus for integrating behavioral health and primary care comes at every level, from the federal agencies, state Medicaid and other state health authorities, numerous foundations, major health systems, health plans and the employers who use them, and individual primary care practices. This is a movement that has been maturing since the 1990s, both with effective clinical models [11] and clear conceptual outlines [7]. New research findings, guidelines, and tools are being added almost daily (See Resource List at the end of the chapter.)

The field of integrated primary care has generated a number of descriptions [12], [13]) and models [14, 15] of how integrated care is done most effectively. Some stress the collaboration between the consulting psychiatrist and the primary care doctor, focusing on a designated population with a target diagnosis [15], while others stress the role of a behavioral health clinician (BHC) supporting the doctor in the flow of her clinical work with consultation and interventions as part of the immediate healthcare team [14]. Each approach has evidence of positive outcomes, though the collaborative care model (CCM) [15] which was developed using controlled therapeutic, care management and medical protocols for clearly defined populations has stronger clinical outcome findings. Each approach has evidence of patient and provider satisfaction and improved access, though the primary care behavioral health (PCBH) model that was built on providing the doctor with a consulting and supporting behavioral health clinician in the flow of daily practice has stronger access and satisfaction outcomes.

Picking a model is not a simple choice between the best clinical outcome for a designated population vs. broad behavioral health infrastructure in the practice. The complexity of the choice is highlighted by two large meta-analyses of implementations of the collaborative care model. In one study using meta-regression of the factors associated with lowering of depressive symptoms, Coventry and his colleagues [16] found that a structured psychological component was the only factor that remained significant in their analysis. Factors that did not show significant results were systematic screening vs. clinician referral, presence or absence of a chronic illness, psychological intervention alone or in combination with medication, and scheduled or ad hoc supervision of the person providing the psychological component. All programs included active engagement with patients to monitor changes in their symptoms and to maintain their engagement in whatever therapy they were receiving. Another large analysis of the CCM [17] found that the most common component across successful models was "a standardized care coordination plan that involved regular interaction (by the care manager) both with patient and physician" (p. 51).

The different terms for the most significant factor (Coventry) or most common factor (Tice) for success in the two studies describe very similar elements. Coventry's "structured psychological component" is similar to Tice's "standardized care coordination plan" in that both describe regular contact (face to face or by telephone) with a designated person on the healthcare team. Both studies use the term "care manager" for this designated person. The staff member in both studies might be a licensed therapist, pharmacist, nurse, or other health professionals who maintained regular contact with both the patient and other members of the team. Coventry, agreeing with Pincus et al. [18], cited some evidence of increased effectiveness if the "care manager" was a licensed mental health clinician but stressed the effectiveness of nurses or other health professionals in this role when supervised by mental health clinicians.

As there would be in any emerging field, there are disagreements about what "model" to choose. The leaders who have been watching their models develop over the longest time, however, are noticing that the models tend to converge in mature practices. These leaders are tending to shift their focus from prescribing how it *should* be done to being champions of measuring the effects of what *is* being done for patients [19]. If we know whether or not patients get better and work in a timely way to make improvements to our clinical practices until patients do begin to improve, most of the leaders in the field will be on board.

This convergence of models is also seen in the guidance that has been created to help practices transition to IPC. There are several tools to help practices manage the process of achieving primary care with integrated behavioral health. The Agency for Healthcare Research and Quality has supported the development of an Integration Academy, a group of experts charged with developing the supportive infrastructure necessary for the spread of primary care behavioral health integration. The website of the academy, www.integrationacademy.ahrq.gov, is a good place to start looking for tools and information in implementing integrated care.

3.3   Organizational Support Needed for the Process of Behavioral Health Integration

Integrating behavioral health into primary care impacts the work of every member of the team, including administrators and administrative staff. That means that administration of the larger health system will need to support the process for it to succeed. Everyone in the practice and on each healthcare team will need to be invited to be a part of the transition that BHI represents. Leadership of the practice and the doctors on each team should articulate the role of behavioral health as a central element in the mission of the organization. It helps if time and resources already have been allotted to address business issues such as billing, sustainability, and job security of current staff. Leadership should be sure that people know that this is not an experiment and that it won't sink the organization financially.

It is important to be realistic about the breadth of the impact beyond the clinical team. Consider just two of many possible examples. The integration of behavioral services will require human resources in the organization to incorporate new staff roles, new training requirements, and new credentials that they may not have seen before. Compliance staff will have to address issues of behavioral health information sharing and documentation that have not been a concern before. Because the implementation of BHI impacts everyone's work in some way, all the people in the organization will need to be reminded of how their contribution to integration supports the organization's coming closer to realizing its mission on behalf of its patients.

The communication processes that build a team out of a squad, both the regular meetings to discuss patients, workflows, roles, and outcomes and the communication in the flow of care, will be crucial as a practice integrates behavioral health. A unified electronic health record is a crucial piece of infrastructure for this communication. Having a unified care plan that lists problems, goals, and treatments for all the care a patient receives in the practice, because of the communication it requires, is another basic element to successful integration. Arranging the physical location of team members so that they encounter each other regularly or can summon each other easily with minimum steps on everyone's part is also part of the communication infrastructure. The efforts that build a culture of teamwork are all important to adding a new person, new role, and new expertise set and clinical perspective to the team.

Behavioral health services in the practice will need to be as clearly delineated as the array of medical services in the practice. Just as the practice does not prescribe antibiotics for every patient who comes with an earache, a protocol will be needed to decide who will be offered the limited resource of the involvement of the BHC. The protocol will be based on evidence, guidance in the field, assessment of what group can most effectively be served, and team members' clinical judgment at the time that the patient is seen. Starting with a defined population that is designated by the doctors, team members, and behavioral health clinicians together allows for the targeting of screening, for more reliable administration of outcome measures, and for better monitoring and outreach procedures to support patients' progress. A clearly delineated population that is not too large keeps the team from being overwhelmed by the new processes. It is crucial to protect the team's meeting time so that they can use the data on patients' progress to improve their routines and techniques. A team of researchers who has done extensive observation of the roles and clinical routines in exemplary integrated primary care practices [20] has documented common phases in the workflows that will need to be developed and tested. They list these phases as identifying, engaging/transitioning to behavioral healthcare, providing treatment, and monitoring/adjusting care. Each of these phases will take substantial conversation, planning, and adjustment before it occurs smoothly.

Having a clearly described population allows the practice to plan for the type of expertise that will need to be added to the team. Most doctors will want access to some consultation with a psychiatric specialist who can share expertise on prescribing medication. While the role of psychological interventions is endorsed in the literature [16, 17], the use of psychotropic medication for some patients is still the second most common tool in successful implementation of BHI [17]. Many of the implementations of the collaborative care model (CCM) use a psychiatric clinician to consult to the primary care doctor on prescribing and to supervise the "care manager" [15]. Other implementations of the CCM have used psychologists in the role of consultant to the doctor and the care manager on all except prescribing [21]. The economics of adding the necessary expertise to the team and having that expertise available more generally to team members over time favor using a psychiatric consultant for prescribing support for the doctor and a health psychologist or Masters-level mental health clinician with experience in primary care as the first full-time hire onto the team itself [17, 22].

Regular screening of patients in the practice for behavioral health conditions is as much a part of integrated primary care as is screening for cancers. Patients in the designated population who are identified as needing behavioral healthcare are offered interventions that are fitted to their needs and are monitored to assess their progress. This usually involves a registry to track all the patients in the population so that their care and their response can be followed and supported. This means that there is an effort to keep in touch with, and to offer behavioral activation and problem solving to, both the patients who come to face-to-face visits and to those who do not. Those patients who don't respond to the initial care approach, whether medication, behavioral protocol, or both, or who have a setback after responding well at first, will need to encounter a team that has a plan for how to address their situation. The second step can include medication adjustment, more contact with the BHC, and/or supported referral to a community resource. The ability to distinguish patients whose symptoms are not improving in order to offer more intensive services is a crucial element in any BHI implementation.

As the team gets more proficient in providing integrated care to the first designated population, the issue of equity will come up. Why are we doing so much for this group and not addressing the needs of others? When the plan for the first group is beginning to run smoothly, new groups can be added, and screening, outcome measurement, and clinical interventions can be more universal. The goal over time is to have behavioral health consultation or supervision for team members, brief behavioral interventions for many patients, and population programming in place for designated subgroups. The evolution of such a complex and highly organized program comes over the course of years, not months. It will need the ongoing support of leadership protecting teams from demands for program development that outpace either the growth in staff resources or the enhancement of team members' expertise.

A patient-centered approach to integration considers patients' understanding of the behavioral aspects of their health and of their care from the beginning. This is true in the transition to IPC. Some practices as they develop their programs develop a brochure, an area of their website, or posters to post in strategic places to explain the new behavioral health services that are available. It is an opportunity to develop language that is engaging to people and minimizes stigma. This language should be used consistently by team members to maximize patient support for the behavioral health aspects of care. Successful implementation often involves training and the development of scripts for team members to use in describing the role of behavioral health services to patients in the practice and in their care. Using scripts and the processes that go into the development of the scripts help to foster a change in the "mental models of care" that is needed for successful integration [23].

3.4 Competencies of Behavioral Health Clinicians

The contributions that behavioral health clinicians can make to a primary care team have been most of the focus to this point. The tone has been very positive. These descriptions have been built on an assumption that needs to be made explicit and examined. It is the assumption that the behavioral health clinician, whether psychiatrist, psychologist, clinical social worker, or other masters level counselor, brings the specific competencies required to work successfully in primary care. It is a crucial point. The primary care landscape is littered with programs that failed because this necessity was not understood. The most central reason for the failure of fledgling integrated primary care programs has been that the new behavioral health clinician tried to practice specialty mental health in a primary care practice.

It is important to distinguish the premises and practice patterns of primary care behavioral health work from those of specialty mental health [24]. The role of the clinician, the focus of care, the relationship to the patient, and the sets of skill employed are different, even when the disciplinary training of both is the same. A specialty mental health clinician (SMHC) carries a caseload of clients for whom she is the therapist. She thinks of herself as a mental health professional who is responsible for the mental health treatment of her caseload. Consultation or supervision that she provides to other professionals is usually by formal arrangement. A primary care behavioral health clinician (BHC) participates in the care of a panel of patients shared by the doctor and the team. She thinks of herself as a healthcare clinician. Consultation with team members is a responsibility that is an essential aspect of team membership. An SMHC focuses care on specific mental health diagnoses or substance use disorders. A BHC addresses mental health and substance use disorders plus the behavioral aspects of chronic illness and other medical conditions. She is a behavioral health generalist who can start with whatever problem the patient is willing to address. The impact on total medical cost of behavioral health work in primary care depends on what sort of interventions are provided. The more these interventions are the same as the psychotherapy of SMHC, the less impact on lowering costs. The more they are targeting behavioral interventions on medical illness, the more the work will be likely to lower other medical costs [25]. A few mental health clinicians learn the premises and practice patterns of primary care behavioral health while in graduate school. The majority learn after they are already licensed to practice. In either case, training to help them make the transition is necessary if they are to provide the additional value to primary care that has been discussed in this chapter [26].

Psychiatric clinicians also need training to orient them to their role when they are consulting in primary care. Psychiatric clinicians are in extremely short supply compared to the need for their services. Psychiatrists working in primary care can have their expertise leveraged to serve many more patients when they work as consultants to primary care doctors. This is a different role than most were taught in their psychiatric residencies. Most were trained to perform "direct consultations" in which they support other physicians by doing face-to-face assessments of patients who were referred by their doctors and offering treatment recommendations to the doctors. Working as a consultant in primary care calls for both additional proficiencies and an adjustment of the attitudes about control and responsibility for patients that they were taught in their psychiatric residencies [27]. Psychiatric clinicians need to learn to consult on specific patients described to them by doctors or behavioral health clinicians as well as doing face-to-face patient evaluations, to recommend medication choices without being the proscribing physician, and to offer teaching or advice more generally on evidence-based practices to a team providing care.

3.5   Addressing the Social Determinants of Health

The more that patients confront challenges in what have been called "the social determinants of health," the more a distinct service that is additional to medical and behavioral health care is required for effective care. It represents the third element of the bio-psycho-social model. The third element of care is targeted not just to improve social challenges or disadvantages but to also enhance the medical and behavioral health aspects care. The roles, titles, and duties of team members who provide this element of care are much more varied than the roles for the medical and behavioral health elements of care. The value of the work of team members providing social elements of care is very well documented. Anyone advocating for the increased involvement in care of one of these roles, whether it is nurse, care managers [28], care coordinators, care navigators [29], community health workers [30], promotores [31], or health coaches [32], will have no difficulty citing evidence for the contribution that the role for which they advocate.

Unfortunately, anyone trying to organize a reliable chart of the credentials and duties of each role is likely to give up in frustration. Role names don't always match with functions. Care management and care coordination are evidence-based functions, but they may or may not be provided by staff members called "care manager" or "care coordinator." Team members in different primary care practices who have the same job title may well have very different role responsibilities requiring different credentials. Team members with similar job descriptions requiring similar credentials may well have different job titles in different health systems or in different states.

The lack of consistency caused the New Hampshire Primary Care Behavioral Health Workforce Initiative to create the term, "care enhancer," as a name for the group of roles on the health team that are not licensed clinicians [33]. Using the concept of care enhancers allowed us to describe possible career ladders within primary care for developing the workforce. It helped us to be able to understand the overall patterns of services on a team and the fit of these services with the needs of their patients.

The functions of care enhancers are broad and, for patients with complex health needs, very important for patient-centered care. Any list of their functions or their skills and services will inevitably be incomplete, yet it is helpful to have lists to help in imagining their contributions. Here is a list of their functions:

1. Create and maintain patient engagement in care within and across health settings.
2. Address issues of health literacy, adherence, and healthy living.
3. Address social and economic barriers patients face in caring for their health and in accessing care.
4. Keep information flowing between the patient, their primary care doctor, the healthcare team, and other providers in the health system.

Care enhancers are able to contribute to one or more of the functions above by being able to offer some combination of the skills and services below:

- Additional time to spend in the care of a designated group of patients
- Flexibility about location of contact—to visit in patients' homes or elsewhere in the health system
- Language skills that make communication with a patient much easier and more reliable
- Shared life experiences with the patient which can facilitate better engagement
- A relationship that increases the engagement the patient to the rest of the team
- Monitoring of the patient's health metrics or the achievement of health goals to share with the team
- Patient education that can be ongoing, more detailed, and better targeted to the health literacy of the patient
- Help for patients to understand and navigate the health system
- Interviewing skills to increase the patient's motivation to achieve health goals
- Communication with other people who are important to the patient's health and treatments, e.g., others in the health system, others in the schools or social service agencies, or family members
- Support so that the patient's personal information and preferences are considered by providers around the health system

The roles of care enhancers include some elements of medical care and some elements of psychosocial care. The goal of what is sometimes called "whole person care" has been understood in the past as combining specific team members, each with the expertise in one of these aspects of care. Often these were the doctor, a behavioral health clinician, and a care enhancer. Yet, the idea of representing the biological, psychological, and social functions of the team by one team member for each function is in one way fundamentally out of step with the history and evolution of primary care. Primary care was built on the importance of the generalist physician to patients. It is distinguished from specialty care, by being the service to which patients can bring any problem they experience as "medical" and expect to find understanding and help, even if subsequently the help they receive involves facilitating their connection with other resources. The primary care doctor's job has been biological, psychological, and social since its inception. The newest attempts to take some of the pressure off of the doctor by expanding the roles of other team members, such as the MA, tend to mirror the multidimensionality of the practice. When an MA meets with a patient, takes their vital signs, reviews their depression screening, and asks questions about possible domestic violence, they contribute to the biological, psychological, and social care for the patient. The recent flowering of roles in the primary care health team makes the categorization as either biological, psychological, or social a lost cause.

Medical, psychological, and social expertise sets are needed to support the multiple aspects of the duties of each of the team members. I find it concerning that new roles for care enhancers with important psychosocial duties are sometimes added while the majority of the behavioral or social expertise they will need to be effective is expected to be provided by a manual developed outside the practice. Montori [34] makes the point that evidence-based approaches created for "this type of patient" often are not a fit for "this patient." Robust expertise sets in psychological, social, and medical aspects of care are important for any health team, and team members who embody this expertise need to be part of the everyday functioning and information exchange of the team. The doctor is the expert in biomedical care on the team. Just as the medical expertise of team members grows if they are able to observe and discuss the doctor's work, the psychological expertise of all team members grows as they are able to observe and discuss the functioning of an expert in psychological care, and the social awareness and expertise of team members grows as they hear the accounts of the interactions of care enhancers with their patients.

The presence on the team of one member with robust psychological or social expertise allows other team members to offer more interventions in that area. They can be confident that if the intervention they devise or that comes from a manual does not succeed, there is a team member with more expertise to help back up and adjust the care. In the case of team members who are transitioning in their care patterns rather than joining the team with new roles, care and support can make the difference in whether they are supportive of integrated team-based care or stressed by it. One study of such a transition found that "Nurses, practice assistants (MAs), and HCAs (CHWs) complain of the psychological burden of providing mental health services in depression care. To avoid exhaustion, they prefer to work part-time" (Gensichen [35], p. 514). This is part of the reason for a longer-term process (see Chap. 11 for training suggestions).

The augmenting of the roles of care enhancers described in Chap. 2 gives tasks formerly done by doctors to other team members, leaving doctors to use more of their time doing tasks that only they are trained to do. In the same way, the BHC can be a trainer and supervisor of the behavioral aspects of the roles of the care enhancers, allowing the BHC to apportion his/her other time working with patients for whose needs their skills are a unique fit.

3.6 Conclusion

A commitment to patient-centered team-based primary care should include a commitment to integrating behavioral health services as part of the primary care practice. It is the key element most often missing in making primary care a comprehensive service for patients. When done well, behavioral health services have been shown to improve clinical outcomes, lower overall medical cost, improve patient and provider satisfaction, and raise the expertise level of physicians and other team members. Behavioral health services can improve chronic illness care as well as care for mental health and substance use problems. Adding effective behavioral health services makes a primary care practice a part of a national movement toward integration. At the same time, it makes the practice better able to meet accreditation standards that are increasingly tied to levels of payment for services.

The transition to the fully realized patient-centered team-based primary care in which patients are partners in designing and managing their own care is not an inevitable outcome of adding a behavioral health clinician or a care enhancer to a practice. Behavioral health clinicians and care enhancers of all stripes are just as likely as medical professionals to be trained in a model of "providing care to" as opposed to "building partnerships with" their patients. New learning is required of every team member if they are to be able engage patients in a partnership in their designing and carrying out their own treatment. This is especially true in the case of patients who are the most challenging to treat and the most complex in their needs.

The transition is challenging and complex. When attempted as part of the larger transition toward patient-centered team-based care, adding behavioral healthcare can be experienced as another key element of a transition to better realize the mission of the organization to better serve its patients. Finally, behavioral health integration can provide a foundation upon which true partnership with patients in their care can be built. In future chapters we will discuss helping the whole team to build successful partnerships with just this population of patients.

References

1. Jabbarpour Y, DeMarchis E, Bazemore A, Grundy P. The impact of primary care practice transformation on cost, quality, and utilization: a systematic review of research published in 2016. Patient-Centered Primary Care Collaborative and Robert Graham Center. 2017. https://www.pcpcc.org/resource/impact-primary-care-practice-transformation-cost-quality-and-utilization

2. Mautner DB, Pang H, Brenner JC, Shea JA, Gross KS, Frasso R, Cannuscio CC. Generating hypotheses about care needs of high utilizers: lessons from patient interviews. Popul Health Manag. 2013;16:S26–33.
3. Friedberg MW, Chen PG, Van Busum KR, et al. Factors affecting physician professional satisfaction and their implications for patient care, health systems, and health policy. Rand Health Q. 2014;3(4):1–122.
4. De Marchis E, Knox M, Hessler D, et al. Physician burnout and higher clinic capacity to address patients' social needs. J Am Board Fam Med. 2019;32:69–78.
5. Borrell-Carrio F, Suchman AL, Epstein RM. The biopsychosocial model 25 years later: principles, practice, and scientific inquiry. Ann Fam Med. 2004;2:576–82.
6. Regier D, Narrow w, Rae D, Manderscheid R, Locke B, Goodwin F. The de facto mental health and addictive disorders service system. Arch Gen Psychiatry. 1993;50:85–94.
7. Blount A. An introduction to integrated primary care. In: Blount A, editor. Integrated primary care: the future of medical and mental health collaboration. New York: W. W. Norton; 1998. p. 1–43.
8. deGruy FV, Etz RS. Attending to the whole person in the patient-centered medical home: the case for incorporating mental healthcare, substance abuse care, and health behavior change. Fam Syst Health. 2010;28:298–307.
9. Vickers KS, Ridgeway JL, Hathaway JC, Egginton JS, Kaderlik AB, Katzelnick DJ. Integration of mental health resources in a primary care setting leads to increased provider satisfaction and patient access. Gen Hosp Psychiatry. 2013;35:461–7.
10. Blount A, Bayona J. Toward a system of integrated primary care. Fam Syst Med. 1994;12(2):171–82.
11. Katon W, von Korff M, Lin E, Walker E, Simon GE, Bush T, Robinson P, Russon J. Collaborative management to achieve treatment guidelines: impact on depression in primary care. JAMA. 1995;273:1026–31.
12. Blount A. Integrated primary care: Organizing the evidence. Fam Syst Health. 2003;21:121–34.
13. Kathol R, deGruy F, Rollman B. Value-based financially sustainable behavioral health components in patient-centered medical homes. Ann Fam Med. 2014;12:172–5.
14. Strosahl K. Integrating behavioral health and primary care services: the primary mental health care model. In: Blount A, editor. Integrated primary care: the future of medical and mental health collaboration. New York: W. W. Norton & Co; 1998. p. 139–66.
15. Unutzer J, Harbin H, Schoenbaum M, Druss B. The collaborative care model: an approach for integrating physical and mental health care in Medicaid Health Homes. Medicaid Health Home Brief; May, 2013.
16. Coventry PA, Hudson JL, Kontopantelis E, et al. Characteristics of effective collaborative care for treatment of depression: a systematic review and meta-regression of 74 randomized controlled trials. PLoS One. 2014;9(9):e108114.
17. Tice JA, Ollendorf DA, Reed SJ, Shore KK, Weissberg J, Pearson SD. Integrating behavioral health into primary care. Institute for Clinical and Economic Review. 2015. https://icer-review.org/material/bhi-final-report/
18. Pincus HA, Pechura C, Keyser D, Bachman J, Houtsinger JK. Depression in primary care: learning lessons in a national quality improvement program. Admin Pol Ment Health. 2006;33:2–15.
19. Unutzer J. Which flavor of integrated care? Psychiatric News. 2016. https://psychnews.psychiatryonline.org/doi/full/10.1176%2Fappi.pn.2014.10b25
20. Davis MM, Gunn R, Cifuentes M, Khatri P, Hall J, Gilchrist E, Peek CJ, Klowden M, Lazerus JA, Miller BF, Cohen DJ. Clinical workflows and the associated tasks and behaviors to support delivery of integrated behavioral health and primary care. J Ambul Care Manage. 2019;42:51–65.
21. Thota AB, Sipe TA, Byard GJ, et al. Collaborative care to improve the management of depressive disorders: a community guide systematic review and meta-analysis. Am J Prev Med. 2012;42:525–38.

22. Huffman JC, Niazi SK, Rundell JR, Sharpe M, Katon WJ. Essential articles on collaborative care models for the treatment of psychiatric disorders in medical settings: a publication by the academy of psychosomatic medicine research and evidence-based practice committee. Psychosomatics. 2013. https://doi.org/10.1016/j.psym.2013.09.002.
23. Cohen DJ, Balasubramanian BA, Davis M, Hall J, Gunn R, Stange KC, Green LA, Miller WL, Crabtree BF, England MJ, Clark K, Miller BF. Understanding care integration from the ground up: five organizing constructs that shape integrated practices. JABFM. 2015;28(Supplement 1):S7–S20.
24. Patterson J, Peek CJ, Heinrich RL, Bischoff R, Scherger J. Mental health professionals in medical settings. New York: Norton; 2002.
25. Blount A, Schoenbaum M, Kathol R, Rollman B, Thomas M, O'Donohue W, Peek CJ. The economics of behavioral health services in medical settings: a summary of the evidence. Prof Psychol Res Pr. 2007;38:290–7.
26. Hall J, Cohen DJ, Davis M, et al. Preparing the workforce for behavioral health and primary care integration. J Am Board Fam Med. 2015;28(Supplement 1):S41–51.
27. Ratzliff AH, Unutzer J, Pasqualy M. Training psychiatrists for integrated care. In: Raney L, editor. Integrated care: working at the interface of primary care and behavioral health. Arlington: American Psychiatric Association Publishing; 2015.
28. Conway A, O'Donnell C, Yates P. The effectiveness of the nurse care coordinator role on patient-reported and health service outcomes: a systematic review. Evaluation Health Prof. 2017;40:18–25.
29. Natale-Pereira A, Enard KR, Nevarez L, Jones LA. The role of patient navigators in eliminating health disparities. Cancer. 2011;117(15. Suppl):3543–52.
30. Kangovi S, Mitra N, Norton L, et al. Effect of community health worker support on clinical outcomes of low-income patients across primary care facilities: a randomized clinical trial. JAMA Intern Med. 2018;178:1635–43.
31. Ferrer RL, Schlenker CG, Romero RL, et al. Advanced primary care in San Antonio: linking practice and community strategies to improve health. J Am Board Fam Med. 2013;26:288–98.
32. Thom DH, Wolf J, Gardner H, et al. A qualitative study of how health coaches support patients in making health-related decisions and behavioral changes. Ann Fam Med. 2016;14:509–16.
33. Blount A, Fauth J, Nordstrom A, Pearson S. Who will provide integrated care: assessing the workforce for the integration of behavioral health and primary care in New Hampshire. Concord: Endowment for Health; 2017.
34. Montori V. Why we revolt. Rochester: The Patient Revolution; 2017.
35. Gensichen J, Jaeger C, Peitz M, Torge M, Güthlin C, Mergenthal K, Kleppel V, Gerlach F, Peterson J. Health care assistants in primary care depression management: role perception, burdening factors and disease conception. Ann Fam Med. 2009;7:513–9.

Resources

Psychiatric Clinicians in Primary Care

AIMS Center Psychiatric Consultant Training: https://aims.uw.edu/resource-library/primary-care-psychiatric-consultation-training-series

Competencies of Behavioral Health Clinicians

https://makehealthwhole.org/. Make Health Whole is a website with the 8 Competencies for Primary Care Behavioral Health presented with video examples and further definition of each.

Miller BF, Gilchrist EC, Ross KM, Wong SL, Blount A, Peek CJ. Core competencies for behavioral health providers working in primary care. In: Colorado consensus conference. 2016.

McDaniel SH, Grus CL, Cubic BA, Hunter CL, Kearney LK, Schuman CC, et al. Competencies for psychology practice in primary care. Am Psychol. 2014;69(4):409.

Hoge MA, Morris JA, Laraia M, Pomerantz A, Farley T. Core competencies for integrated behavioral health and primary care. Washington, DC: SAMHSA-HRSA Center for Integrated Health Solutions; 2014.

Clinical Practices and Culture in Exemplary Settings

An exhaustive study of the clinicians and practice patterns of primary care sites that are national examples of excellence conducted by the National Academy for the Integration of Behavioral Health and Primary Care, supported by the Agency for Healthcare Research and Quality. https://integrationacademy.ahrq.gov/products/professional-practices

Choosing the people who will make be the team members you need: https://hbr.org/2018/10/rethinking-how-medicaid-patients-receive-care

Support for Developing Integrated Primary Care

AHRQ Integration Academy. The Playbook: A Guide to Integrating Care in Primary Care and Other Ambulatory Settings. https://integrationacademy.ahrq.gov/playbook/about-playbook

AHRQ Integration Academy. Self-Assessment Checklist for Integrating Behavioral Health and Ambulatory Care. https://integrationacademy.ahrq.gov/playbook/integrating-behavioral-health-and-ambulatory-care-self-assessment-checklist

AIMS Center Collaborative Care Implementation Guide. https://aims.uw.edu/collaborative-care/implementation-guide

Meadows Mental Health Policy Institute. 2016. Best Practices in Integrated Behavioral Health: Identifying and Implementing Core Components. https://bit.ly/2Hcbb5z

SAMHSA-HRSA Center for Integrated Health Solutions. A Quick Start Guide to Behavioral Health Integration for Safety-Net Primary Care Providers. https://www.integration.samhsa.gov/resource/quick-start-guide-to-behavioral-health-integration

Literature on Behavioral Health Integration

A current, searchable collection of literature, including journal articles, books and substantive reports done by the National Academy for the Integration of Behavioral Health and Primary Care, supported by the Agency for Healthcare Research and Quality. https://integrationacademy.ahrq.gov/products/literature-collection

Chapter 4
Getting from "Delivering Care to Patients" to "Partnership with Patients"

The best care results from the conscientious, explicit, and judicious use of current best evidence and knowledge of patient values by well-trained, experienced, clinicians. (Committee on Quality Health Care in America, Institute of Medicine. (2001), Crossing the Quality Chasm: A New Health System for the 21st Century. p. 76)

Patient and family engaged care (PFEC) is care planned, delivered, managed, and continuously improved in active partnership with patients and their families (or care partners as defined by the patient) to ensure integration of their health and health care goals, preferences and values. It includes explicit and partnered determination of goals and care options, and it requires ongoing assessment of the care match with patient goals. (Adapted from Institute of Medicine, Transforming Health Care Scheduling and Access: Get it Now, 2015, Frampton et al. [1])

4.1 The Rising Expectation of Patient Participation

The IOM's dictum that the patient should be the source of control in the pursuit of their healthcare was revolutionary to much of the field when it came out in 2001. It set a bar for practice that was a step in the direction that the evidence of improved outcomes with increased patient participation was leading. At the same time, most HP's had (and still have) little experience of what achieving that bar would mean in practice. What would the interaction of HP and patient be? Would it take a lot of extra time in discussion? What if patients made poor decisions and didn't get healthier? How could whatever change was needed be done in the current system with its time pressures and its focus on payment for outcomes?

In summarizing the rules articulated in the "Quality Chasm" report as they related to patients, the IOM offered the first quote above. A well-trained, experienced clinician should use the best current evidence and their knowledge of the patient's values. The implication is that the clinician is weighing multiple factors in designing or directing care. The patient's values constitute one of those factors. It would seem that even the IOM report authors, when they came to imagining their

© Springer Nature Switzerland AG 2019
A. Blount, *Patient-Centered Primary Care*,
https://doi.org/10.1007/978-3-030-17645-7_4

dictum on the patient as the source of control in practice, imagined the clinician leading the care.

Fourteen years later, another report from the IOM seems to have interpreted the "source of control" in a way that is best described as a partnership with the clinician. At this point, the family, or the patient's core social network in their care, receives emphasis as a crucial element. The "patient" from 2001 has become the "patient in their social context" in 2015. We will look at the implications of routine involvement of the patient's family in their care later in this chapter. For now, it will be challenging enough to address the shift of the patient from a source of values and preferences that the HP takes into account to a partner in the planning and carrying out of healthcare.

Partnership implies some level of parity between two people with a common task or goal. Yet there is a gulf between doctors and many of their patients that is not easy for either to bridge. On one side of the gulf is a "well-trained and experienced clinician" who can make "conscientious, explicit, and judicious use of current best evidence." On the other side is a person needing the help of that clinician to understand what is wrong, to advise on steps the person should take, and to provide treatment to improve their condition.

Both the training of doctors and the strictures of evidence-based medicine that they are expected to follow make crossing the gulf difficult. Doctors are taught to take responsibility. The reminders of the physician being responsible for the quality and completeness of the treatment interaction are scattered across the process. In their practice they may be working with other professionals, but they are expected to know what each member of the group is doing for the patient, and their signatures drive the ability to bill for the care in most cases. If there is a bad outcome, the focus will be on them. In many hospital settings, there is the tradition of "morbidity and mortality rounds." This is a process in which a group of doctors (and not the rest of their teams) get together to dissect the chain of events that led to a bad outcome. This is done for the purpose of constructing better practice protocols for the future, but to do that, there is inevitably an element of assigning responsibility for what went wrong. It seems reasonable to liken much of medical training to boot camp in the military. For doctors in training, however, it is boot camp in making medical decisions and taking responsibility.

The reduction of variability and the increase in the use of evidence in making medical decisions are prominent as goals of the Quality Chasm report. To reach those goals, medical practitioners need decision support. Someone has to synthesize the evidence for practicing clinicians who cannot provide clinical care and at the same time keep up with the ever-growing and ever-changing cascade of evidence. We have entered what might be called "the era of the guideline." Guidelines are everywhere. Each guideline was made by a group of experts who looked at the available evidence and prescribed a general or specific way that a given condition should be treated based on their review. Pressure to follow guidelines has gradually increased as financial incentives and disincentives have focused on paying for health rather than paying just for services. When doctors make treatment recommendations while following guidelines, the amount of training, clinical science, and medical authority informing those recommendations is truly prodigious.

Doctors are not the only ones in the doctor-patient relationship who are likely to have been powerfully socialized to the expectation that doctors deliver care to people. Years of experience in pediatric as well as adult healthcare, in the USA or in most other countries in the world, teach patients that they are to bring their medical problems to the doctor, cooperate while the doctor does an examination and looks at the results of tests, listen to the doctor's instructions, and carry out those instructions. While patients may have complaints about how their doctor carries out his or her role, few have an expectation that the doctor will take a different role.

The arrangement of roles in the doctor-patient relationship that both parties have been trained to expect has inherent structural problems for fostering the compliance of many patients. One person (doctor) or a group of people (team) is usually much more knowledgeable than the other person (patient) or group of people (family). Particularly in the case of a long-term problem, like a chronic illness, one will have to teach the other what to do and monitor whether they carry out what they have been taught. Teaching someone else something for their own good has a plethora of unpleasant echoes for many people. That is what happened in the adult-child relationship that patients experienced in school or with their parents, a time that many people found unpleasant, disenfranchising, and even demeaning. No matter how benevolently doctors experience their side of the relationship, many patients experience echoes of those old adult-child relationships. They find themselves drawn to acts of autonomy and independence. If the doctor sets out a plan that represents the actions by the patient most likely to lead to improved health, patients who are experiencing reminders of earlier adult-child relationships often chose not to follow the doctor's plan as an expression of autonomy. Actions by a patient that HPs experience as noncompliant or non-adherent, can be experienced by the patient as "making my own decisions."

When we add differences in income, social status, perceived power, and education between the doctor and many patients, we understand the common finding that so many patients are hesitant to participate actively with their doctor in their healthcare. The more we study the perception of the doctor-patient relationship on the part of patients of lower income and educational attainment, the more we find patient perception of a coercive relationship based on a dramatic asymmetry of power. We will look at this pattern in more detail in Chap. 5.

The difference in knowledge between doctors and their patients is one important consideration when thinking about the possibility of patients being partners in designing their care, but it may not be, in itself, the most important difference. Doctors and their patients seem to have different ways of thinking and talking about illness, even if the patient is well educated about what he or she needs to do to stay as healthy [2]. When doctors and patients were asked separately to rate the patients' health on a five-point scale from poor to excellent, they agreed in their ratings or were only one level off 86% of the time. In a study of over 500 physician-patient dyads in several primary care practices, when both were asked separately for the reason for any lack of perfect health of the patient (e.g., severity of illness, obesity, lack of exercise, tobacco), the multiple possible reasons chosen by the doctor and those chosen by the patient showed no agreement at all 75% of the time. It seems that while doctors and patients show general agreement on how healthy the patient is, the likelihood that they agree on what the problems are is small. In addition, there is a minority of patients (14%) whose basic assessment of how healthy they are is substantially different from their doctors'[3].

In a study of conversations between patients and doctors about the patients' self-management of their chronic illness (diabetes), Robin Kruse and her colleagues [4] studied the different ways each group talked about the subject. The approaches were different enough so that instead of describing their findings in terms of different levels of knowledge, they termed the whole process "parallel play." Parallel play is a type of interaction in which two young children who developmentally are not yet able to play together with one mutual game or toy play physically in the same space, each with his or her own game or toy. Kruse et al. found that doctors, who were usually following guidelines, wanted to use checklists to be sure they covered certain topics in the visit. Most of these topics were related to some numerical measure of the state of the patient's illness. When one of the measured test values was out of the recommended range, doctors wanted to discuss what barrier impeded the patient from getting the number down or up into the recommended range. Patients, on the other hand, wanted to tell the story of how their efforts at coping with their illness had been going. They tended to measure their assessment of how they were doing by how they felt, and how they felt tended to be the driver of any changes they made in self-management.

In the study there was almost no conversation that connected the two approaches. They stayed parallel. A connection would have been a conversation about how getting the numbers into the recommended range might impact the patient's feeling better or what the experience would be like for the patient when their illness was not going well and the numbers were getting worse. One of the reasons that this kind of conversation was not common may have been that in the case of chronic illnesses like diabetes, hypertension, and heart disease, self-management changes that could affect the measurements on tests often have little or no impact on how a patient feels at the time the behavior change happens. Changes in the subjective experience of the illness often come much later.

Where doctors looked for individual barriers that prevent a patient's improving their numbers, patients tended to see barriers that were related to their obligations to the needs or demands of others [4]. Changing their daily schedules or their diets was seen as possible by patients only as much as they could make the changes without overly stressing their partners and families. This finding highlights the impact which patients' attachments to their families can make in their health decisions, both in supporting or impeding healthy behaviors. This role is often invisible to health professionals who prefer to approach patients as autonomous beings who make all their own health decisions. The question to patients about the role of their family's or close friends' opinions or needs on the patients' health choices is rarely asked, even in the many instances in which family members or friends are in the exam room for the visit.

Doctors are well aware of how hard it can be to guide patients in successfully managing their chronic illnesses. Most do not conceptualize the parallel or nonintersecting nature of the communication in which they engage with many of their patients as Kruse describes it. For any who do agree with the description Kruse and her colleagues offer, a way of bridging the parallel nature of the communication won't necessarily be obvious.

To the doctor or other HP, the prospect of broadening the conversation to discuss barriers in the context of patients' relationships can be difficult. It takes more time. The same is true for changing from using checklists to sitting with patients for the narrative about their self-management in the context of their lives. Kruse and her colleagues, like the IOM, end by saying that doctors may need to change the basic organization of care to be able to speak with patients in ways that are a better fit for them. Unfortunately, they do not provide a pathway to achieving that goal. In the rest of this chapter, we will look at current methods of bridging the gulf and promoting approaches to partnership. In later chapters we will examine less common adaptations of care that can be carried out by the whole health team to build partnership with even the most complex or challenging patients.

4.2 Describing the Divide

Kruse and her colleagues conducted a fairly small study. Their sample is not large enough to represent the actions of primary care doctors generally, much less of all professionals in healthcare. It does, however, frame the problem of the inevitable gulf between the training and scientific knowledge of professionals, on one hand, and the multifaceted personal experience of patients on the other. The table below provides a somewhat oversimplified definition of the roles in the two models of healthcare relationships, one in which professional expertise is the most valued element and one in which partnership is the most valued aspect. When professional expertise and knowledge are most valued, the professional is expected to lead the process. The relationship becomes quite different when partnership is most valued, even though professional experience and knowledge never cease to be crucial to success (Table 4.1).

4.3 Bridging the Divide

A central challenge is how to effect the transformation from the HP in the lead to partnership without causing precipitous changes that destabilize the primary care practice. A change that demands sudden shifts in behavior, definition of roles, time allotment, or team membership for professionals or for patients simply isn't going to be workable in the pressured environment of current primary care practice. Following a stepwise approach to making the transition, both conceptually and in practice, may be the most useful way to envision the pathway from one model to the other. We will outline the conceptual steps first and then talk about the practice that goes with each step.

Table 4.1 Roles change when partnership is achieved

	The HP leads	Patient-HP partnership
Patient role	Be a good "historian" about signs and symptoms Understand recommendations Follow recommendations	Share physical and affective experience so the professional can make the best informed recommendation Elicit information from professional needed for patient to make their decision about how to proceed
Professional role	Elicit information (history) from the patient and discover information (exam and tests) needed to identify and monitor the patient's condition(s) and guide treatment. Communicate assessment and plan clearly	Function as a "guide" to best possible health. (A guide knows the territory and learns the preferences and capabilities of the traveler to lead a successful journey. Helps design pathways to grow the abilities of traveler to function as autonomously as possible in the landscape)
Treatment planning	HP follows guidelines. Uses judgment and skill to make a plan when guidelines are not adequate. Offers teaching to improve patient's ability to follow recommendations	Guidelines and professional skills are one sort of information in planning. Patient's knowledge of own physical and emotional experience is equally important. Professional and patient make a mutual decision about how to maximize health and minimize any disruptive impact of the care on the quality of the patient's life based on patient's values and preferences

HP's can begin by adjusting their communication to be a better fit for the understanding of the patient. "Health literacy" is a concept that facilitates the HP paying more careful attention to the language, cultural beliefs, learning style, and education of the patient. This enables adjustments in the way the HP communicates information to the patient to promote better understanding by the patient.

"Motivational interviewing" (MI) is a technique that helps the HP manage their own urge to tell the patient what to do about their health. This is done in a way that respects and enhances the patient's health decision-making. By refusing to push the patient in a direction, while assertively engaging with the patient, offering information as the patient is interested in hearing it, and dispassionately supporting the patient's examining the pros and cons of changing or staying the same, HPs can facilitate patients making health decisions that the HPs could never lead or push them to make.

"Shared decision-making" (SDM) is an approach that encourages HPs to invite patients to join in making decisions about treatment, particularly in cases in which the evidence endorses multiple courses of action. The same approaches used in "health literacy-enhanced" communication are used to provide decision aids that allow patients to make more informed decisions.

"Minimally disruptive medicine" (MDM) is an approach that can be useful when patients have complex medical situations, such as coping with multiple chronic illnesses. MDM acknowledges the workload of coping with illness and following a complex treatment plan that the patient faces. It uses an understanding of complex adaptive systems to understand the way small increases in workload or other stresses can move the relationship of the patient's resiliency in the face of the physical and emotional challenges of the illness and treatments out of balance. This causes both to decline. Each illness is likely to have its own guidelines for treatment, which, when they are combined, create a large number of recommended treatments. MDM helps HPs work with patients to elicit their informed preferences with the goal of minimizing the "footprint" of treatment in the patient's daily life and to build other indigenous supports in the patient's life.

Coaching patients to behave in a more enfranchised way when interacting with their doctor or HP is an approach that helps to overcome the socialization of patients toward passivity in their relationships in healthcare. As patients learn how to ask for the information they want, to express their affective reactions to care, to overcome their timidity or embarrassment, and to negotiate more directly for what they want in care, they make a bridge toward partnership with their doctor.

"Relationship-centered care" (RCC) is an approach designed to humanize the doctor-patient relationship. It urges HPs to be more genuine and open in their communication with patients and to appreciate the patients' reciprocating in kind. It encourages partnership that grows out of authentic interactions between human beings working together to maintain or improve the patients' health.

"Family-informed care" (FIC) describes the incorporation of information about the family of the patient in treatment planning and the ability and willingness to make the incorporation of family members a feature of the final treatment plan. Family members can therefore have roles as informants, caretakers, supporters, or recipients of interventions designed to improve outcomes for the patient.

The sequence of these approaches moves from improving communication of information to the patient from the HP, to shifting the HP's role as directing care in a way that influences the patient to make healthier decisions, to offering the patient a role in deciding treatment direction in situations when the evidence says multiple choices are approximately equal, to an approach in which the doctor and the patient together step away from the rule of guidelines to make choices most consistent with the patient's values for how much they want to let care impact their lives, to coaching the patient to act the role of a more enfranchised partner in their care, to facilitating the development of an authentic human relationship between HP and patient, beyond the boundaries of their prescribed roles in healthcare. Each step will impact the experience of the HP-patient relationship as it impacts the behavior of each member of the relationship. While it is not possible to offer a practice manual for each approach here, it seems reasonable to try to provide a more complete description of the evidence for and the practices involved in each approach.

4.4 Improving the "Health Literacy" of the Patient

"Health literacy" is a concept with both clinical and public health implications. It is a separate concept from "literacy" but built on the evidence that the independent effect of literacy in healthcare outcomes is strong [5]. The role of literacy in health tends to be underemphasized when assessing the impacts of life conditions such as the "social determinants of health[1]" on a population's health status [6].

The IOM defines health literacy as:

> The degree to which individuals have the capacity to obtain, process, and understand basic information necessary to make appropriate health decisions. (IOM [7])

The public health aspect of this definition includes access to schooling and to other ways in the culture and media environment that people obtain the three core elements that are considered foundational to health literacy. Those are basic literacy, numeracy, and health knowledge [8, 9]. The literature from the USA has commonly focused on how clinical settings can build on the foundation that patients bring by assessing health literacy as a way to increase clinician sensitivity for interacting with patients and adjusting communication language and the level of complexity of teaching aids to target the health literacy level of a patient or a population of patients. The goal in this literature generally is to improve the patient's ability to take in information, thereby being able to comply with medical treatment plans more successfully which can lead to improved health outcomes [8] (see Health Literacy in Resources).

Literature from health systems outside the USA (UK, Australia, and Canada) and the definition of the World Health Organization (WHO) have tended to focus on health literacy as an asset rather than simply a way to reduce health risk [8]. They stress the impact that improved health literacy can have on allowing patients to participate in decisions about their healthcare. In this literature, the word "empowerment" is more prominent than in the US literature. The WHO's definition of health literacy, in its differences from the IOM definition, is a good example:

> Health literacy represents the cognitive and social skills which determine the motivation and ability of individuals to gain access to understand and use information in ways which promote and maintain health. Health literacy implies the achievement of a level of knowledge, personal skills and confidence to take action to improve personal and community health by changing personal life styles and living conditions. (Nutbeam [8])

This definition of health literacy envisions patients who not only participate in and impact decisions about their own healthcare but grow to understand the impacts of the social determinants of health in their lives and to take actions to change those determinants.

The resources available to help clinicians foster successful compliance (see Health Literacy in Resources) can also be supportive of patient participation in their healthcare decisions. They are likely not sufficient, however, to build the confidence and skills at obtaining information and negotiating treatment plans that would create the enhanced patient role in their own health and healthcare envisioned by the WHO definition. These resources also tend not to focus on helping patients work collaboratively within a community to have impact on the social determinants of health in their lives. The T.E.A.M. steps outlined in the second half of this book provide a new way that practices can foster this sort of health literacy.

---

[1] The Social Determinants of Health as listed by Healthy People 2020 [55] are economic stability, the neighborhood and built environment, access to healthcare, social and community context, and education.

4.5 Enhancing Motivation

Motivational interviewing (MI) can be another bridge for the divide described above as the "parallel play" of doctor and patient [4]. MI causes the professional who is using the approach to focus on the consciousness of the patient using empathic communication to build the relationship in order to help the patient explore and resolve ambivalence they may have about a given change in health behavior. In MI, the professional uses certain basic counseling skills, though often the HP-patient relationship is not defined as "counseling." The HP engages the patient by asking open-ended questions, offering affirmations for the patient's thoughts or actions toward making healthy decisions, uses reflective listening to let the patient know they are being heard and to help keep the conversation on the change that the patient is considering, and periodically provides summary statements to indicate appreciation for the work being done and whatever progress is being made [10]. The HP is careful to assess whether the patient is just encountering the topic of change, thinking about it but not ready to do anything to make the change, or is somewhere in the process of trying to make the change. The "Stages of Change" model is the commonly used conceptual structure to guide this assessment and change conversation [11]. The change could be something discreet and difficult, such as controlling substance use [12]. In primary care, MI is commonly used to help patients resolve their ambivalence about making a change in one or more of the many health behaviors that are needed to manage their illness successfully.

In a brief summary such as this, MI can seem to be a way to exert influence in one direction in the HP-patient relationship. To that purpose, techniques from MI have been borrowed for use in many aspects of primary care. In those contexts, a particular technique can be helpful to influence a patient toward better compliance or other health behavior. Where the HP is trained in MI and uses the approach well, the experience tends to be more reciprocal. Each person in the HP-patient relationship is influenced. As HPs learn to avoid directing or guiding the patient, they learn to empathize with the patient's experience and health dilemmas in very immediate ways. That empathic behavior and understanding in turn tends to make it easier for patients to experience their own ability to make health decisions, as opposed to continuing with unhealthy behavior out of fear of failure or determination not to be directed by another person in what they do.

4.6 Shared Decision-Making

Shared decision-making (SDM) in medical care is just what the name implies, the health professional, usually the doctor, and the patient each have a role in making a decision about what sort of tests or treatment to pursue for the patient. In most situations the doctor presents the choices to the patient and does everything possible to be sure that the patient understands what actions each choice entails and what the risks and possible rewards for each choice are. The patient picks among the choices, and the doctor and the patient go forward on the path that the patient chooses.

The idea of the patient making decisions in their own care is by no means new. Patients regularly sign consent for treatments of all sorts in many medical settings. It is commonplace for patients to be asked to express a preference about care measures they would want done in an emergency or at the end of life. Patients are able to delegate these choices to a medical proxy, usually a family member or trusted friend, to be consulted should the patient be unable to make a choice themselves about their care. These choices tend to come up in situations of acute medical need. They are largely the right to accept or refuse treatments, rather than to pick between treatments. In these instances, the patient is not a partner in planning their care as much as they are a person who may be able to opt out of care determined for them. In acute settings, the patient's choice is sometimes ignored when medical personnel are not made aware of the patient's preference or decide that a different choice is necessary. The right to refuse treatment is very important. Examples of the extensive and sometimes cruel overuse of treatments, without sharing decisions with the patient or the family, have been highlighted graphically in stories of the end-of-life care [13].

SDM is an extension of the right of patient control of their care into more common, less dramatic, and more nuanced decisions that are part of the longitudinal doctor-patient relationship in primary care and outpatient specialty care. It is built not so much on the idea of protecting patient rights as on the hope of building patient investment in their health and healthcare. Since patients' health behaviors, i.e., how well they adhere to recommended treatments and how consistently they engage in habits of healthy living, constitute the largest determining factor in their health outcomes, any process that can build their investment in self-managing their illnesses would seem to be worth pursuing. One of the drives for SDM by physicians is the belief that patients who are involved in determining their care are more likely to be proactive in managing their own chronic diseases [14]. The evidence in controlled studies of SDM tends to bear out these assumptions. Patients who are able to make decisions about their treatment that reflect their personal preferences often experience more favorable outcomes. They are likely to be less anxious about treatments, to recover more quickly, and to be more adherent to treatment regimens [15].

SDM can be good for the health system as well. Patients who understand the risk-reward picture of procedures proposed by their doctors are more likely to choose the conservative course. They are happier with their doctor, less unnecessary care is delivered, and, while it is not the avowed goal of shared decision-making, costs tend to be lower [16, 17].

One of the most obvious challenges of this ideal situation is the complexity of the decision in many situations. Evidence for quantifying risks or rewards is often not well studied or is contradictory. It is common for patients to have difficulty understanding the contingencies of the choices they are facing. Decisional aids that simplify the explanation of the treatment or test and the likelihood of positive or negative outcomes can be very helpful to many patients. For this seemingly good outcome to be common, however, the conversations between patients and doctors have to become more complex than is commonly the case. Doctors need to move from the usual practice of describing treatment alternatives to careful discussion of risk-benefit trade-offs [18].

Multiple authors distinguish between "effective decisions" and "preference-sensitive decisions" in advocating for SDM [19, 20]. "Effective decisions" are treatments or actions that are overwhelmingly positive in outcome in relation to any harm. They suggest that there are several ways of determining what would be considered an "effective decision," one of the best being that the course of action has an A or B level recommendation by the US Preventive Services Task Force. In those cases, they consider SDM to consist of "decision support," i.e., helping the patient make the "right" decision. Decision support in those contexts consists of provision of clear information through carefully prepared decisional aids, motivational interviewing, and using the stages of change model.

"Preference-sensitive" decisions are decisions about medical treatments or tests in which there is some equivalence between possible actions or between an action and no action. Defining these decisions depends on evidence as much as defining "effective decisions." As evidence accrues and changes, some decisions that had been considered "effective" are redefined as "preference sensitive." The decision about when some women should start regular mammograms is a good example.

SDM is not a value for many patients. Whether this is because patients like to have their doctor in the lead or whether they are simply unable to imagine how they might actively participate in their care, many prefer to have the doctor leading their care. The doctor leading the care for a patient who prefers this model is actually a better situation than having the doctor pushing for the patient's involvement in decisions to the discomfort or confusion of the patient. The concordance of the patient's and their doctor's attitudes about who should lead the patient's care seems to be more important for good outcome than a universal model of shared decisions [21]. In other words, sometimes the partnership for doctors and patients is in choosing a model for the doctor-patient relationship, rather than in sharing the decisions within that model.

SDM has been described by some to be the pinnacle of patient-centered care, the goal for completing the transition called for by the Quality Chasm report [22]. It can be seen as extending the right of the patient to be involved in their care. Because the engagement of patients in making their health decisions requires doctors to be knowledgeable about the current evidence, it may reduce overuse of treatments or tests of doubtful value, increase the use of interventions of proven value, reduce variations in care delivery, and over time increase the investment of a population in their healthcare [23].

The focus on SDM internationally has been substantial for more than 20 years with a literature of thousands of articles [23]. Unfortunately, the percentage of adoptions of SDM that lead to what experts in the field consider effective realizations of the approach based on direct observations of doctors and patients is comparatively small [24]. Interventions to improve the adoption of SDM by healthcare professionals have yielded less than dramatic results. It is true that any intervention to promote SDM, whether made to enhance the patient's ability to participate, to promote the doctor's use of the approach, or focused on both simultaneously, makes some difference in the occurrence of shared decision behaviors. As one might expect, the most effective interventions have targeted both the doctor and the patient, offering decisional aides to help patients understand their choices, and offering training for doctors to increase their experience of self-efficacy in being able to effectively utilize SDM [23]. Yet the "divide" that we have been describing between patients and doctors doesn't seem to go away just because a new approach is implemented in a practice. The barrier of lack of time for the careful discussion of multiple choices, plus the risks and rewards of each choice, continues to concern doctors considering adopting SDM. Plus, the socialization of doctors and patients to the "doctor in the lead" model is difficult to overcome. To achieve the many benefits of SDM, both doctors and patients need clear information about its value and how to interact to carry it out, plus, many patients and their doctors need an increased experience of self-efficacy to have the confidence to make the change in their usual approach. For doctors, it is the change in their approach to healthcare. For patients, it is a change in their approach to their relationship with their HP and to their health.

4.7 Minimally Disruptive Medicine

Minimally disruptive medicine (MDM) is an approach designed for treating complex or multimorbid patients. It is a more recent approach than SDM that attempts to incorporate the practices and values of SDM. In addition, MDM adds goal elicitation, broader patient partnership, patient capacity assessment, workload assessment, capacity coaching, and patient-reported outcome tracking [25]. MDM takes what might be called a fundamentally humble stance on the part of the HP. The approach helps HPs appreciate the amount of work that is required every day on the part of patients to manage their chronic illnesses, estimated at 2 hours per day on average [26]. MDM introduces new considerations for an HP in what treatment planning should entail. Adding to the evidence-based approach to patient needs and an informed knowledge of patient wants and preferences, it adds a consideration of a patient's capacity for meeting demands of their illness, their lives, and the workload of their treatments. These are done with the goal of offering patient-centered care, aimed at caring for and supporting the whole person, in their context, with the minimum footprint of healthcare on their daily lives.

The theory undergirding this approach is based on an understanding of complex adaptive systems. This informs an understanding of problem development and problem resolution. The theory highlights the interactive aspects of a person's illness challenges and environmental challenges in explaining the common development of "emergent syndromes" that do not seem to be the result of any one causal factor. The concept of "emergent syndromes" is a name for the way a complex situation in which a patient is managing illnesses, their behavioral stresses, and their life responsibilities can change substantially from inbalance to out of balance, from managed to unmanaged, by the addition on one new challenge. The "Cumulative Complexity

Model" [27] describes the interaction of illness factors, life factors and treatment factors, and the way they interact to impact the patient's capacity to cope with the workload of their illness and live situation. It guides the clinician in making an assessment of the fit of treatments to the patient's capacities. Because multiple complex treatment regimens can become an additional stress factor, simplifying and reducing the time and effort required by a patient's regimen becomes in itself an intervention on behalf of the stressed system that is the patient in their relational environment. Minimizing of treatment regimens is done in collaboration with the patient, based on their understanding of the options and their goals for their life. HPs take account of patient's capacity to maintain treatment regimens in suggesting courses of action.

Simplifying treatment regimens requires the team of provider and informed patient to step back from the multiple guidelines that may be applicable to the patient's situation in order to create workable regimens that the patient can maintain in their current life context. Together they work to match the workload of coping with the illness and carrying out the patient's regimens with the patient's capacity in their current situation, always ready to increase or decrease the workload as the patient's situation and their coping evolve. MDM has been used to provide a lens for understanding success and failure in several areas of healthcare. One example is an analysis of the problem of high rates of hospital readmissions less than 30 days after discharge [28].

In designing the right care for patients in the MDM model, the HP is encouraged to prioritize feasibility. They should strive for a process that is sensible to and is experienced as sustainable by both patient and HP. They should attempt to involve available resources, to encourage the team and the patient to reach out to community for aids such as public health services, faith-based and other social networks, and community education opportunities. The common factor in these recommendations is building of a social network of nourishing relationships for the patient.

The MDM model makes a beginning effort to take the impact of relationships into account. It briefly mentions challenging or stress-inducing relationships as needing mitigation [25]. Its analysis, when describing the relationship of different team members to the patient, "makes special efforts to embrace and leverage some of the psychobehavioral factors that interact between and among these players; again, because they seem to matter" (Leppin et al. [25], p. 57). In this area, the model seems underdeveloped. The psychoneuroimmunology literature has clearly established the biological/immunological impact of stressful interpersonal relationships and the positive results when these stresses become supportive [29, 30]. The impact of a doctor's behavior, such as showing empathy, on health outcomes seems to have immunological impacts, beyond being simply influencing the patient's adherence [31]. The team needs to be able to monitor and address instances in which a team member has a stressful relationship with the patient for many reasons. Still, a view that only looks at the relationship of team members to the patient probably overestimates the impact of the professionals and underestimates the impact of a patient's family relationships [32]. Having a team member who is skilled at working with couples and families to help mitigate stressful relationships and improve effective mutuality seems a reasonable part of this approach, assuming that the process does not add significantly to the treatment footprint.

The relative newness of the MDM model as compared to more tested approaches such as SDM may account for the observation that the literature does not contain an array of studies assessing the broad implementation of its practices. When a model with exciting new ways of approaching care and good results in initial controlled studies begins to be more widely taught and recommended, issues of model fidelity begin to be important. At that point, the initial results in early studies may no longer apply to all the settings that purport to be using the model (see Couët et al. [24] about SDM).

4.8   Coaching Patients to Increase Their Participation in Their Care Decisions

The idea advanced by the IOM that the patient should be the source of control is supported by clinical evidence. Kaplan, Sheldon, and Ware [33] summarized clinical trials that compared elements in the communication patterns of physicians and patients with the patients' health outcomes, both outcomes perceived by the patient and those measured by the physician. One of the impetuses for the study was the evidence that patients wanted more involvement in their care than they usually were offered [34, 35]. The authors were suspicious of "patient satisfaction," the most common outcome measure of the patients' experience of the doctor-patient relationship, as a measure of the quality of care. It is not impossible that a patient could be very satisfied with healthcare that does not meet current standards for quality [36] leading to poorer outcomes than patients had a right to expect. In fact, sometimes the more satisfied patients turn out to be less healthy than less satisfied patients [37]. It is easy to imagine a doctor who did not mention issues such as smoking or drinking or weight loss to patients and who therefore made the patient visit a more comfortable interaction, as having more satisfied and less healthy patients.

Kaplan and her colleagues analyzed audio recordings of patients' visits with their doctors. They studied care for four conditions in different settings: diabetes, hypertension, ulcers, and breast cancer. In the experimental condition, each patient was given access to their medical record along with crafted teaching aids on disease management for their condition to help them interpret what they saw in their record. They were coached on strategies for increasing their participation in visits with their doctors, strategies such as negotiating skills, asking questions, and how to focus on their medical care during the conversation. They were given techniques for lowering their own barriers to communication, barriers such as embarrassment, anxiety, and intimidation. The researchers found that while the patients' perceived health improved more than the physical metrics measuring their health, both improved significantly for the experimental condition over usual care. Physicians were blinded to the group to which each patient they met was assigned.

The results seemed to highlight a possible bridge in the usual "parallel play" described by Kruse et al. They found that patients who were more assertive experienced significantly more improvement in their health markers (blood pressure, blood sugar), their functional status (days lost from work, functional limitations index), and their evaluation of their own overall health (number of reported health problems, overall health rating). In the breast cancer group, the physical measure was the level of symptoms in reaction to chemotherapy, which was significantly better in the group that got the training.

In both the group that got the training and in the usual care group, patients who were more assertive in relating to their doctors at baseline had better outcomes over the course of the study. They continued to be more assertive to their own benefit. Of the group that received the coaching, both more and less assertive patients at baseline showed significant improvement in their health markers, their functioning, and their perceptions of their health after the training. The more assertive patients in the usual care group did not show improvements from baseline.

What I am calling "assertive" behavior by patients was measured in the study as being active in seeking information, being more directive toward the doctor, being more expressive of emotion (both positive and negative), and speaking for a larger percentage of the visit. The doctors' behaviors in response to these assertive patient behaviors were the complement of the patients' behaviors. These doctors' behaviors were less controlling, more information giving, and talking for a lower percentage of time in visits with the more enfranchised patients, who then did better on all three outcome dimensions.

In working with the patients who got the training, the doctors of these patients also showed more negative emotion. Negative emotion was not so much in the form of anger as in showing more frustration and tension during the interaction. Kaplan et al. expressed the finding this way, "On the surface counterintuitive, the positive relationship between negative affect and patient's health status might very well be evidence of 'healthy friction' or role tension between physicians and patients, in which patients' assertions of control compete with physicians' normal role-related dominance of the visit and create some role strain for both" (Kaplan et al. [33], p. S123).

The doctors as well as the patients have to be given credit for the improvement of the group of patients who learned and used the new skills they got from the training intervention. Not every doctor could make the adaptations that the patients' new behavior called for. In the visits in which the doctors made the adaptation better, the patients were cued to be more confident and responsible in their medical visits, which in turn led to these patients being more enfranchised in and attentive to their self-care. The study authors point out, "Physicians may influence the outcomes of those patients not only through the medical care process, but also by shaping how patients feel about the disease and their ability to control or contain its impact on their lives" (p. S124).

Patient coaching shows a good deal of potential, and some health systems have adopted it as a regular service. In these settings, instead of a focused training for patients, the health system commonly offers an additional team member who can help the patient plan for their visits with the doctor and organize their questions to the doctor. These people also coach and help patients negotiate other barriers to care such as following-up on referrals and obtaining other resources [38]. This additional person may be called a "navigator," "care coordinator," or other names in different health systems. Models vary in the degree to which the patient is coached to interact more successfully with their doctor as opposed to the new team member explaining and reinforcing the doctor's instructions to the patient. There are also people called "health coaches" who tend to be focused on helping the patient adhere to their regimen and improve their habits of healthy living rather than on their enfranchisement in their relationship with their doctor [39]. Navigators and staff with similar roles are often found in specialty medical settings in which patients' likelihood of being confused or overwhelmed is high, such as oncology or cardiology services. As time goes on, additional team members helping patients be more successful at coping with the workload of their care are proliferating. The trend to expand the team by adding a care coordinator to keep patients from "falling through the cracks" as they move from one health setting to another, such as is called for in the Quality Chasm report, has now yielded a dizzying array of roles. At this point there is little consistency between health systems in the duties that go with a particular job title. There is also no reliable way of predicting which roles will tend to support the partnership of the patient as a part of the team, on one hand, and which will focus on simply delivering care more effectively to a patient on the other. The stepped approaches outlined in this chapter can be made part of the skill sets of all team members, even though most were originally conceived as improving specifically the doctor-patient relationship.

4.9   Relationship-Centered Care

An approach that seems to hold out the possibility of fundamental change in the doctor-patient relationship is relationship-centered care (RCC) [40]. RCC focuses on the fact that healthcare is conducted through relationships. It holds that if healthcare is "humanized" and if it occurs in a more authentic relationship between a healthcare professional (HP) and the patient, it will be more effective. It rests on four principles:

1. Relationship in healthcare ought to include dimensions of personhood as well as roles.
2. Affect and emotion are important components of relationship in healthcare.
3. All healthcare relationships occur in the context of reciprocal influence.
4. RCC has a moral foundation (Beach et al. [41]).

   In the terms of this chapter, RCC might seem to be the completion of the transition to patient-centered care. When they look at the current reality of patient-centered care, most authors in RCC say that it is different from "patient-centered" care because "1. RCC focuses on how patients and HPs relate to one another 2. RCC views relationships as therapeutic and as the medium of care 3. RCC values patients and HPs as active participants who bring important aspects to the relationship 4. RCC focuses on HPs being present for themselves and others and 5. RCC recognizes that interactions influence the course and outcomes of care" (Soklareidis et al. [42], p. 113).

RCC endorses actions that are considered to be part of patient-centered care (e.g., viewing patients as experts, tailoring the approach to each patient based on knowledge of the patient) and adds additional elements aimed at the basic experience of the doctor-patient relationship (e.g., valuing the achievement of mutual respect and unconditional positive regard, being aware on one's own feelings and biases). In its attention to relationship as the foundation of care, RCC attends not just to the patient-clinician relationship but to clinician-clinician relationships, practitioner-community relationships, and the clinician's relationship to self [41]. This broad view of the centrality of relationships has led to RCC being adapted to use in improving relationships in the whole healthcare organization, beyond the relationships between professionals and patients [43].

4.10   The Challenge of Changing Relationships and the "Be Spontaneous" Paradox

One of the challenges for a HP attempting to change their relationship with patients is that, to the degree that an approach calls for them to "feel" something different, instead of simply acting differently, they may have difficulty knowing how to comply. RCC can present a particularly striking example of this dilemma, "RCC emphasizes the importance of authenticity, in the sense that clinicians should not, for example, simply act as if they have respect for someone; they must also aim actually to have [internally] the respect that they display [externally]" (Beach et al. [41], p. S4). How does one "aim actually to have" an internal experience that might more commonly be thought of as the *result* of one's interactions in a relationship? HPs or others who encounter descriptions of approaches such as RCC might well have a hard time imagining their internal experiences of and reactions to their patients changing in the ways that would allow them to work within the model.

Approaches to bridging the gulf between the HP-led care and partnership with patients that are founded on changing the professionals' experience of their own relationship with their patients run the risk of creating paradoxical instructions for the HPs involved. This sort of problem has been described in systems-based analyses of communication as the "be spontaneous" paradox [44]. The "be spontaneous" paradox is a name for a class of instructions that are made impossible to carry out by the fact that the recipient was instructed to do them. The example of the instruction, "You should be spontaneous," is easy to understand and impossible to follow. If you are instructed to be spontaneous, whatever you do cannot be considered spontaneous. You were told to do it. You didn't do it spontaneously. Consider this paradox in a slightly broadened way. There are numerous categories of behavior that are only "genuine" if they are spontaneous. The list is quite long. If there is a suggestion that a person should be enthusiastic, genuine, supportive, transparent, or happy, we are in "be spontaneous" territory. In essence, any instruction that asks for a response that "comes from the heart" is likely to be paradoxical in its structure.

When commands or injunctions that are paradoxical are allowed to stand, either unchallenged or without a meta-comment upon the process, a likely scenario for blame is created. A meta-comment is a comment upon a piece of communication, contextualizing the communication by taking a new perspective on its form or function. A challenge to a paradoxical instruction such as "be more spontaneous with your patient" might be "I will decide what I feel I should do with my patient." A meta-comment would be "I can't be spontaneous if I am instructed to do so. Then it isn't spontaneous."

In situations in which there is no meta-comment and the paradox makes complying impossible, the blame for the impossible instruction, if there is any, may be cast by the person giving the instructions. More commonly, however, the blame will be self-generated by the person receiving the instructions. Instead of noticing that there was no way to fulfill an instruction to "be empathetic," the receiver is more likely to blame themselves for not "feeling" what they believe they should feel to comply with the instruction. Sometimes, as a way to deal with the guilt of not being fully empathetic, for example, an HP will blame the patient: "Who could empathize with that guy after what he did?" Sometimes they will blame themselves. More commonly, the solution is to blame the model or approach that is putting them into the uncomfortable situation.

HPs and the people who teach them, as they work to learn the skills and practices that are part of the models discussed in this chapter, need to be aware of the "be spontaneous" paradox and to avoid teaching in ways that create such dilemmas. Asking someone to "act empathic" is possible when asking them to "be empathic" is not. When people act empathic in multiple iterations in one relationship or in several relationships, it is likely that the "feeling" that was called for in the model starts to arise. The model can be fulfilled, including its demand of "authenticity," as long as a team member learning the model is encouraged to act in ways that portray authenticity and leave the experience of authenticity to develop after they have used that behavior many times. The advice of Alcoholics Anonymous to "fake it 'til you make it," that an alcoholic should act like a socially responsible sober person until they truly experience themselves as one [45], is built on good social science [46].

4.11 Family-Informed Care

Family-informed care is an as yet underdeveloped tool for improving the healthcare of adults. Most of the research on the role of families having an impact on the healthcare of one member focuses on situations in which the family is likely to have a major role in the person's health decision-making. These are usually situations such as care for children, adolescents, the elderly, and the disabled. The evidence supporting the family's role in healthcare of these populations is very strong and plentiful [47, 48]. There is much less research on situations in which the family has no formal caretaking or decision-making role, though what has been done shows the possibility of the family having a substantial role. Over one third of cancer patients in one study reported that their primary source of medical information was their family or friends [49]. Possibly more subtle but pervasive influence can be exerted because the family is so often the group in which patients develop their "explanatory models" [50] of their illnesses [51].

The role of the family has become much more prominent in descriptions and standards of patient-centered care over the last 20 years. The difference in the prominence of the family in the two quotes at the beginning of this chapter is typical of the change over that time. The increase in the family's prominence in the design of patient-centered care in most settings has not been accompanied by a corresponding increase in the consideration of family factors or the inclusion of family members in the primary care of adult patients.

In 2002, Weihs, Fisher, and Baird published a comprehensive summary of the evidence on the research on the family in the healthcare of chronic illnesses. Their work was published with the imprimatur of the Institute of Medicine. They began by reviewing the evidence of the greater impact of family relationships as opposed to those described by the generic term, "social relationships." "Family relationships have greater intensity that most other social relationships and research suggests that there is a substantive, positive relationship between specific bonds within families and chronic disease management that is different from the association between support from others and chronic disease management" (Weihs et al. [48], p. 8). They define the family as broadly as is necessary for the multiple forms that families take in contemporary society, assuming that to be families, relationships "persist over time, they are emotionally intense, and they involve high levels of intimacy in day-to-day life" (p. 9). For a family, defined this way, chronic disease of one member is likely to be a long-term stressor, the intensity of which will be related to "the magnitude of changes required of the patient and family members in their day to day activities and in the way they relate to each other … The level of stress generated by the illness is the capacity of the patient within the circumstances of the family and their approaches to life to make these changes … Finally, the availability of medical assistance and community resources can mitigate or exacerbate the stress of the illness" (p. 9).

While the number of studies of the impact of families on the outcomes of chronic illness for adults are few, the findings of those studies support the increased emphasis on families in the evolving PCMH literature. In studies of patients with chronic disease attending oncology, rheumatology, and gastroenterology clinics in one institution, the overall quality of family functioning predicted psychological and self-care adjustment of the patients [52]. Among patients hospitalized with their first myocardial infarction, marital dissatisfaction predicted a second MI within a year as well or better than any biological marker [53]. In a large study, sometimes called the "Johns Hopkins Hypertension Study," a single home visit with the family and the newly diagnosed patient with hypertension (HTN) to develop a personalized plan so that the family could assist with medication and support lifestyle changes led to improved adherence to medication and dietary restrictions, reduced blood pressure, more successful weight control, and reduced mortality at 2- and 5-year follow-ups, compared to controls [54].

It is clear that families can significantly affect outcomes for adults coping with chronic illnesses. Any routine, well-designed ways of including the families in care can increase the supportive aspects of the family's influence. The regular engagement with families can increase the potential for certain team members to provide targeted interventions in certain families to reduce the likelihood of family stresses leading to poorer outcomes. Weihs, Fisher, and Baird's review of the literature found consistent linkages between family process and disease management on targeted chronic illnesses. These linkages showed the protective influence of family closeness, mutuality and connectedness, caregiver coping skills, mutually supportive family relationships, clear family organization, and direct communication about the illness and its management. Risk factors shown were intrafamilial conflict, criticism and blame, psychological trauma related to diagnosis and treatment of disease, external stress, lack of an extrafamilial support system, disease interruptions of family members developmental tasks, and perfectionism and rigidity (p. 15).

Most of the research on including families as a part of care in primary care settings for adults is old and therefore likely to seem less credible than the current research in the PCMH model. The reconfiguration of the healthcare team that "provides a 'place' for the family over time and a setting in which the family is known as it faces each stage of disease management can make the delivery of health services more 'family-friendly' and possibly more effective" was called for in 1993 [55]. "Patient and family engaged care" that involves an active partnership between patients and their families was called for in 2017 [1]. The Institute of Medicine is still promulgating this call, in part, because there has been little progress on the routine implementation of a reasonable role for families devised in the meantime, despite the evidence on the influence families can have on the successful management of chronic illnesses. One reason for this lack of progress may be the conceptual and ethical models of the autonomous patient that can appear to be an element of the "patient as the control of their healthcare" from the IOM's ten rules for "Crossing the Quality Chasm" [56]. Part, also, is likely to be related to doctors' discomfort in interviewing multiple family members in a patient's visit, particularly if conflicting opinions that could demand unpredictable amounts of extra time might arise. While we won't be able to address the challenges of interviewing as a part of primary care of adults in this volume, we can say that this is a skill and that it is reasonable to expect a behavioral health member of the team to be able to provide and to teach. In addition, practices following the T.E.A.M. Way routinely will be clearer about the patient's desires in relation to the role of family members in the care of those patients. In these practices, the whole health team will understand the specifics of their enfranchisement in relation to communicating with those family members. The potential for a clear and easy involvement of family members in the chronic illness care of adult patients is likely to a future development in the current march toward team-based patient-centered care.

4.12 Conclusion

It is the intent of this chapter to make clear the benefits of partnership for patients and HPs, to show approaches that can be part of a pathway to partnership, and to be realistic about the challenges involved. This could allow for more realistic planning for building a culture of partnership in a practice or health system. It is clear that making a partnership of the sort imagined in the more recent IOM publications can be very difficult. The knowledge divide between professionals and patients varies depending on the patient and the situation, but it can be very challenging. And the divide between HPs and patients consists of much more than simply difference of medical knowledge. There is the divide of the different ways that doctors and patients experience and discuss the patient's illness, the "parallel play" of the chronic care visit. There is the challenge of patients who are socialized to the "doctor in the lead" relationship in healthcare. There are the challenges of finding the extra time required for more detailed conversations and the challenges of effecting changes in the role of the HP for in order to move toward partnership. For some patients, sometimes referred to as "complex patients," there is the even more daunting challenge of their lack of the experience of enfranchisement or self-efficacy needed to participate in their health decisions, even when invited to do so. The notion that clinicians should be guided by the best evidence and a knowledge of patient values, as quoted at the opening of the chapter, when considering these patients, looks a good deal more complex than one might think from the success shown by the methods described in this chapter.

In working toward partnership, it is important to keep the patients and their challenges in the equation when picking approaches to implement. In the next chapter we will describe a group of patients who are not uncommon in primary care who have great difficulty utilizing primary care and taking care of their health as well as we would hope. At the same time, these patients find dealing with primary care and with healthcare in general to be extremely challenging for them. During the second half of the book, we go into a set of methods that can be incorporated as routine behaviors in the clinical work of the whole care team. These methods are designed to augment and facilitate partnership with the majority of patients in primary care and to make partnership possible for the group of patients who currently are not able to participate. Patients with complex behavioral and medical illnesses, patients with low education and income, patients from cultures with substantially different assumptions about illness and treatment, and patients with severe trauma histories, all are part of the group that primary care HPs find challenging and, conversely, who find interacting with primary care and the medical system in general to be a challenge that keeps them from receiving successful care.

References

1. Frampton S, Guastello S, Hoy L, Naylor M, Sheridan S, Johnston-Fleece M. Harnessing evidence and experience to change culture: a guiding framework for patient and family engaged care. National Institute of Medicine. 2017. https://nam.edu/harnessing-evidence-and-experience-to-change-culture-a-guiding-framework-for-patient-and-family-engaged-care/
2. Kuzel AJ, Woolf SH, Gilchrist VJ, Engel JD, LaVeist TA, Vincent C, Frankel RM. Patient reports of preventable problems and harms in primary health care. Ann Fam Med. 2004;2(4): 333–40.
3. Elder NC, Imhoff R, Chubinski J, et al. Congruence of patient self-rating of health with family physician ratings. JABFM. 2017;30:196–204.
4. Kruse RL, Olsberg JE, Shigaki CL, Oliver D, Vetter-Smith M, Day T, LeMaster J. Communication during patient-provider encounters regarding diabetes self-management. Fam Med. 2013;45:475–83.
5. Parker RM. Health literacy: a challenge for American patients and their healthcare providers. Health Promot Int. 2000;15:277–91.
6. Hayes MV, Ross IE, Gashner M, Gutstgein D. Telling stories: news media, health literacy and public policy in Canada. Soc Sci Med. 2007;64:1842–52.
7. Institute of Medicine. Health literacy: a prescription to end confusion. Washington, DC: National Academies Press; 2004.
8. Nutbeam D. The evolving concept of health literacy. Soc Sci Med. 2008;67:2072–6.
9. Paasche-Orlow MK, Wolf MS. The causal pathway lining healthy literacy to health outcomes. Am J Health Behav. 2007;31:S19–26.
10. Miller WR, Rollnick S. Motivational Interviewing, Helping People Change. 3rd ed. New York: Guilford Press; 2012.
11. Prochaska JO, DiClemente CC. The Transtheoretical approach: towards a systematic eclectic framework. Homewood: Dow Jones Irwin; 1984.
12. Miller WR, Rollnick S. Motivational Interviewing: Preparing People to Change Addictive Behavior. New York: Guilford Press; 1991.
13. Rauch J. How not to die. The Atlantic. May, 2013: 65–69.
14. Bodenheimer T, Lorig K, Holman H, Grumbach K. Patient self-management of chronic disease in primary care. JAMA. 2002;288:2469–75.
15. Guadagnoli E, Ward P. Patient participation in decision-making. Soc Sci Med. 1998;47:329–39.
16. Devine EC, Cook TD. A meta-analytic analysis of effects of psychoeducational interventions on length of postsurgical hospital stay. Nurs Res. 1983;32:267-274.
17. Stiggelbout AM, Van der Weijden T, De Wit MPT, et al. Shared decision making: really putting patients at the centre of healthcare. BMJ. 2012;344:1–6.
18. Onel E, Hamond C, Wasson JH, et al. Assessment of the feasibility and impact of shared decision making in prostate cancer. Urology. 1998;51:63–6.
19. Elwyn G, Dehlendorf C, Epstein RM, Marrin K, White J, Frosch DL. Shared decision making and motivational interviewing: achieving patient-centered care across the spectrum of health care problems. Ann Fam Med. 2014;12:270–5.
20. O'Connor AM, Legare F, Stacey D. Risk communication in practice: the contribution of decision aids. BMJ. 2003;327:736–40. https://www.ncbi.nlm.nih.gov/pmc/articles/PMC200814/
21. Cvengros JA, Christensen AJ, Hillis SL, Rosenthal GE. Patient and physician attitudes in the health care context: attitudinal symmetry predicts patient satisfaction and adherence. Ann Behav Med. 2007;33:262–5.
22. Barry MJ, Edgman-Levitan S. Shared decision making – the pinnacle of patient-centered care. N Engl J Med. 2012;366:780–1.
23. Lagare F, Stacey D, Turcotte S, et al. Interventions for improving the adoption of shared decision making by healthcare professionals. Cochrane Database Syst Rev. 2014. http://onlinelibrary.wiley.com/doi/10.1002/14651858.CD006732.pub3/full

24. Couët N, Desroches S, Robitaille H, Vaillancourt H, Leblanc A, Turcotte S, et al. Assessments of the extent to which health-care providers involve patients in decision making: a systematic review of studies using the OPTION instrument. Health Expectations. 2015;18:542–61.

25. Leppin AL, Montori VM, Gionfriddo MR. Minimally disruptive medicine: a pragmatically comprehensive model for delivering care to patients with multiple chronic conditions. Healthcare. 2015;3:50–63.

26. Jowsey T, Yen L, Mathews WP. Time spent on health-related activities associated with chronic illness: a scoping literature review. BMC Public Health. 2012;12:1044.

27. Shippee ND, Shah ND, May CR, Mair FS, Montori VM. Cumulative complexity: a functional, patient-centered model for patient complexity can improve research and practice. J Clin Epidemiol. 2012;65:1041–51.

28. Leppin AL, Gionfriddo MR, Kessler M, et al. Preventing 30-day hospital readmissions: a systematic review and meta-analysis of randomized trials. JAMA Intern Med. 2014;174: 1095–107.

29. Kiecolt-Glaser JK, Fisher LD, Grocki P, Stout J, Speicher C, Glaser R. Marital quality, marital disruption, and immune function. Psychosom Med. 1987;49:13–34.

30. Uchino BN, Cacioppo JT, Kiecolt-Glaser JK. The relationship between social support and physiological processes: a review with emphasis on underlying mechanisms and implications for health. Psychol Bull. 1996;119:488–531.

31. Rakel DP, Hoeft TJ, Barrett BP, et al. Practitioner empathy and the duration of the common cold. Fam Med. 2009;41:494–501.

32. Rossland A, Heisler M, Piette JD. The impact of family behaviors and communication patterns on chronic illness outcomes: a systematic review. J Behav Med. 2012;35:221–39.

33. Kaplan SH, Greenfield S, Ware JE. Assessing the effects of physician-patient interactions on the outcomes of chronic disease. Med Care. 1989;27:S110–27.

34. Haug MR, Lavin B. Public challenge of physician authority. Med Care. 1979;17:429.

35. Vertinsky JB, Thompson WA, Uyeno D. Measuring consumer desire for participation in clinical decision-making. Health Serv Res. 1974;15:121.

36. Woolley FR, Kane RI, Hughes CC, et al. The effects of doctor-patient communication on satisfaction and outcome of care. Soc Sci Med. 1978;12:123.

37. Patrick DL, Scrivens E, Charlton J. Disability and patient satisfaction with medical care. Med Care. 1983;21:1062.

38. Belkora J, Edlow B, Aviv C, Sepucha K, Esserman L. Training community resource center and clinic personnel to prompt patients in listing questions for doctors: follow-up interviews about barriers and facilitators to the implementation of consultation planning. Implement Sci. 2008;3:6.

39. Adelman AM, Graybill M. Integrating a health coach into primary care: reflections from the Penn State ambulatory research network. Ann Fam Med. 2005;3:S33–5.

40. Tresolini CP. Pew-Fetzer task force on advancing psychosocial health education. Health Professions Education and Relationship-Centered Care. 1994. Pew Health Professions Commission, GoogleBooks.com: San Francisco.

41. Beach MC, Inui T, The Relationship-Centered Research Network. Relationship-centered care: a constructive reframing. J Gen Intern Med. 2006;21:S3–8.

42. Soklareidis S, Ravitz P, Nevo GA, Lieff S. Relationship-centered care in health: a 20-year scoping review. Patient Exp J. 2016;3:130–45.

43. Suchman AL, Sluyter DJ, Williamson PR, editors. Leading change in healthcare. London: Radcliffe Publishing; 2011.

44. Watzlawick P, Bavelas JB, Jackson DD. Pragmatics of human communication. New York: W. W. Norton; 1967.

45. Miller WR. Living as if. Philadelphia: Westminster Press; 1985.

46. Carney DR, Cuddy AJC, Yap AJ. Brief nonverbal displays affect neuroendocrine levels and risk tolerance. Psychol Sci. 2010;21:1363–8.

47. Ryan P, Sawin KJ. The individual and family self-management theory: background and perspectives on context, process, and outcomes. Nurs Outlook. 2009;57:217–25.

48. Weihs K, Fisher L, Baird M. Families, health, and behavior. Fam Syst Health. 2002;20:7–46.
49. Lewis N, Gray SW, Freres DR, Hornik RC. Examining cross-source engagement with cancer-related information and its impact on doctor-patient relations. Health Commun. 2009;24:723–34.
50. Kleinman A, Eisenberg L, Good B. Culture, illness, and care: clinical lessons from anthropologic and cross-cultural research. Ann Intern Med. 1978;88:251–8.
51. Siminoff LA. Incorporating patient and family preferences into evidence-based medicine. BMC Med Inform Decis Mak. 2013;13:S6.
52. Arpin K, Fitch M, Browne GB, Corey P. Prevalence and correlates of family dysfunction to chronic illness in specialty clinics. J Clin Epidemiol. 1990;3:373–83.
53. Medalie JH, Goldbourt U. Angina pectoris among 10,000: psychosocial and other risk factors as evidenced by a multivariate analysis of a five-year incidence study. Am J Med. 1976;60:910–21.
54. Morisky DE, DeMuth NM, Field-Fass M, Green LW, Levine DM. Evaluation of family health education to build social support for long-term control of high blood pressure. Health Educ Q. 1985;12:35–50.
55. Mittleman MS, Ferris SH, Mackell JA, Ambinder A, Cohen J. An intervention that delays institutionalization of Alzheimer's disease patients: treatment of spouse caregiver. The Gerontologist. 1993;35:792–802.
56. Institute of Medicine. Crossing the quality chasm: a new health system for the 21st century. Washington, DC: National Academies Press; 2001.
57. Healthy People 2020. www.HealthyPeople.gov

Resources

Patients Advocating for Patient Participation

https://thelizarmy.com/
http://www.epatientdave.com/

Health Literacy Resources

From the Office of Disease Prevention and Health Promotion: https://health.gov/communication/literacy/quickguide/healthinfo.htm
Chronic pain tools for patients with low reading levels. http://pmt.ua.edu/publications.html
Agency for Healthcare Research and Quality health literacy toolkit for health systems. https://www.ahrq.gov/professionals/quality-patient-safety/quality-resources/tools/literacy-toolkit/index.html
Videos on Culture and Health Literacy: https://www.thinkculturalhealth.hhs.gov/resources/videos
Agency for Healthcare Quality and Research offers a guide for improving patient-provider communication https://www.ahrq.gov/professionals/systems/hospital/engagingfamilies/strategy2/index.html.

Motivational Interviewing Resources

Motivational Interviewing Network of Trainers website with links to a great many resources: http://motivationalinterviewing.org/motivational-interviewing-resources

The Ineffective Physician and The Effective Physician: https://video.search.yahoo.com/search/vid eo?fr=tightropetb&p=the+ineffective+physician#id=1&vid=1278e1c1e056216608ff888a44b 71dba&action=click; https://video.search.yahoo.com/search/video?fr=tightropetb&p=videos +of+motivational+interviewing#id=5&vid=670307f45b4db2c085ab9411dd4a0b0b&action=c lick

"Stages of Change Model" in medical settings. Outline: http://www.currentnursing.com/nursing_ theory/transtheoretical_model.html

Shared Decision-Making Resources

For Professionals

AHRQ. The SHARE approach. 2017. https://www.ahrq.gov/professionals/education/curriculum-tools/shareddecisionmaking/index.html

Tools from Massachusetts General Hospital. http://www.massgeneral.org/decisionsciences/ research/Choice_Report.aspx

Ottawa Hospital Patient Decision Aides and the Healthwise Knowledgebase. https://decisionaid. ohri.ca/azinvent.php. The Healthwise Knowledgebase is intended for professional evaluation and not intended for distribution directly to patients or consumers.

PCORI database of articles on the benefits of patient engagement: https://www.pcori.org/literature/ engagement-literature?f%5B0%5D=field_article_phases%3A470&f%5B1%5D=field_arti-cle_phases%3A473#search-results

Decisional Aids for Patients

https://shareddecisions.mayoclinic.org/. Mayo Clinic Shared Decision-Making National Resource Center. 1/27/18 offers tool kits for 8 conditions.

Best access to multiple medical decision aids websites: http://www.dartmouth-hitchcock.org/ supportive-services/patient-resources.html

Minimally Disruptive Medicine

Blog and connecting point for those interested—www.minimallydisruptivemedicine.org

Chapter 5
When the Doctor-Patient Divide
Is a Chasm

5.1 Understanding Multiply-Disadvantaged Patients

In 2011, Atul Gawande, noted surgeon and author, changed the consciousness of the healthcare system, particularly those studying healthcare costs, when he first reported on the work of Dr. Jeffrey Brenner in Camden, N. J. In his article, "The Hotspotters" in *The New Yorker* [1], he described the interactions between Brenner and some of his patients in the most disadvantaged areas of Camden. The data about such patients had been well documented [2], but Gawande told the individual stories of these patients in a way that made sense of their dilemmas and their costs. "The Hotspotters" gave people names and life stories who otherwise are called "complex," "high-utilizing," "multimorbid," "low-income," "minority" patients. Giving the story of individuals who were extremely high utilizers added an element that the data often fails to convey: hope. His stories described the kind of care that made a substantial difference in their lives in addition to a difference in their costs to the healthcare system.

Perhaps one reason that the patients that Gawande described and that Brenner treated seemed so underrepresented in the literature was that they were described in different literatures under different categories. There was a literature on high-utilizing patients and another on multimorbid patients, particularly those with both behavioral health and medical diagnoses, who are often brought together under the label of "complex" patients. There was a literature on low-income patients and their interactions with the health system. There was another literature on the treatment of patients from minority or immigrant groups by the health system. Each literature tended to focus on people defined by the category that it studied. Few studies were careful about how else their group had been defined in other literatures. This practice tended and still tends to underplay the fact that patients in one studied group are also members of other groups studied in other literatures.

There is one more group description that commonly can be applied to Dr. Brenner's patients: trauma victims. In a study done by Brenner's team [39] that

© Springer Nature Switzerland AG 2019

A. Blount, *Patient-Centered Primary Care*,
https://doi.org/10.1007/978-3-030-17645-7_5

involved in-depth interviews with many of these patients, the high-utilizing, multimorbid, complex, low-income, mostly minority patients his team interviewed in depth had high scores on a measure of adverse childhood experiences [3]. They had experienced abuse and/or chaotic home lives of an intensity that has been shown to correlate with greatly increased risk of mental and physical problems in later life.

Not every patient who fits one of these groups (disadvantaged, complex, trauma victim) belongs in the others. It doesn't take a lot of time to find an example of a patient who only fits in one or two of them. Still, the overlap is much more substantial and much more common than is represented in any of the literatures on any of the groups (see Appendix). In this chapter, we will look at what is known about the relationship of high-cost, high-morbidity patients (complex patients), low-income patients with low educational attainment (disadvantaged patients), and patients with histories of trauma. Patterns of behavior or problems that may seem unexplained, when a patient is considered in one group, will begin to make better sense when they are considered as a member of a second or third. All of this is done so that healthcare procedures and methods that have been shown to be helpful to one group can be brought to bear for patients recognized as members of others. This should make the case for a synthesis of current approaches to providing care for these groups and for a new approach to building partnerships with them.

5.2 Complex Patients

There are a number of published systems for designating "complex" patients [4–10]. In addition, it is common for individual health systems or even individual primary care practices to create their own approaches to designating patients as "complex." All of the systems have in common an attempt to identify a subgroup of patients for additional monitoring and services. Most focus on the confluence of high medical cost and multiple chronic illness [11]. After eliminating the "high utilizers we can't do anything about," e.g., cancer patients needing a bone marrow transplant, we are left with the high utilizers described here [12]. Many use the addition of a psychiatric diagnosis as a heavily weighted element because of the great increase in cost that is associated with the comorbidity of a chronic illness and anxiety or depression [13, 14]. They try to meet a dual goal of designating patients who are likely to derive significant health benefits and to require less costly overall healthcare when the additional monitoring and support services of a program for complex patients are brought to bear.

When high-utilizing patients are studied, they prove to be more likely to have psychiatric or substance use problems in addition to the chronic illnesses with which they are coping. When they are compared with moderate utilizers with the same acuity of chronic illness, the high utilizers are younger, and they have higher burdens of anxiety, depression, and substance use [15]. This is a finding from a study that controlled for the effects of medical morbidity, adverse events, age, race, gender, employment status, and health insurance coverage. An anxiety diagnosis contributed the most to identifying high-utilizing patients, and a diagnosis of anxiety, depression, or substance use correlated most powerfully with patients with medical illness complexity and utilization.

The question of how to identify complex patients, when considered in more detail, can be addressed with another question, "Complex to whom?" One approach is to specify types of complexity. Consider the categories used by Frankel, Bourgeois, and Erdberg [16] of clinical complexity, presenting with conditions that are difficult to identify and treat; operational complexity, the difficulty in coordinating the multiple health professionals needed to deliver optimal treatment; and management complexity, the difficulty a patient presents as health professionals try to exert influence on their health behavior and adherence. In this model, and others like it, the complexity is in the experience of the healthcare team. Their job of providing care is complex.

Perhaps a more sophisticated definition of complexity at this writing is the Patient Centered Assessment Method (PCAM) [17]. It is an example of the way a good deal of research, wisdom, and experience can been condensed into a one-page assessment of a patient's complexity that grew out of work in Minnesota [18]. In this model, the complexity is seen as in the patient's social, health system, and medical circumstances. The task of the team is not just to assess the numbers of medical diagnoses but to "understand that proportion of the patient's despair, demoralization, discouragement, and withdrawal that is related to 'complexity' derived from non-medical factors that inhibit quality of life and can block improvement from routing medical or mental health care" ([4], p. 302). In the rest of this volume, calling a patient "complex" will signify a patient coping with medical, behavioral health and social circumstances that complicate their interaction with the health system and make usual medical or mental healthcare likely to be ineffective or less effective than would be expected of patients with their medical diagnoses alone.

The PCAM is filled out by a health profession about the patient. It asks about 4 general areas of a person's health situation using 12 questions. The PCAM assesses current health and well-being by asking about the physical health needs that should be investigated, physical problems impacting mental well-being, problems with lifestyle behaviors, and other concerns about the patient's mental well-being. It assesses social environment by asking about the safety and stability of the person's home environment, about the impact on their well-being of their daily activities, about their social network, and about their financial resources. It assesses the person's health literacy and communication with their health professionals by asking how well they understand their health situation and how well they engage in conversations with their health professionals. And finally, it asks about service coordination by asking for a rating of other needed services and how well-coordinated current services are.

The PCAM is much more sophisticated than might appear on the surface, allowing a clinician with no access to health cost data about a patient, to make reliable decisions about which patients to consider complex and how to assess levels of complexity. It is remarkably accurate in predicting patterns of a patient's interaction with the health system such as length of stay in the hospital [19]. Perhaps more importantly, it can guide a health team on where to put efforts and resources in making care more successful for complex patients.

5.3 Disadvantaged Patients

Asking about finances is important for understanding a patient's relationship with the health system, not to assess their ability to pay their medical bills but because income correlates with health. Findings in the USA and other industrialized countries indicate a monotonic relationship between income and a number of health outcomes such as birth outcomes, life expectancy, chronic disease rates, quality of life ratings, and mortality [20]. In other words, the poorer you are, the sicker you are, and the shorter your life will be. Barnett and her colleagues put the relationship of socioeconomic status (SES) to health in their study in a particularly vivid way, "Young and middle-aged adults living in the most deprived areas had rates of multimorbidity equivalent to those aged 10–15 years older in the most affluent areas." Their review of ten studies showed a 24% higher rate of multimorbidity in the most deprived areas over the most affluent. While the most powerful predictor of multimorbidity is age, for all ages lower than 85, patients in more deprived areas had higher levels of multimorbidity than those in more affluent areas. In the more deprived areas, the likelihood that a person with multimorbidity had a mental health as well as a physical diagnosis was more than double the likelihood in the more affluent areas. And having a mental health disorder was strongly associated with having more physical disorders. Income seems to determine how likely a person would be classified as complex in the way of grouping patients described above.

Low income and low education on one hand and race and ethnicity on another intersect in recursive and reciprocal ways [21] in influencing health risk, morbidity, and mortality. Much of the literature comparing socioeconomic status with health outcomes does not distinguish between racial and ethnic groups. Because certain racial and ethnic groups are overrepresented among low-income populations, research on the health burdens of low SES on one hand and race/ethnicity on the other is describing many of the same people. It does seem clear, however, that additional disadvantage for many is attributable to discrimination and racism leading to additional stressful life experiences and psychological distress. These populations show a greater likelihood of reacting with hostility, anxiety, depression, and hopelessness [22]. In studies that have controlled for income, African Americans have a higher likelihood of high allostatic load scores at all ages but particularly at ages 35–64. African American women had higher scores than their male counterparts [23]. Allostatic load is the wear and tear on the body caused by chronic exposure to stressful experiences or situations. When situations are experienced as dangerous or unsettling, the "fight-or-flight" response can stay chronically activated leading to changes in the functioning of the immune system which over time can cause organ damage, impaired response to new dangers, and heightened vulnerability to disease. High allostatic load is a feature of people who have experienced multiple traumatic events as well as people who live with high levels of stress on a day-to-day basis.

However the research is grouped; people in lower SES groups and certain racial and ethnic minorities appear to face both higher rates of traumatic events and higher levels of stress [22]. Interviews with a number of young adults who grew up in low-income neighborhoods in a major American city (Philadelphia) showed levels of adverse childhood experiences at rates much higher than the national average. Nationally 45% of adults report one or more adverse childhood experiences, as defined by the ACE screen, before the age of 18 [24]. A sample of low-income, mostly minority adults (African American, Hispanic and Native American) in an urban environment reported adverse childhood experiences at extremely high levels [25]. Their reports included the items on the ACE screen and additional adverse experiences such as single-parent homes; lack of parental love, support, and guidance; death of family members; exposure to violence; criminal behavior; economic hardship; personal victimization; and discrimination. Of the 119 adults interviewed, 511 adverse experiences of those on the ACE screen or the list above were reported [25].

A term used in some of the research on this group that brings together the concept of a person's comparative income and social status as impacts on their options and stresses in life is "disadvantaged." And the impact to trauma greatly increases that disadvantage.

5.4   Trauma Victims

Traumatic events, particularly occurring in childhood, have a powerful impact on future physical and mental health. The study of the impact of trauma brings together neurobiological, immunological, and genetic evidence on one hand and epidemiological evidence on the other [33] for a picture that forms a plausible "back story" for the patients that are being designated as "complex." The impact of trauma has been brought into focus through the use of a measure of adverse childhood experiences [3]. The "ACE" measure asks about patients' history of abuse (emotional, physical, and sexual), witnessing domestic violence and parental marital discord, and growing up with mentally ill, substance-abusing, or criminal household members [26]. The use of the ACE measure has shown a dose-response relationship between the number of types of adverse experiences remembered and a varied array of illnesses and dysfunction as adults. The list of the problems and conditions that increase in likelihood as the number of adverse childhood experiences goes up is long and varied. Early trauma impacts such basic elements of development as the size and function of several areas of the brain [27–29] and the expression of the genome [30]. These impact the function of the immune system leading to hyperarousal and increased stress response to events and relationships [31]. People with higher adverse childhood experiences have correspondingly higher psychiatric

disorders, substance use disorders, psychosocial disturbances, and physical illnesses. They show higher depression, anxiety, panic, suicide attempts, PTSD, hal-
lucinations, dissociative disorders, and borderline personality disorders [33]. ACE
scores correlate with substance abuse: smoking, alcohol use, illicit drug use, and
injection drug use [33]. The same correlation exists with psychosocial disturbances
such as difficulty controlling anger, intimate partner violence, difficulty with long-
term attachment, likelihood of stormy interpersonal relationships, problems regu-
lating mood, early intercourse, and high lifetime number of sexual partners [33].
ACE scores correlate with cognitive problems such as memory for events. The
number of adverse childhood events correlates with physical illnesses such as cardiovascular disease, hypertension, hyperlipidemia, asthma, metabolic abnormali-
ties, diabetes, obesity, infection, and other physical disorders with or without
corresponding medical findings [3, 32]. Finally, many of the elements are additional traumas in themselves, while others contribute to a life of continual disadvantage. They include poor work performance, financial stress, adolescent pregnancy,
risk of sexual violence, risk of intimate partner violence, and poor academic
achievement.

The habit of Western science to dichotomize the mind and body is one reason
that the observations of the impacts of trauma have only recently begun to coalesce.
The study of the impacts of trauma has been a pivotal part of the converging of the
study of "psychiatric" and "medical" illness. In fact, it is reasonable to reconceptu-
alize the types of impacts listed above (neurobiological and genetic, immune system
functioning, psychiatric illnesses, psychosocial difficulties, and physical illnesses)
as different points of observation on what is one long-term, highly complex process.
And, while the argument against attributing causation to patterns of correlation is
always important to consider, Anda and his colleagues [33] argue that the massive
quantity of evidence about the impact of trauma meets Sir Bradford Hill's nine criteria for establishing an argument for causation [34]. But one does not need to make
a case for causation in order to make a case for the likelihood of a trauma history
among patients designated as "complex" by standards of multimorbidity or high
utilization.

Clinicians have observed the confluence of psychiatric, psychosocial, and physical problems for years, often without a theory of what could explain this pattern.
They observed that some patients were more disabled by their illnesses than others
who had similar clinical pictures. They saw that some patients came to medical care
much more often than others who were equally sick. They saw that some patients
with chronic illness were more likely to also have depression or anxiety or to be
using substances. In each case, it was not common for clinicians to inquire about a
trauma history as the factor that united these observations [35]. It is probably fair to
say that the level of awareness of the impact of trauma in many quarters has changed
only marginally in the last 20 years.

Patients who tend to be what the British term "frequent attenders," who seem,
despite their higher levels of care and attention, to be more disabled by their illnesses than their peers, can be frustrating to clinicians. This is particularly true

because many of these patients who come so often do not reliably follow the treatment plans offered to them or they go to multiple medical settings so their treatments are not coordinated. One telling name for this group is patients who are "over-serviced and underserved" [36]. Another is a description of the patients as identified by their doctor's reaction to seeing their names on the schedule for the day, calling them "heartsink" patients [37].

While there has not been a lot of research aimed at studying the impact of a trauma history on socioeconomic status (SES), it is reasonable to put together some of the factors that are associated with childhood trauma to support the suspicion that there is a correlation between the two. Factors such as a higher likelihood of disability, higher burdens of medical and psychiatric illness, higher probability of substance use disorders, problems with anger management, and interpersonal relationships, a higher likelihood of illness due to immune system dysregulation, difficulties with long-term relationships, and higher likelihood of homelessness lead to a picture of a population that has significantly increased challenges in getting and keeping employment adequate to maintain a reasonable standard of living. Studies that elaborate the difference in health status of higher- and lower-income people, including different rates of obesity, mental health problems, unsafe neighborhoods, and access to care, often fail to include differing rates of traumatic experiences [38]. These increased rates of trauma reciprocally potentiate impact of the other elements cited in these inventories.

As we consider the lives of these three overlapping groups of patients, the term "multiply-disadvantaged" seems an appropriate description. It is a term that can bring together patients otherwise termed "low-income," "low-education," "complex," "high-utilizing," "underserved," or "trauma" survivors. These are patients who are likely to wear their disadvantage physically and functionally, in their immune system, in their psychological challenges, in the conditions of their day-to-day lives, and in their burden of illness. Keeping in mind the full resonance of the term can also give access to noticing how much a patient has accomplished in spite of their challenges, the strengths they have developed, the relationships they have maintained, and their contributions to other people. Those are distinctions that will be needed when we come to talking about how to make partnerships with multiply-disadvantaged patients.

5.5   The Health System and Multiply-Disadvantaged Patients

"Multiply-disadvantaged" is a fitting term for the patients that Atul Gawande described in *The New Yorker* article mentioned earlier. His term, "hotspotters," is a term from the perspective of the health system, one that was very important because it helped the medical world and the public to conceptualize patterns of high utilization and high cost that previously were not widely recognized. Mautner and her colleagues [39] offer a picture of the interaction of these same multiply-disadvantaged patients with the health system from the patients' perspective. Over half of the patients interviewed reported interactions with the healthcare system that they found upsetting, disrespectful, or demeaning. These patients were likely to report that their subsequent interactions with the health system were influenced by these experiences. They were less likely to follow the treatment suggestions they were given and sometimes less likely return for care. Many reported trying to change providers, though that was probably not something that was easy in their situation.

Just as their negative interaction with the health system tended to impact their health behavior, positive experiences made a difference in their health behavior in the opposite direction. Those who reported feeling "cared for," despite the likelihood that their functioning would deteriorate because of their diabetes, hypertension, and depression, said that they felt better over time. Their health status improved. These patients particularly focused on their interactions with the care management team in Brenner's program for the outreach and relationships offered more than for specific services.

Caruso [40] interviewed very-low SES patients at a rural health center in New England about their experience with the health system. She isolated six themes in their experiences with physicians that seem to be an elaboration of the themes found by Mautner. She found that her respondents experienced the power asymmetry between themselves and their physicians as reminiscent of previous experiences that they had experienced as oppressive or stigmatizing. They sometimes avoided future visits after an unpleasant medical encounter. Their emotional reactions to unpleasant interactions in an environment of power asymmetry contributed to their being less likely in the future to ask for needed information or express their opinions. They commonly chose not to make some disclosures that they felt were too dangerous to make to authority figures such as their physicians. And, as with Mautner's interviewees, physicians who were personable increased patients' comfort with care, and physicians who asked about patients' dissatisfaction or other possible ruptures in the doctor-patient relationship tended to ultimately strengthen the relationship with accompanying likelihood of improvement of the effectiveness of their care.

When Bernheim and her colleagues [41] interviewed physicians who treated multiply-disadvantaged patients, they found the same patterns in mirror image. The physicians tended to characterize patients as "stoic," "guarded," and "distrustful," though some physicians described them as "appreciative." The physicians, half of whom were of racial minority background, reported that when they made adaptations in their usual care patterns with these patients, they did it for the patients' benefit. They were likely to prescribe fewer and less expensive medications, make fewer specialty referrals, try to get more done in one visit (and thereby seem more hurried), and postpone testing when possible. They altered their usual routines to try to adapt to what they expected about the patients, that because of their low incomes, they needed costs kept to a minimum; that because of their low education levels, they would have difficulty understanding their treatment regimen, or that because of their chaotic lives, multiple visits for care would be especially difficult.

All of these changes in care have been named in research into the disparities in healthcare afforded to disadvantaged patients and racial or ethnic minorities [42]. The expectation of lower education, lack of interest in their health, or lack of adherence becomes embodied in medical practice in ways that have been demonstrated in the studies. This leads to the finding that physicians encountering patients of lower income or education are commonly less patient-centered than with more affluent patients [43, 44]. They are more directive and use less relationship-building approaches such as counseling, empathy, or talk of emotions [45]. In a study by Garrison and his colleagues [46], it was a found that pediatricians working with the parents of Medicaid patients in sites in less affluent areas elicited and answered fewer questions about children's psychosocial issues from parents than in sites in which most patients had private insurance. They were also quicker to refer these patients to mental health services for problems that they addressed and managed in their practices for families in more affluent suburban practices.

In the case of medical services for multiply-disadvantaged patients, the difference in income and education can become a daily fact of life for doctors and for patients. It becomes an assumption about the relationship, not something to notice occasionally when it happens to occur. But what is experienced as an asymmetry of knowledge by the doctor is often experienced as an asymmetry of power by the patient. Over time, this asymmetry can lead to a lack of trust that influences both doctors and patients.

Some patients come from ethnic communities that have experienced domination and/or oppression by other groups. For these patients the reminder involved in the stark contrast of knowledge and income (power) can be even more sinister. Whether people are cued toward being passive in the face of a perceived authority or assume mal-intent in interactions in which they are not confident of their doctor's motives, this cuing is an unacknowledged part of many medical visits. Doctors who choose to serve in low-income or underserved communities can find many of their patients reacting in ways that are openly wary of them or feigning cooperation to get what the patients think they need. For those patients, the doctor's expertise is sometimes useful, but his or her motives are not trusted. In these situations, patients can express beliefs about doctors "just being in it for the money" or colluding with each other against them; "they all talk to each other."

Healthcare providers and multiply-disadvantaged patients, presumably doing their best in the situation as they each understand it, can be said to engage in a reciprocal and mutually reinforcing pattern; they "cooperate" to make care less effective. Multiply-disadvantaged patients who are less healthy are also less likely to engage actively in a visit. They are more likely to internalize stigma about themselves and their knowledge of health information. They need more experiences of support and positive relating than more advantaged patients to receive the intended benefit from their care. Yet they commonly receive more directive and less supportive care from providers. Health professionals mistakenly assume that these patients are less active in visits because they want less information and care less about their health than more affluent patients. The reciprocal interaction pattern that leads to physician/patient relationship being less patient-centered and more directive is often exacerbated in the case of minority patients such as African Americans [47].

Nurses, medical assistants, and administrative staff observe and sometimes amplify the pattern of mutual frustration between doctors and multiply-disadvantaged patients. This has been shown in the case of patients who come to their primary care site with problems like substance abuse and multiple chronic illnesses that are due in part to their own poor health behaviors. They are more likely to smoke, to be obese, to abuse substances, and to be poor at following a medical regimen, each of which will contribute to the impact of their diabetes, asthma, heart disease, and other illnesses. The judgment that "it is their own fault" can be part of a cooler or more perfunctory interaction style by nurses and medical assistants as well as doctors [48, 49]. Patients who use illicit drugs are likely to be expecting discrimination, and for those who do experience discrimination, it correlates with poorer physical and mental health [48].

5.6   Taking Stock

The usual divide between doctors and their patients in their different perspectives on health and healthcare and in their different purposes during a medical visit makes the goal of creating a partnership with patients in their healthcare a significant challenge. How much more challenging, then, is the chasm between doctors and multiply-disadvantaged patients, if partnership is still to be one of the goals of care? It is my hope that clarifying the challenge will lead to a better likelihood of addressing it successfully. Currently there are a number of ways of improving the engagement between doctors and their patients and of adapting care to make a better fit for patients which have been shown to make a difference in the processes and outcomes of care for this population. These will be discussed in the next chapter. In the following chapter and beyond, I will talk about a new approach to the routine interactions of care that can change the expectations on the part of health professionals and those of multiply-disadvantaged patients. The new interactions and expectations can lead to reciprocal and mutually reinforcing process that improves the health of these patients and the work experience of the healthcare team.

Appendix

Increased incidence of:	Complex patients (multimorbid and/or high utilizing)	Disadvantaged patients	Trauma histories (high ACEs or PTSD)
Depression	Ford et al. [15], Violen et al. [50], Barnett et al. [51]	Barnett et al. [51]	Danese et al. [52], Löwe et al. [53], Larkin et al. [54]
Anxiety	Ford et al. [15], Violen et al. [50], Barnett et al. [51]	Barnett et al. [51]	Löwe et al. [53], Larkin et al. [54]
Medically unexplained symptoms	Edwards et al. [55]		Löwe et al. [53], Larkin et al. [54]
Substance use disorders	Mautner et al. [39]	Myers [21]	Larkin et al. [54]
Multiple chronic illnesses	Smith et al. [8], Ford et al. [15], Violan et al. [50], Barnett et al. [51]	Barnett et al. [51], Smith et al. [8]	Felitti et al. [3], Anda et al. [33]
Diabetes	Noyes et al. [7], Barnett et al. [51]	Barnett et al. [51], CDC [56], Adler and Newman [57]	Larkin et al. [54], Roberts [58]
Osteoarthritis	Violan et al. [50]	Adler and Newman [57]	Larkin et al. [54]
Lung disease	Barnett et al. [51]	Barnett et al. [51], Adler and Newman [57]	Felitti et al. [3], Larkin et al. [54]
Metabolic risk markers	Violan et al. [50]	Adler and Newman [57]	Danese et al. [52]
Hypertension	Noyes et al. [7]	Adler and Newman [57]	Su et al. [59]
Heart disease	Violan et al. [50]	CDC [56], Adler and Newman [57]	Larkin et al. [54], Sumner et al. [60]
Homelessness or insecure housing	Mautner et al. [39]	Mersky et al. [61]	Mersky et al. [61], Herman et al. [62]
Problems with social determinants of health:	Mautner et al. [39]	Adler and Newman [57], Mersky et al. [61]	Mersky et al. [61]
Being considered "complex"		Barnett et al. [51]	Anda et al. [33]
Coping with poverty	Barnett et al. [51], Mautner et al. [39]		Nurius [73]
History of trauma (ACEs)	Mautner et al. [39]	Mautner et al. [39]	
Female gender	Violan et al. [50]	Mersky et al. [61]	Breslow [63], Uddin [64]
Problems with care:			

continued

continued

Increased incidence of:	Complex patients (multimorbid and/or high utilizing)	Disadvantaged patients	Trauma histories (high ACEs or PTSD)
Difficulty forming trusting relationships or partnerships	Mautner et al. [39]	Willems et al. [44], Street [65], Fox and Chelsa [66]	Green et al. [67]
Problems for HPs:			
HP is more frustrated with relationship with patient	Mautner et al. [39]	Mautner et al. [39]	Purkey et al. [68], Mautner et al. [39]
HP experiences extra stress from providing care and needs support	Bodenheimer and Berry-Millett [5]	Raja et al. [69]	Green et al. [67]
Underestimate incidence of trauma	Felitti et al. [3]	Felitti et al. [3]	Felitti et al. [3], Löwe et al. [53]
Aspects of effective care:			
HP is committed to helping patient become a partner in the plan of their care	Mautner et al. [39]	Fox and Chelsa [66], Raja et al. [69]	Netting and Williams [70]
HP takes a strength-based approach		Fox and Chelsa [66]	Green et al. [67], Purkey et al. [68]
Need a team to provide care	Frankel and Bourgeois [71], Dorr et al. [72], Smith et al. [8], Netting and Williams [70]		Mautner et al. [39]

References

1. Gawande A. The hotspotters. The New Yorker. Jan 24, 2011.
2. Braveman PA, Cubbin C, Egerter S, Williams DR, Pamuk E. Socioeconomic disparities in health in the United States: what the patterns tell us. Am J Public Health. 2010;100(1):186–96.
3. Felitti V, Anda R, Nordenberg D, Williamson M, Spitz A, Edwards V, Koss M, Marks J. Relationship of childhood abuse and household dysfunction to many of the leading causes of death in adults: the Adverse Childhood Experiences (ACE) study. Am J Prev Med. 1998;14:245–58.
4. Baird MA, Peek CJ, Gunn WB, Valeras A. Working with complexity in integrated behavioral health settings. In: Talen MR, Burke-Valeras A, editors. Integrated behavioral health in primary care: evaluation the evidence, identifying the essentials. New York: Springer; 2013. p. 299–324.

5. Bodenheimer T, Berry-Millett R. Care management of patient with complex health care needs. Robert Wood Johnson Foundation. 2009. https://www.rwjf.org/en/library/research/2009/12/care-management-of-patients-with-complex-health-care-needs.html

6. Johns Hopkins University. Johns Hopkins University ACG system: white paper – technical. 2012. www.hopkinsacg.org

7. Noyes K, Liu H, Temkin-Greener H. Medicare capitation model, functional status, and multiple comorbidities: model accuracy. Am J Manag Care. 2008;14(10):679–90.

8. Smith SM, Soubhi H, Fortin M, Hudon C, O'Dowd T. Managing patients with multimorbidity: systematic review of interventions in primary care and community settings. BMJ. 2012;345:1–10.

9. Von Korff M, Wagner EH, Saunders K. A chronic disease score from automated pharmacy data. J Clin Epidemiol. 1992;45:2.

10. Pratt R, Hibberd C, Cameron IM, Maxwell M. The Patient Centered Assessment Method (PCAM): integrating the social dimensions of health into primary care. J Comorb. 2015;5:110–9.

11. Long P, Abrams M, Milstein A, Anderson G, Apton KL, Dahlberg ML, Whicher D, editors. Effective care for high-need patients: opportunities for improving outcomes, value and health. Washington, DC: National Academy of Medicine; 2017.

12. Newton WP, Lefebvre A. Is a strategy focused on super-utilizers equal to the task of health care system transformation? No. Ann Fam Med. 2015;13:8–9.

13. Katon WJ, Egede LE. Major depression in individuals with chronic medical disorders: prevalence, correlates and association with health resource utilization, lost productivity and functional disability. Gen Hosp Psychiatry. 2003;29:409–16.

14. Melek S, Norris D. Chronic conditions and comorbid psychological disorders. Milliman research report. 2008. http://us.milliman.com/insight/research/health/pdfs/chronic-conditions-and-comorbid-psychological-disorders/

15. Ford JD, Trestman RL, Steinberg K, Tennen H, Allen S. Prospective association of anxiety, depressive, and addictive disorder with high utilization of primary, specialty and emergency medical care. Soc Sci Med. 2004;58:21456–2148.

16. Frankel SA, Bourgeois JA, Erdberg P. Comprehensive care for complex patients: the medical-psychiatric coordinating physician model. New York: Cambridge University Press; 2013.

17. Maxwell M, Hibberd C, Pratt R, Peek CJ, Baird M. Patient centered assessment method. 2013. www.pcamonline.org

18. Peek CJ, Baird MA, Coleman E. Primary care for patient complexity, not only disease. Fam Syst Health. 2009;27:287–302.

19. Yoshida S, et al. Validity and reliability of the Patient Centered Assessment Method for patient complexity and relationship with hospital length of stay: a prospective cohort study. BMJ Open. 2017;7:e016175.

20. Adler NE, Boyce T, Chesney MA, Cohen S, Folkman S, Kahn RL, Syme SL. Socioeconomic status and health: the challenge of the gradient. Am Psychol. 1994;49:15–24.

21. Myers HF. Ethnicity and socio-economic status-related stressed in context: an integrative review and conceptual model. J Behav Med. 2009;32:9–19.

22. Hatch SL, Dohrenwend BP. Distribution of traumatic and other stressful life events by race/ethnicity, gender, SES and age: a review of the research. Am J Community Psychol. 2007;40:313–32.

23. Geronimus AT, Hicken M, Keene D, Bound J. "Weathering" and age patterns of allostatic load scores among Blacks and Whites in the United States. Am J Public Health. 2006;96:826–37.

24. Sacks V, Murphey D. The prevalence of adverse childhood experiences nationally, by state, and by race or ethnicity. Bethesda: Child Trends; 2018.

25. Wade R, Shea JA, Rubin D, Wood J. Adverse childhood experiences of low-income urban youth. Pediatrics. 2014;134:e13–20.

26. Dong M, Anda RF, Felitti VJ, Dube SR, Giles WH. The relationship of exposure to childhood sexual abuse to other forms of abuse, neglect and household dysfunction during childhood. Child Abuse Negl. 2003;27:625–39.

27. Anderson CM, Teicher MH, Polcari A, Renshaw PI. Abnormal T2 relaxation time in the cerebellar vermis of adults sexually abused in childhood: potential role of the vermis in stress-enhanced risk for drug abuse. Psychoneuroendocrinology. 2002;27:231–44.
28. Carrion VG, Steiner H. Trauma and dissociation in delinquent adolescents. J Am Acad Child Adolesc Psychiatry. 2000;39:353–9.
29. De Bellis M, Thomas L. Biologic findings of post-traumatic stress disorder and child maltreatment. Curr Psychiatry Rep. 2003;5:108–17.
30. Perry BD, Pollard R. Homeostasis, stress, trauma, and adaptation. A neurodevelopmental view of childhood trauma. Child Adolesc Psychiatr Clin N Am. 1998;7:33–51.
31. Sanchez MM, Ladd CO, Plotsky PM. Early adverse experience as a developmental risk factor for later psychopathology: evidence from rodent and primate models. Dev Psychopathol. 2001;13:419–49.
32. Musselman DL, Evans DL, Nemeroff CB. The relationship of depression to cardiovascular disease. Arch Gen Psychiatry. 1998;55:580–92.
33. Anda RF, Felitti VJ, Bremner JD, Walker JD, Whitfield C, Perry BD, Dube SR, Giles WH. The enduring effects of abuse and related adverse experiences in childhood: a convergence of evidence from neurobiology and epidemiology. Eur Arch Psychiatry Clin Neurosci. 2006;256:174–86.
34. van Reekum R, Streiner DL, Conn DK. Applying Bradford Hill's criteria for causation to neuropsychiatry: challenges and opportunities. J Neuropsychiatry Clin Neurosci. 2001;12:318–25.
35. Stein MB, McQuaid JR, Pedrelli P, Lenox R, McCahill ME. Posttraumatic stress disorder in the primary care medical setting. Gen Hosp Psychiatry. 2000;22:261–9.
36. Peek CJ, Baird MA. Point-of-care complexity assessment helps primary care clinicians identify barriers to improved health and craft integrated care plans. AHRQ Innovations Exchange. 2009.
37. O'Dowd TC. Five years of heartsink patients in general practice. BMJ. 1988;297:528–30.
38. Cunningham PJ. Why even health low-income people have greater health risks than higher-income people. To the Point (blog), Commonwealth Fund. 2018.
39. Mautner DB, Pang H, Brenner JC, Shea JA, Gross KS, Frasso R, Cannuscio CC. Generating hypotheses about care needs of high utilizers: lessons from patient interviews. Popul Health Manag. 2013;16:S26–33.
40. Caruso M. The patient-physician relationship from the perspective of economically disadvantaged patients (Dissertations & Theses). 361. 2017. http://aura.antioch.edu/etds/361
41. Bernheim SM, Ross JS, Krumholz HM, Bradley EH. Influence of patients' socioeconomic status on clinical management decisions: a qualitative study. Ann Fam Med. 2008;6(1):53–9.
42. American Psychologic Association, APA Working Group on Stress and Health Disparities. Stress and health disparities: contexts, mechanisms, and interventions among racial/ethnic minority and low-socioeconomic status populations. 2017. Retrieved from http://www.apa.org/pi/health-disparities/resources/stress-report.aspx
43. Agency for Healthcare Research and Quality (AHRQ). National healthcare quality and disparities report. Rockville. 2016. July 2017. AHRQ Pub. No. 17-0001.
44. Willems S, De Maesschalck S, Deveugele M, Derese A, De Maeseneer J. Socio-economic status of the patient and doctor-patient communication: does it make a difference? Patient Educ Couns. 2005;56:139–46.
45. Fiscella K, Goodwin MA, Strange LC. Does patient educational level effect visits to family physicians? J Natl Med Assoc. 2002;94:157–65.
46. Garrison WT, Bailey EN, Garb J, Ecker B, Spencer P, Sigelman D. Psychiatr Serv. 1992;43:489–93.
47. Peek ME, Odoms-Young A, Quinn MT, Gorawara-Bhat R, Wilson SC, Chin MH. Race and shared decision-making: perspectives of African Americans with diabetes. Soc Sci Med. 2010;71:1–9.
48. Ahern J, Stuber J, Galea S. Stigma, discrimination and the health of illicit drug users. Drug Alcohol Depend. 2007;88:188–96.

49. Marteau TM, Riordan DC. Staff attitudes towards patients: the influence of causal attributions for illness. Br J Clin Psychol. 1992;31:107–10.
50. Violan C, Foguet-Boreu Q, Flores-Mateo G, Salisbury C, Blom J, et al. Prevalence, determinants and patterns of multimorbidity in primary care: a systematic review of observational studies. PLoS One. 2014;9(7):e102149. https://doi.org/10.1371/journal.pone.0102149.
51. Barnett K, Mercer SW, Norbury M, Watt G, Wyke S, Guthrie B. Epidemiology of multimorbidity and implications for health care, research, and medical education a cross-sectional study. Lancet. 2012;380:37–43.
52. Danese A, Moffit TE, Harrington H, et al. Adverse childhood experiences and adult risk factors for age-related disease. Arch Pediatr Adolesc Med. 2009;163:1135–43.
53. Löwe B, Kroenke K, Spitzer R, Spitzer C. Trauma exposure and posttraumatic stress disorder in primary care patients. J Clin Psychiatry. 2011;72:304–12.
54. Larkin H, Shields J, Anda R. The health and social consequences of adverse childhood experiences (ACE) across the lifespan: an introduction to prevention and intervention in the community. J Prev Interv Community. 2012;40:263–70.
55. Edwards T, Stern A, Clarke DD, Ivbijaro G, Kasney LM. The treatment of patients with medically unexplained symptoms in primary care: a review of the literature. Ment Health Fam Med. 2010;7:209–21.
56. Center for Disease Control and Prevention National Center for Health Statistics. Diabetes prevalence and glycemic control among adults aged 20 and over, by sex, age, and race and Hispanic origin: United States, selected years 1988–1994 through 2011–2014 [trend tables: table 40]. Health, United States, 2015 – poverty. 2015. Retrieved from https://www.cdc.gov/nchs/data/hus/2015/040.pdf
57. Adler NE, Newman K. Socioeconomic disparities in health: pathways and policies. Health Aff. 2002;21(2):60–76.
58. Roberts AL, Agnew-Blais JC, Spiegelman D, Kubzansky LD, Mason SM, Galea S, Hu FB, Rich-Edwards JW, Koenen KC. Posttraumatic stress disorder and incidence of type 2 diabetes mellitus in a sample of women: a 22-year longitudinal study. JAMA Psychiat. 2015;72:203–10.
59. Su S, Wang X, Pollock JS, Treiber FA, Xu X, Snieder H, McCall WV, Stefanek M, Harshfield G. Adverse childhood experiences and blood pressure trajectories from childhood to young adulthood: the Georgia Stress and Heart study. Circulation. 2015;131:1674–81.
60. Sumner JA, Kubzansky LD, Elkind MSV, Roberts AL, Agnew-Blais J, Chen Q, Cerdá M, Rexrode KM, Rich-Edwards JW, Spiegelman D, Suglia SF, Rimm EB.
61. Mersky JP, Janczewski CE, Nitowski JC. Poor mental health among low-income women in the U.S.: the roles of adverse childhood and adult experiences. Soc Sci Med. 2018;206:14–21.
62. Herman DB, Susser ES, Struening EL, Link BL. Adverse childhood experiences: are they risk factors for adult homelessness? Am J Public Health. 1997;87:249–55.
63. Breslow N. Gender differences in trauma and posttraumatic stress disorder. J Gend Specif Med. 2002;5:34–40.
64. Uddin M, Aiello AE, Wildman DE, Koenen KC, Pawelec G, de Los Santos R, Goldmann E, Galea S. Epigenetic and immune function profiles associated with posttraumatic stress disorder. Proc Natl Acad Sci. 2010;107:9470–5.
65. Street RL. Communicative styles and adaptations in physician-parent consultations. Soc Sci Med. 1992;34:1155–63.
66. Fox S, Chelsa C. Living with chronic illness: a phenomenological study of the health effects of the patient-provider relationship. J Am Acad Nurse Pract. 2008;20:109–17.
67. Green BL, Saunders PA, Power E, et al. Trauma-informed medical care: CME communication training for primary care providers. Fam Med. 2015;47:7–14.
68. Purkey E, Patel R, Phillips SP. Trauma-informed care: better care for everyone. Can Fam Physician. 2018;64:170–2.
69. Raja S, Hasnain M, Vadakumchery T, Hamad J, Shah R, Hoersch M. Identifying elements of patient-centered care in underserved populations: a qualitative study of patient perspectives. PLoS One. 2015;10(5):e0126708.

70. Netting FE, Williams FG. Geriatric case managers: integration into physician practices. Care Manag J. 1999;1(1):3–9.
71. Frankel SA, Bourgeois JA. Integrated care for complex patients. New York: Springer; 2018.
72. Dorr DA, Wilcox AB, Brunker CP, Burdon RE, Donnelly SM. The effect of technology-supported, multidisease care management on the mortality and hospitalization of seniors. J Am Geriatr Soc. 2008;56(12):2195–202.
73. Nurius PS, Logan-Greene P, Green S. Adverse childhood experiences (ACE) within a social disadvantage framework: distinguishing unique cumulative, and moderated contributions to adult mental health. J Prev Interv Community. 2012;40:278–90.

Resources

"Hotspotters"

https://www.newyorker.com/magazine/2011/01/24/the-hot-spotters

For Patients Concerning Trauma

Gift from Within. A site for survivors of trauma and victimization. www.giftfromwithin.org
National Center for Posttraumatic Stress Disorder, http://www.ncptsd.org
National Child Traumatic Stress Network, http://www.nctsn.org
Sidran Institute. For Survivors and Loved Ones – printable handouts. http://www.sidran.org

Trauma Informed Care

http://www.traumainformedcareproject.org/resources.php

Chapter 6
Bridging the Chasm:
The Current State of the Art

6.1 The Challenge

In the last chapter, we described the challenges of building partnerships with multiply-disadvantaged patients. These are patients who have multiple chronic illnesses including psychiatric diagnoses. They are thought of as "complex patients' by people studying patterns of healthcare utilization". Many of them have low incomes and low levels of education. Many have histories of trauma as children and/ or as adults. They present a challenge for primary care and for the health system, just as primary care and the health system present a challenge for them. Even as primary care settings work toward patient-centered care that helps patients be part-ners on their healthcare team, these patients are more likely to encounter health professionals who are more directive and less collaborative when working with them. Doctors may adjust their usual approaches away from partnership believing it is better for these patients [1, 2]. Many of these patients already have experiences with the health system in which they felt disrespected or poorly treated. For their part, these patients are more likely than other patients to be distrustful, withholding, passive, or nonadherent. They are prone to overutilizing to get what they feel they need or underutilizing to avoid the unpleasantness of interacting with the health system. Without experience and knowledge about caring for multiply-disadvantaged patients, it is easy for primary care sites to develop a mutually reinforcing interac-tion pattern with them that fails to bring out the best of either side. These patients need our best as healthcare professionals. If we learn to be successful in caring for them, it helps us be better in caring for all our patients.

Health settings around the country have made important progress in being able to successfully care for multiply-disadvantaged patients. Some of these methods have been described in the literature on complex patients, some in the literature on caring for low-income or disadvantaged patients, and some in the literature on car-ing for patients with trauma histories. This chapter will attempt to assemble descrip-tions of these efforts into a synthesis that could be called the "state of the art."

© Springer Nature Switzerland AG 2019
A. Blount, *Patient-Centered Primary Care*,
https://doi.org/10.1007/978-3-030-17645-7_6

Perhaps "state of the art" is a bit too ambitious to describe what we can produce, knowing that it is impossible to track all the types of effective approaches that are being practiced or are in development. Still, it should be a synthesis that has not been attempted commonly, one that should be useful on the way to building a new approach to patient-centered care and partnership with multiply-disadvantaged patients.

6.2   It Starts with Relationship

Improving the doctor-patient relationship in the service of better healthcare communication, or better communication in the service of better doctor-patient relationships, is getting a lot of attention [3–6]. The quality of relationships with all team members makes a great deal of difference to multiply-disadvantaged patients. The patients in Jeffrey Brenner's clinic in Camden, NJ [7], who were designated as complex due to their multimorbidity and high utilization, who were low income, and many of whom reported trauma histories, said that their experience of whether or not their doctor "cared" about them made a difference in whether they tried to follow the advice and treatment plan that they were given. The patients Caruso interviewed (2017) talked about how helpful it was if the doctor was "personable" and, over time, how important it was that the doctor addresses problems that arose in the relationship. People who don't feel enfranchised to disagree with the doctor are particularly appreciative when the doctor notices that there may be a rupture in the relationship and addresses it in a way that is open and accepting.

The skills of empathic and open communication, of "relationship-centered care," are important as a part of building the relationship. While less disadvantaged patients will tolerate a medical visit that attends only to diagnosis and treatment in order to get medical care, during such as a visit with the doctor in the lead, being directive about treatment advice, and offering little opportunity to express emotion, multiply-disadvantaged patients are more likely to experience the visit as a demonstration of the asymmetry of power in the room. To people who have suffered the challenges of multiple illnesses, the travails of poverty and/or discrimination, and traumatic past experiences, a medical visit without a positive relationship with the doctor can be one more reminder of how little control they have in their lives. When a patient experiences lack of control or autonomy in their medical visit, the likelihood that they will exercise the control and autonomy it takes to improve their health practices is very low.

The language describing the ideal doctor-patient relationship in some approaches seems more about what a doctor should feel rather than what she should do to establish and maintain a productive relationship with a patient. An example is a list suggested as required for the healthcare relationship, "emotional connection, mutual respect, genuine interest, patient perspective and psychosocial context, and shared commitment to positive outcome" [3]. It is easy to imagine these being attributes of a successful visit, but what if you are a clinician considering what to do to improve the care you provide? For some health professionals, language such as "emotional connection" or "genuine interest" can be inspiring, but for many it is daunting. What if they don't feel that way? Are they wrong?

Some authors have made empathy the central guiding principle in an attempt to improve healthcare communication [4]. The concept of "empathy" can be a perfect example of a prescription for what the doctor is supposed to feel. For those who understand empathy in its dictionary definition as "the psychological identification with or vicarious experiencing of the feelings, thoughts, or attitudes of another" (Dictionary.com), this could even seem to be in conflict with the values of professionalism and objective judgment in a medical visit. As we said in Chap. 4, prescribing how a person should "feel" is putting them in an inherently paradoxical position, since feelings are considered spontaneous reactions or signals of state [8] which cannot be produced on command.

Models that focus on the primacy of the doctor-patient relationship in designing ideal medical visits can lead to more pressure on the doctor than the reality of primary care practice demands. It is not uncommon for another member of the team to have a more intense, more empathic connection with a patient, particularly with multiply-disadvantaged patients. The behavioral health clinician or care enhancer may well spend much more time with the patient than the physician. For their part, these patients are more likely to bring a family member or friend to the visit. This can help with problems of health literacy, but it can also moderate the intensity or disadvantage they feel when meeting alone with the doctor. In one study, patients with low health literacy, more depressive symptoms, and four or more comorbid illnesses were more likely than adult patients in general to bring a "companion" to the medical visit. Patients reported that they were more likely to understand the doctor's advice (77%) and to discuss difficult topics with the doctor (44%) in visits when they brought a companion. Those patients also were more satisfied with their PCPs [9].

Suchman and his colleagues took on the topic by trying to distill an empirically derived model of empathic communication in medical interviews [10]. If it is possible to specify what empathic communication looks like in practice, that may allow practitioners to behave in empathic ways without the requirement that they first have a specific set of emotional experiences. Suchman and his colleagues ask only for a commitment to better communication with patients and a willingness to try to achieve that communication. Their definition of empathic communication has both cognitive and behavioral aspects. It is "the accurate understanding of the patient's feelings by the clinician and the effective communication of that understanding back to the patient so that the patient feels understood" (Suchman et al. [10], p. 678). By studying tapes of primary care interviews, they observed that patients frequently gave clues about their emotional experience without articulating that experience directly. Though it was less common, sometimes patients expressed their emotional reactions directly. In both situations, the doctors were likely to redirect the conversation to the process of investigating medical history and symptoms in search of a diagnosis or toward monitoring patients' adherence to a treatment plan.

Identifying moments that have an emotional charge, even if the emotion is not expressed, becomes the first step in Suchman's model. *Keeping the focus* on those moments rather than redirecting the interview becomes the next step using statements such as "I see" or "tell me more about that." This implicitly tells the patient that discussing their emotional reactions is an acceptable part of the interview and makes it more likely that the emotion behind the hint will be expressed. When emotion is expressed, it allows the clinician to *reflect* the emotion that the patient is communicating, e.g., "that must have been painful for you" and to offer *praise* for the elements in the patient's account that the clinician would like to support, e.g., "you really stuck with it, even though it was hard for you." Empathy, when it is defined in this way, can be operationalized, allowing the process of empathic communication to be taught to and used by any member of the healthcare team. These skills can be taught in fairly brief workshop formats [11].

While some consider the determination of team members to act "as if" they felt empathetic to be a recipe for inauthentic care, the requirement that an emotional experience precede a behavior is an arbitrary preference that does not represent the way things often work in life. An example is the common experience of newly trained members of a profession as they begin practicing their profession, that they are imposters. The feeling of being an imposter pretending to be a professional attenuates and disappears the more the person "acts out" the role. In the same way, empathy is just as reasonably achieved through the behavior leading to the emotional experience, rather than the other way around.

When we consider the common report among multiply-disadvantaged patients: that they have experienced interactions with the healthcare system that left them feeling disrespected and treated poorly, that they respond better to a doctor who is personable, that they are acutely aware of the asymmetry of power and status in a medical interview, and that they greatly appreciate a doctor who recognizes when they are not engaged in the process and is open to addressing the issues involved, the process of empathic communication that Suchman outlines seems a sine qua non for building a bridge to this population.

6.3   The Team Makes the Difference

Multiply-disadvantaged patients are part of a larger group of high-utilizing, high-cost patients that the health system is trying to serve more effectively at less cost. The statistics on utilization and cost are compelling. The top 1% of "spenders" use more than one fifth of all medical spending. The top 5% account for more than half [12]. In the face of these patterns, federal, state, and private funders of healthcare, plus foundations that fund innovative attempts to improve healthcare, have put significant resources into finding ways to reduce this excessive spending. While some patients with serious acute illnesses or at the end of their lives are getting appropriate, if very expensive care, the shared assumption is that if other high-cost patients can be engaged in health services that are a better fit to their needs, some of the more expensive services such as multiple emergency room visits and inpatient stays can be avoided. It is also assumed that this will improve the health and quality of life of the patients.

One approach has been to create special programs for complex, high-utilizing patients in which doctors have significantly smaller patient panels to care for. This allows them to provide more intensive services, such as spending more time for each patient at visits and between visits. In some models, doctors take on some of the care management functions that are given to other members of the team in other practices. The relationship that is so important to engaging the patients is provided almost completely by the physician. This has proved to be very effective in lowering costs and reducing utilization, though not always improving the well-being of the patients [13, 14]. The problem with this approach on a regional or national level is one of available workforce. Such an arrangement could be said to exchange the resource that is being overutilized from dollars to doctors.

The far more common approach has been to add new members to the health team to augment the services that the doctor and the current members of the team are supplying. Staff in this role are variously called care managers, care coordinators, case managers, or navigators. We are using the term "care enhancers" to cover all of the names that may be assigned to this role. They try to help patients (and the people who are their support systems) manage their illnesses and their psychosocial problems more effectively with the goal of improving their health status and lowering their need for medical services. Care enhancers are commonly trained as nurses or social workers, though the training requirements are variable, just as the duties in different programs are variable. In general, experts believe that care management should be a part of primary care for multiply-disadvantaged patients [15], though that is not always financially feasible without redirecting funds from other parts of the health system. Some successful programs have added a care enhancer serving multiple small primary care practices or based in hospitals outreaching to high-utilizing patients. Wherever it is based, active involvement of the primary care doctor seems to be an element necessary to the success of a care management program (Bodenheimer and Berry-Millett), and the care manager should be experienced by the patient to be part of the primary care health team [16]. The care management described here should not be confused with services by the same name (sometimes called "disease management") which are not part of the healthcare team in primary care. When nurses provide care management by telephone, without the involvement of the primary care physician, directed at only one specific illness, it generally does not improve patient outcomes [17]. In general, more successful programs have tended toward "high-touch" involvement, meaning face-to-face interaction between the care enhancer and the patient. Ultimately, successful care management is based on the quality of relationship between the patient and the care manager as much or more than on the array of services the care manager offers [18].

Because advancing age is the greatest risk factor for multimorbidity, because long-term care can be calculated as a part of medical costs, and because Medicare is the most accessible source of nationwide cost data, studies that focus solely on the absolute dollars spent on patients' care tend to produce a group in which the elderly are substantially overrepresented [14]. The more care management programs focus on elderly patients, the more "medical" they are likely to seem. One summary of the problems addressed by a care management programs lists falls, lack of mobility, chronic pain, incontinence, hearing loss, depression, visual impairment, and dementia [19], the problems of the elderly. When looking at a study about high-need patients for a health system, it is important to be clear about what percent of the population in the study is elderly or might be in more intensive services than simply being a patient in primary care.

Focusing on high-need patients in primary care brings a picture in which psychosocial variables take a more central role in the picture. These will be younger patients with high needs for whom cost is impacted by social and behavioral health variables. The National Academy of Medicine (formerly the IOM) has published a report on high-need patients [14] that describes the central role of "high-impact social variables" and "high-impact behavioral variables." The high-impact social variables the report identifies are low socioeconomic status, social isolation, community deprivation, and housing insecurity. The high-impact behavioral health variables are substance abuse, serious mental illness, cognitive decline, and chronic toxic stress. Chronic toxic stress is a name for the chronic burden of trauma that significantly increases the risk of disease and other behavioral health disorders. This focus on the impact of psychosocial elements also tends to happen as programs mature, even if these elements were not nearly so prominent in the design of the programs. Program designers are often unaware of the true degree to which psychosocial factors, especially trauma, impact illness and functioning until they see the program run for a while.

In a review of approaches to helping patients with multimorbidity, Smith et al. [20] report that two programs were significantly more effective than the rest in improving patient outcomes. They theorize that this was because these programs focused on only two comorbidities, depression and a chronic illness (diabetes, heart disease, or hypertension), rather than general multimorbidities [21, 22]. The narrow focus also allowed easier measuring of results since they could use disease-specific measures. It might be just as reasonable to talk about the fact that the comorbid picture included depression and that the methodologies used are ones that were developed for depression and adapted to include chronic illness rather than the reverse. The Katon team used the Collaborative Care Model with intensive involvement by a team member who, in this case, was a specially trained nurse. The Collaborative Care Model (CCM) was developed by Katon and his colleagues at the University of Washington as an adaptation for treating depression of the Chronic Care Model for treating chronic illness [23]. The CCM provides psychiatric specialist consultation to primary care doctors and uses licensed mental health professionals or specially trained nurses in the behavioral health clinician role on the team [24]. This team member outreaches by phone or in person, if necessary, to maintain contact with patients in the program. In this study the approach to both depression and chronic illnesses was patient centered in the sense that the patients set the goals for the focus of their work with the BH clinician and the rest of the team. The BH clinicians used motivational interviewing and support with proactive outreach between frequent face-to-face visits (every 2–3 weeks) to achieve the findings which were significantly improved medical outcomes as well as improved depression outcomes.

The Katon et al. [22] study highlights the importance of the role of the behavioral health clinician in building a bridge to engage multiply-disadvantaged patients. Helping with behavioral health challenges (mental health disorders, substance use disorders, poor health habits, and toxic stress) is crucial to finding some relief for these patients from their biological and social as well as their psychological problems. The more generalist BH clinicians are a daily part of the teams, going to huddles, being available to consult about care during the day, the better they can be resources to other team members for the whole range of needs presented by complex patients.

Having behavioral health generalists on the team, as opposed to specialists in substance abuse or depression, means that the "no wrong door" aspect of primary care can be available to complex patients in the makeup of their health team. For example, a patient coping with depression, who is drinking too much, and has poorly managed diabetes needs help in all three areas. It is not predictable where the patient will have the most concern and therefore where they would want to begin in working with a BH clinician. If they start by cutting back their drinking, or by improving their diet, or by getting more exercise, or by working to improve their mood, they are taking a step in the right direction for all their concerns. As people find even small successes on one front, they tend to become more hopeful and motivated to attempt improvements on others. For patients with many morbidities, being expert at engagement and being able to begin by focusing wherever the patient is willing to start is a particularly valuable skill of the behavioral health clinician on the team.

6.4   The CareOregon Experience

CareOregon is a nonprofit health plan serving low-income Oregonians. It actively partners with the primary care practices that serve its members to support better care. In a report on its website written in 2014, Rebecca Ramsey, the Director of Community Care for the health plan, tells the story of how CareOregon came to its innovative approach to caring for multiply-disadvantaged patients [25]. She tells how they "improved disease management and access to preventive care, built more data driven processes, brought behavioral health consultants (clinicians) on the team and expanded our capacity to reach different populations. However, we still didn't quite get there – the high cost and very complex patients remained elusive." Ramsey's "high-cost and very complex patients" turn out to be similar to the patients that Brenner treated and that Caruso interviewed, multiply-disadvantaged patients.

In her description of the CareOregon plan, Ramsey describes the process that the leadership of the plan went through to better understand the patients which they had been unable to reach. After a "pilgrimage" to visit other programs around the country, they began their pilot by instituting a new approach using outreach workers to go into the community and work with these patients. The choice of their first two workers was very important. "We hired individuals with amazing engagement skills, social justice understanding, compassion, exceptional interpersonal skills and extensive knowledge of vulnerable populations." Though they were employees of the health plan, the outreach workers were each located in a primary care practice as part of the health team there. They assumed that patients would need individualized plans and that a detailed understanding of the barriers to healthcare for each patient would be necessary. "They found that there were mild cognitive impairments, developmental disabilities, health literacy issues, housing instability, childhood trauma, post-traumatic stress disorder, anxiety, depression, addiction, etc. It was what we were expecting but of a far larger magnitude.... We were blown away by how prevalent the experience of childhood and lifetime trauma was in our patients."

The work of the pilot program was very successful. Their doctors were happy, both for the support in reaching these patients and for the way that these patients seemed more engaged and receptive in their clinic visits. Emergency room use and hospitalization for these patients went down. The pilot project became a program-wide innovation. Two outreach workers increased to 17 serving 17 clinics. The role was renamed "Health Resilience Specialist." To fill the role, they have hired skilled behaviorists who are embedded as part of the health team in a primary care practice. They spend much of their time focused on the social determinants of health and are trained in trauma-informed care and evidence-based trauma-recovery interventions [14]. These specialists are teamed with community health workers who are peers, in the sense that they are people with lived experience of some of the travails of the population they are trying to reach. As of 2014, they had seen a 34% decline in hospital and emergency use by the patients served. They expected savings somewhere between 150% and 290% of the cost of the new program.

The core element in the training both the Health Resilience Specialists and the other staff members of the primary care practices is trauma-informed care (TIC). This training is designed to help the Health Resilience Specialists and the staff in the primary care clinics learn to "avoid being hierarchical and to motivate patients so they had a stake in their own care." For high-cost, high-need patients, CareOregon uses trauma-informed care as a bridge to building partnerships with patients.

6.5   Trauma-Informed Care

Trauma-informed care (TIC) is well named. It is not a treatment for trauma but a set of principles and approaches for adapting other sorts of care to make them more likely to be helpful to people whose lives have been affected by traumatic experiences. Five principles that are commonly used to guide TIC are safety, transparency and trustworthiness, choice, collaboration and mutuality, and empowerment [26]. "Safety" means making settings for delivery of care safe and conveying to patients a commitment to making sure that they experience the processes and procedures of care to be safe. "Transparency and trustworthiness" means making the operations and practices of a setting transparent and giving patients meaningful roles in making decisions about their care. "Choice" is the recognition that meaningful decision-making involves being able to choose between alternatives and between care and no care without losing the services of the setting. "Collaboration and mutuality" describe using the commitment to shared decision-making and to offering meaningful choices as a way to create engaged relationships with patients. "Empowerment" means that any aspect of care, in as much as possible, will highlight and focus on patients' strengths rather than focusing solely on illnesses and deficits. In order to put these principles into practice in a program, it is necessary that the staff and designers of any program realize how prevalent trauma is in the patients they serve. They need to be able to recognize the ways that trauma affects individuals, its impact on the nervous and immune systems of victims. This means they are aware of the likelihood of those patients becoming overwhelmed, experiencing intense feelings of vulnerability, and initiating behaviors that allow themselves to withdraw from (or be ejected from) settings that feel unsafe. When creating a program embodying TIC, these realizations should be put into practice by training any member of the staff so that when someone behaves in the ways just described, their reaction is not "what's wrong with you?" but "what has happened to you?"

TIC has been associated with settings providing mental health and/or substance abuse services, particularly for women or adolescents, but attention to its role in improving care for multiply-disadvantaged patients in primary care is growing [27–30]. Davis and Maul add details to the picture of TIC in action. They note that active listening is a large part of building relationships, that clinicians ask permission to help rather than assuming it is their role, and that some team member often spends time helping the patient prepare for their visit with the doctor and talks to them afterward to help them decompress and to solidify important points from the visit. Besides building on strengths, team members try to identify triggers for an individual patient in the routines of care and to modify those routines or alleviate their impact. Finally, actions that patients present that seem maladaptive (such as substance abuse, missing appointments, or aggressive behavior) are scrutinized for their possible value as ways for patients to alleviate problems that are more disturbing (to the patient) at the time such as anxiety or dissociation.

One more learning from service providers in the mental health world needs be a part of TIC in primary care: the understanding of the existence of vicarious trauma in people providing care and the need for self-care and mutual activities of support among the healthcare team. Working closely on a multidisciplinary team serving a range of patients in any primary care setting tends to increase the closeness of the team because of the amount of contact, discussion, and mutual effort involved. Working closely serving multiply-disadvantaged patients requires in addition that each team member to be aware of the mood and functioning of other team members, be willing to discuss their own mood and functioning if asked, and make time for discussion to share personal reactions and sometimes to ask for help or relief. The behaviors that are helpful for patients, such as active listening, asking permission before offering help, respecting the choices of the other, and understanding the impact of trauma without asking a person to tell the story of their traumatic experiences, are all useful in relating to colleagues on the team. Choosing to be a healthcare provider identifies one as slightly more likely than the population as a whole to have a personal history of traumatic experiences [31]. This should be a shared understanding in the background as team members seek to support each other.

6.6   A Story from the Mountains of North Carolina

In 2010 Margaret R. Pardee Hospital in Hendersonville, NC, in partnership with the family medicine residency of the Mountain Area Health Education Center, also in Hendersonville, began an innovative program to try to offer an alternative to the high number of uninsured patients who were using the ED for all or most of their healthcare [32]. They identified 255 patients who had used the ED at least 6 times in the previous year. Out of that group, they were able to contact 147. (Hendersonville is in a rural mountainous area in which many people didn't have or would not give a working phone number.) The group of 147 yielded 70 that professed an interest in the program and 36 who completed the enrollment process which involved showing documentation of their income and completing common behavioral health screening forms. All of those in the group had incomes that were 200% or less of the federal poverty designation. Two dropped out early and so the effort produced 34 patients who participated.

The participating patients were older than the high-utilizing cohort as a whole. Their median age was 45, while the whole cohort's median age was 32. They had exactly the same rate of utilization as the whole cohort (0.58 visits per month) in the 12 months previous to the beginning of the program. In that time the care of the participants had been significantly more expensive than the cohort as a whole, $1167 vs. $628 monthly. The participants were 44% female, while the cohort was 51% female.

The program that the 147 who could be contacted were presented involved a regular drop-in group medical appointment (DIGMA), immediate telephone access to a nurse care manager during business hours on week days, a life skills and support meeting with the care manager each day of a DIGMA in the hour before the group meeting started, and an opportunity for individual sessions with members of the care team in the half hour after the DIGMA. The DIGMA was held twice a week on Tuesdays and Fridays from 12 to 1. The location of the meeting was in a building that housed a free health clinic and offices of other social service organizations.

The team leading the DIGMA consisted of three experienced professionals: a family physician, the nurse care manager, and a primary care behavioral health clinician. There were two BH clinicians who were part of the team, though only one attended at each meeting. The team would huddle before the meeting and prepare by discussing patients and reviewing their medical records. They identified which records to review based on who they saw in the waiting room.

This drop-in medical group was different from other groups offered for patients in primary care in that it was not focused on particular medical problems. This means that it did not have the patient education curriculum that is often a part of groups focused on particular chronic illnesses or problems. As with most groups in primary care, it was not a therapy group, in that there was no focus on individual behavior or group processes occurring during the meeting. The time was used to allow patients to present, in turn, any medical, behavioral, or social issues they wished the group and the care team to address. Over time, the group took on a structure that became familiar to participants and developed group norms involving mutual support and feedback to participants to help them help themselves. There was no limit in the number of groups a participant could attend and no pressure to attend more than they felt they needed. So, twice each week patients had the opportunity for an hour of individual or small group life skills meeting with the care manager, participation in the larger DIGMA with the whole team, and an individual meeting with a care team member for medical care, care management, or therapeutic discussion. The use of these resources was entirely up to the patient. Team members observed a pattern in which patients would regularly use the program when they were in a period of instability with their health, social situation, or psychological symptoms. As their lives stabilized again, they came much less often. On average, patients had slightly less than one outreach call with the care manager for each time they had a face-to-face contact at the program site.

The impacts of the program were assessed after a year in operation. The average monthly cost of care in the ED per participant had dropped from $1167 for the year before the program to $230 during the year of the program. Only one member of the group of participants had any employment at the beginning of the program, but 14 were employed full or part time at the end. Seven members of the group were homeless at the beginning of the year, and only one was still without stable housing at the end. The projected cost of ED care for the year for the whole group of participants, had no program occurred, would have been $476,000 at the beginning of the year, but the actual cost for the year was $93,800. The saving of $382,200 was many times more than the cost of time of the care team.

What was it about this program that made such a difference in cost and in the quality of participant's lives? The program allowed much greater time to build relationships with patients than would be possible in an appointment-based system. The patients, not the professionals, made the decision about when they would and would not use services. When they did need something, contact was easily available, and in-person visits were usually possible in only a day or two. Patients reported that the easy access to telephone contact or a visit with a person they already knew was the main factor in their being able to wait when they had a concern, rather than heading for the ED. It would seem that the biopsychosocial array of skill sets of the team members was a good fit to the biopsychosocial needs of the participants. Patients got to tell their stories, in as much as they wanted to, to people they thought would understand. Participants supported and were supported by their peers and built bonds that were both within and outside the program. The patients identified themselves as a group of folks "on the fringe" of society, which became an identification that ultimately contributed to group cohesion. In that way patients' experiences of stigma were reduced. While the program did not report assessing for histories of trauma, if the evidence in the last chapter is convincing, there is every reason to believe that trauma was a significant part of the past experience of many of them.

Reading the account of the program by Crane and his colleagues [32], one comes away with the sense that the principles of TIC, safety, transparency and trustworthiness, choice, collaboration and mutuality, and empowerment were very much a part of the program as it was delivered.

6.7 The Team at the State of the Art

A reasonable formulation of the current state of the art in creating a bridge to partnership with multiply-disadvantaged patients could be something like the following: trauma-informed primary care, routinely using empathic communication methods, with a focus on shared decision-making and attention to patient motivation and reservations about treatment, delivered by a multidisciplinary team with at least a doctor, a care manager, and a behavioral health clinician, providing continuity of relationships for patients, quick access to a responsive member of the team, and good linkages with other social services for help with the social determinants of health. There will inevitably be other team members as well, medical assistants and/or nurses, reception staff, and possibly scribes, community health workers, pharmacists, consulting specialists, and more. The team should have time to meet and discuss challenging situations and, though we have spent little time on it so far, have access to current meaningful data to assess the impact of the interventions they develop. Finding a role in the primary care effort for people who have been successful in their own struggles, for the "alumni" of the program, helps further engagement for future participants and buttresses the progress made by the alumni.

To make the state-of-the-art primary care possible, the payment method will need to be adjusted toward supporting the general health of multiply-disadvantaged patients rather than paying either for each service or for changes in the metrics of single diseases. Long et al. [14] suggest that the care manager would be supervised by the behavioral health clinician with "dotted line" supervision to the doctor on the team or to the doctor who is championing the care management effort for the practice. The longer teams work together, however, the more blurred these lines can be expected to become, and the more the exchange of expertise in the team will be described as mutual by team members. The mutuality in team relations would be part of the environment supporting mutuality with patients.

6.8 What Is Missing?

We have been working to build a bridge to partnership with multiply-disadvantaged patients across the chasm in communication and trust that was outlined in Chap. 5. We are trying to meet the goal articulated by the Institute of Medicine for even this most challenging group of patients:

Patient and family engaged care (PFEC) is care planned, delivered, managed, and continuously improved in active partnership with patients and their families (or care partners as defined by the patient) to ensure integration of their health and health care goals, preferences and values. It includes explicit and partnered determination of goals and care options, and it requires ongoing assessment of the care match with patient goals. (Frampton et al. [33])

It may very well be that the current state of the art gets us there, but how do we get to the current state of the art? How will we enact "transparency and trustworthiness?" How do we weave "empowerment" and a strength-based approach into the routines of care? How will we help patients who feel vulnerable and disenfranchised, who have difficulty getting through a primary care visit without intense stress, to be able to formulate and express health goals? How will we help multiply-disadvantaged patients become activated to pursue their health goals without being directive or coaching in ways that are experienced by then as playing on the asymmetry of power between themselves and their team? What regular processes can we design to be sure that the values and goals of the patient and family members they choose to be involved, even when they are elicited, are not ignored by other doctors or healthcare workers with whom they come in contact? How do we assure that the patients' goals are known to and incorporated by all of the care providers in their healthcare network?

One currently available pathway to transformation of an organization is literature and technical assistance to move a primary care practice into a trauma-informed organization [34, 35]. This model, created for inpatient psychiatric, outpatient mental health, substance abuse, and other social service organizations, can be adapted for primary care. Perhaps the best resource in that effort is the Center for Health Care Strategies supported by the Robert Wood Johnson Foundation (see Resources).

In the rest of this volume, we will offer another approach, one that adapts some of the changes that are coming in healthcare, such as patients having easy access to all their records, into a method for achieving and even growing the state of the art. We will examine routines of care that enact transparency, support empathic behaviors by team members, build empowerment, and further relationship between multiply-disadvantaged patients and team members. We will discuss ways of using attributions toward patients that help them to move beyond empowerment toward activation in improving their health. Finally, we will talk about using basic elements that are already a part of care, such as a treatment or care plan, to achieve the goal of making patients' understanding of their needs and their health goals known to and potentially used by all of the care providers in their healthcare network.

References

1. Pollack KI, Alexander SC, Grambow SC, Sulsky JA. Oncologist patient-centered communication with patient with advanced cancer: exploring whether race and socioeconomic status matter. Palliat Med. 2010;24:96–8.

2. Willems S, De Maesschalck S, Deveugele M, Derese A, De Maeseneer J. Socio-economic status of the patient and doctor-patient communication: does it make a difference? Patient Educ
   Couns. 2005;56:139–46.
3. Boissy A, Gilligan T, editors. Communication the Cleveland Clinic way. New York: McGraw-
   Hill; 2016.
4. Lee TH. An epidemic of empathy in healthcare. New York: McGraw-Hill; 2016.
5. Steiner R, Morse J, Myers IJ. Re-framing primary care and patient-centered medical homes
   in the lens of complexity, culture and relationship-centered care. Virginia Beach: Convergent
   Publishing; 2015.
6. Windover AK, Isaacson JH, Pien LC, Merrell J, Moore AS. Relationship-centered healthcare communication: an advanced topic guide. North Charleston: Create Space Independent
   Publishing Platform; 2014.
7. Mautner DB, Pang H, Brenner JC, Shea JA, Gross KS, Frasso R, Cannuscio CC. Generating
   hypotheses about care needs of high utilizers: lessons from patient interviews. Popul Health
   Manag. 2013;16:S26–33.
8. Bateson G. A social scientist views the emotions. In: Knapp P, editor. Expression of the emotions in man. New York: International University Press; 1963. p. 230–5.
9. Rosland A-M, Piette J, Choi HJ, Heisler M. Family and friend participation in primary care
   visits of patients with diabetes or heart failure: patient and physician determinants and experiences. Med Care. 2011;49:37–45.
10. Suchman AL, Markakis K, Beckman HB, Frankel R. A model of empathic communication in
    the medical interview. JAMA. 1997;277:678–81.
11. Roter DL, Hall JA, Kern DE, Barker LR, Cole KA, Roca RP. Improving physicians' interview-
    ing skills and reducing patients' emotional distress. A randomized clinical trial. Arch Intern
    Med. 1995;155:1877–84.
12. Dzau VJ, McClellan MB, McGinnis JM, et al. Vital directions for health and healthcare: priori-
    ties from a national academy of medicine initiative. JAMA. 2017;317:1461–70.
13. Furman D. Alignment healthcare: changing healthcare one patient at a time. Presentation at
    the July 7th National Academy of Medicine Models of Care for high need patients meeting,
    Washington, DC. 2015.
14. Long P, Abrams M, Milstein A, Anderson G, Lewis Apton K, Lund Dahlberg M, Whicher D,
    editors. Effective care for high-need patients: opportunities for improving outcomes, value,
    and health. Washington, DC: National Academy of Medicine; 2017.
15. Bodenheimer T, Berry-Millett R. Care management of patient with complex health care needs.
    Robert Wood Johnson Foundation. 2009. https://www.rwjf.org/en/library/research/2009/12/
    care-management-of-patients-with-complex-health-care-needs.html
16. Schoen C, Osborn R, Squires D, Doty M, Pierson R, Applebaum S. New 2011 survey of
    patients with complex care needs in eleven countries finds that care is often poorly coordinated.
    Health Aff. 2011;30(12). https://www.healthaffairs.org/doi/abs/10.1377/hlthaff.2011.0923
17. Piteikes D, Chen A, Schore J, Brown R. Effects of care coordination on hospitalization, qual-
    ity of care and healthcare expenditures among Medicare beneficiaries: 15 randomized trials.
    JAMA. 2009;301:603–18.
18. Dorr DA, Wilcox A, Jones S, Burns L, Donnelly SM, Brunker C. Care management dosage. J
    Gen Intern Med. 2007;22:736–41.
19. Counsell SR, Callahan EM, Clark DO, Tu W, Buttar AB, Stump TE, Ricketts GD. Geriatric
    care management for low-income seniors. JAMA. 2007;298:2623–33.
20. Smith SM, Soubhi H, Fortin M, Hudon C, O'Dowd T. Managing patients with multimor-
    bidity: systematic review of interventions in primary care and community settings. BMJ.
    2012;345:1–10.
21. Bogner H, de Vries HF. Integration of depression and hypertension treatment: a pilot, random-
    ized controlled trial. Ann Fam Med. 2008;6:295–301.
22. Katon W, Lin E, von Korff M, et al. Collaborative care for patients with depression and chronic
    illnesses. N Engl J Med. 2010;363:2611–20.
23. Bodenheimer T, Wagner EH, Grumbach K. Improving primary care for patients with chronic
    illness. JAMA. 2002;288:1775–9.
24. Ratzliff A, Unutzer J, Katon W, Stephens A. Integrated care: creating effective mental and
    primary health care teams. Hoboken: John Wiley & Sons; 2016.

25. Ramsey R. Health resilience specialists: the key to providing quality care to high-risk patients. 2014. http://healthyamericans.org/health-issues/prevention_story/health-resilience-specialists-the-key-to-providing-quality-care-to-high-risk-patients/
26. Harris M, Fallot R, editors. Using trauma theory to design service systems. San Francisco: Jossey-Bass; 2001.
27. Davis R, Maul A. Trauma-informed care: opportunities for high need, high cost Medicaid populations. Center for Health Care Strategies. 2015. www.chcs.org. Downloaded 28 May 2018.
28. Earls MF. Trauma-informed primary care: prevention, recognition, and promoting resilience. N C Med J. 2018;79:108–12.
29. Green BL, Saunders PA, Power E, et al. Trauma-informed medical care: a CME communication training for primary care providers. Fam Med. 2015;47:7–14.
30. Machtinger EL, Cuca YP, Khanna N, Rose CD, Kimberg LS. From treatment to healing: the promise of trauma-informed primary care. Womens Health Issues. 2015;25:193–7.
31. Candib L, Savageau J, Weinreb L, Reed G. Inquiring into our past: when the doctor is a survivor of abuse. Fam Med. 2012;44:416–24.
32. Crane S, Collins L, Hall J, Rochester D, Patch S. Reducing utilization by uninsured frequent users of the emergency department: combining case management and drop-in group medical visits. J Am Board Fam Med. 2012;25:184–91.
33. Frampton S, Guastello S, Hoy L, Naylor M, Sheridan S, Johnston-Fleece M. Harnessing evidence and experience to change culture: a guiding framework for patient and family engaged care. Washington, DC: National Institute of Medicine; 2017.
34. Bloom S, Farragher B. Restoring sanctuary: a new operating system for trauma-informed systems of care. Oxford: Oxford University Press; 2013.
35. Esaki N, et al. The sanctuary model: theoretical framework in chapter 6: strategy, sanctuary and turnaround. In: Mortell M, Hansen-Turon T, editors. Making strategy count in the health and human service sector: lessons learned from 20 organizations and chief strategy officers. New York: Springer Publishing; 2014.

Resources

Doctor-Patient Communication

Mauksch L. Patient centered observation form. University of Washington, Department of Family Medicine. 2011. www.oafp.org/assets/Family-Medicine-PCO-Form.pdf

Trauma Informed Care

Trauma Informed Care Project – www.traumainformedcareproject.org
National Center for Trauma Informed Care & Alternatives to Seclusion and Restraints – https://www.samhsa.gov/nctic
Wisconsin Department of Health Services site on TIC – https://www.dhs.wisconsin.gov/tic/principles.htm
Access to materials by Sandra Bloom, creator of the Sanctuary Model – www.sanctuaryweb.com

TIC in Primary Care

Center for Health Care Strategies, Inc. www.chcs.org
National Council for Behavioral Health site. https://www.nationalcouncildocs.net/trauma-informed-care-learning-community/tic-in-primary-care

Chapter 7
"T" Is for Transparent

7.1 Opening a New Channel for Communication

IOM rules for the new healthcare [1]:

4. "Shared knowledge and free flow of information." Patients should have "unfettered" access to their own medical information and to clinical knowledge relevant to their health.

7. "The need for transparency." Their health system should make all information available that is relevant to patients making informed decisions including possible alternative treatments. This should also include information about stakeholders, effectiveness, and costs of the health system and its components.

The "chasm" of miscommunication between doctors and other health professionals on one hand and some of their most complex patients is often substantially bigger than the health professionals can imagine. During my many years working as a behavioral health clinician and behavioral science teacher in primary care, I sometimes heard stereotypes about doctors from patients, descriptions that seemed completely at odds with my experience of the family physicians, both faculty and residents, that I worked with. "They are only in it for the money." "They all talk to each other and they never go against each other." "They don't care a bit about us if we aren't rich." "We are just guinea pigs for them." I tried to understand how this difference in perception of their doctors between myself and these patients would arise, especially since the family doctors I knew were, as a group, the most idealistic professionals I ever met. Occasionally the explanation might have been that the patient was angry at not being prescribed the pain medication or benzodiazepine they thought they should have. Often the patients had been through negative experiences in the hospital or at an emergency department and were generalizing to my primary care colleagues (see Chap. 5). It was clear, however, that these patients still experienced their contacts with their doctors as alienating. Nothing about the idealism or benevolent communication skills of my family physician colleagues seemed to impact the negative generalizations that these patients maintained.

© Springer Nature Switzerland AG 2019
A. Blount, *Patient-Centered Primary Care*,
https://doi.org/10.1007/978-3-030-17645-7_7

When I talked to the family medicine residents I was teaching about the level of disaffection of some patients in primary care, they were polite, but I am sure they thought I was being overly dramatic. They had encountered few if any patients whose behavior would give credibility to my descriptions. The patients who made these bitter statements to me, a professional who was not a physician, showed a much more compliant and less bitter side of themselves when they met with their doctors. They often failed to adhere to elements of their treatment plans, but they did not show overt alienation in their visits with their doctors. These were usually people who had lots of contact with doctors. They had multiple chronic illnesses. Many were disabled. They had behavioral health problems and often had a history of trauma and substance abuse.

The research that was centrally important in Chap. 5 [2] confirmed my experience that often patients with complex medical and behavioral health issues, with low socioeconomic status and poor education, and with histories of traumatic childhood and adult experiences feel alienated and distrustful. They can experience contact with their physician as an uncomfortable interaction between people of very different social class and position power. Because they are hesitant to share their ideas, requests, or reactions with their doctors, their doctors often have little clue about the depth of the communication chasm. These patients are not transparent with their doctors. The doctors, for their part, are more likely to be directive and less likely to use approaches such as shared decision-making with these patients and so are less transparent with this population [3, 4]. Bridging the communication chasm is crucial to caring for these patients. It appears that transparency is needed in both directions. To foster transparency in both directions, the health professionals have to go first.

7.2   A Call for Transparency

Transparency is addressed by rules #4 and #7 of the 10 rules for a new healthcare articulated in the Crossing the Quality Chasm report by the Institute of Medicine [1]. The logic is simple: how can a patient be the source of control for their healthcare if they don't have the necessary information? "Have no secrets. Make all information flow freely so that anyone involved in the system, including patients and families, can make informed choices and know at any time whatever facts could be relevant to a patient's decision making." (IOM [1], pp. 79–80). The conception of transparency in the IOM report was that doctors or other health providers would share the information that the patient would need to be able to participate in making decisions about their care. The question of how health professionals would determine what information patients needed in order to contribute to the decisions about their care was not fully worked out. The rule, as articulated in the report, was clearly presented as an ideal rather than as a protocol that could be implemented by any practice that chose to follow it.

The Quality Chasm report was as much focused on transparency concerning the details of the functioning of a health system as it was about the transparency that describes a patient's access to his or her medical information. If the patient is going to be the source of control, they need all the information necessary to choose well who will provide their care. Good choices make for informed "consumers" and stronger relationships. The report points out that the information about medical errors that could come from institutional transparency could help in improving patient safety and in lowering rather than raising litigation against health settings. Over time, elements of this sort of transparency have become more common. A patient can now access information about a doctor and their record with the state medical board. Medicare has a system of grading hospitals, nursing homes, and other healthcare settings, and some rating surveys include measures of patient satisfaction in the data used to determine a site's grade. There is also a movement to try to compel transparency about charges for specific types of care or specific tests in various settings. While a determined and knowledgeable consumer can get a lot of information for making comparisons, at this point comparison of hospitals and other health settings across a standardized meaningful set of measures is not easy or intuitive for most people. The data that is expected to be shared is often not the data on which patients make decisions in choosing care providers, and the scarcity of resources in many areas makes the promise of informed choice irrelevant.

The Quality Chasm report lists two benefits that can come from a patient being able to see their own health record. Firstly, it assumes that a patient might see details of their medical history that were incorrect or incomplete and be able to correct any errors that the record contained. This is seen as a way to increase patient safety. Secondly, the report predicts that patients would be aided in understanding their treatment plan and be reminded toward better adherence to their medical regimen. When the report considers what other sorts of information a patient would see if they had access to their medical information, it lists results of laboratory tests, medications being taken, and the correct doses. This is seen as an improvement in the communication with the patient by the doctor and the health system.

7.3   Opening the Record

At about the same time that the Quality Chasm report was coming together, a meeting took place as part of the Salzburg Global Seminar (SGS) in Austria. The SGS is a nonprofit organization that sponsors multi-year programs that convene current and future leaders from across the globe to work for sustainable change for the common good. Fellows, as they are called, are brought to Schloss Leopoldskron, a grand house/hotel outside of Salzburg at which several scenes of "The Sound of Music" were filmed. In 1998, a meeting about the role of transparency in the doctor-patient relationship was convened there. This was by no means the first place that the patient having access to their records was discussed [5], but it was likely the first time that the idea was vetted before a group of such influential medical leaders. At that meeting the idea offered was of an Internet-based patient record that was accessible to both patient and clinician. The record could be written by both the clinician and the patient. Patients would be able to add to the record to correct information, to track and explicate problems, to prioritize needs, and to make suggestions for diagnoses or treatment plans [6]. There would be ways for patients to keep track of their own adherence to their medical regimens and for health clinicians to provide reminders. The medical record would be linked to patient education materials about the specific illnesses or problems of each patient. Patients could review transcripts of their visits and offer anecdotal feedback through secure email systems. The description at that time was that patients would have "nearly complete" access to their information, though it did not say on what basis some information would be held back. All information would be confidential, held within the medical system on one hand and the group with whom the patient chose to share information on the other. The vision articulated at the Salzburg gathering was published in the medical literature in 2001 [7].

In 2010, another meeting of the same project occurred in the same venue. This program presented the evolution of the idea and what had been achieved in the time since 1998. At that time, Dr. Tom Delbanco, a central player in the drive toward transparency of patient records, reviewed the design of an early pilot program called "OpenNotes" [8, 9]. OpenNotes is a system for allowing patients easy access to the notes of their medical visits written by their doctors. It is portrayed as a movement rather than a specific software program (www.OpenNotes.org). Multiple vendors of EHRs offer or are developing the capability for open notes.

The pilot test of open notes was conducted in adult primary care practices of three health systems, an urban academic medical center in Boston, a rural health system in Pennsylvania, and an inner-city health system in Seattle serving indigent patients. All three systems had or were just implementing electronic patient portals through which patients could access test results, medication lists, appointment schedules, and exchange secure messages with their doctors. Doctors were offered the possibility of their patients being able to read their own visit notes for 1 year with the option to continue with the service after the year was over if they wanted to. Participation by PCPs was voluntary, and the PCPs who declined to participate and their patients became the control group. One hundred and fourteen chose to participate and 140 declined. The patients invited to join the project were patients of the participating doctors who had accounts on the patient portal. Doctors could remove patients from the invitation list if they felt there might be harm caused by their having this access. The participating doctors overall removed about 5% of the eligible patients, with the majority of these designated by doctors whose patient panels included a high percentage of patients with serious mental illness or substance abuse diagnoses.

Participating and nonparticipating doctors and their designated patients were surveyed ahead of implementation to see what they expected from the opportunity for open notes. Seventy to 80% of the participating doctors across the three sites thought OpenNotes was a good idea and expected it would help patients maintain or improve their health. A range of 20–30% of the nonparticipating doctors agreed that it might help patients with self-management. Over 90% of patients cared for by participating and nonparticipating doctors thought it was a good idea. About 50% of participating doctors thought that it could cause patients confusion or worry, and about 90% of the nonparticipating doctors shared this concern. About 15% of patients thought that might be possible.

At the end of the year, the patients experience with OpenNotes exceeded the expectations of even the most optimistic proponents. Over 80% had read at least one note. They reported that reading their notes made them feel more in control (77–87%, depending on the setting) and improved their medication adherence (60–78%). Some had privacy concerns (26–36%), but about as many took the opportunity to share their medical information with family and other health advisors (20–42%). The nonparticipating doctors' prediction that patients would face increased confusion or worry didn't materialize. Increased worry or confusion was reported by 0–8%. Doctors' fears that visits would be longer did not happen (reported by 0–5% of doctors), and increases in time answering questions outside of visit also rarely occurred (0–8%). About 60% of patients, having had a taste of transparency going in one direction, wished that they could put comments about their doctors' notes in the record. At the end of the year, 99% of patients wanted to continue with open notes, and no doctors dropped out of the program [10].

Since that pilot, the OpenNotes approach has spread among healthcare's leading centers. These centers have added capabilities so that in many settings, other members of the healthcare team who are enfranchised to write in a patient's record can expect that their notes will be read as well. In 2015, there were 85,000 patients who had access to open notes [11]. In June of 2018, that number was 22.7 million (OpenNotes.org). The general experience of doctors, that open notes improves care with little increase in the demands on them, except for the few who report spending a bit more time in writing their notes, tends to make it hard for sceptics who have not tried it to make a convincing case. The overwhelming opinion of patients that open notes is a good thing, both before they get access and after they have it, has made having this capability an important marketing point for health systems that are early adopters.

7.4 Open Notes for Multiply-Disadvantaged Patients

We have been particularly concerned with how transparency can be a core element in building a bridge to partnership with multiply-disadvantaged patients. The designers of the open notes pilot were concerned about the effect it would have on patients with low education and low health literacy, especially if they had complex health needs. Wouldn't these patients be put off by complex medical terminology or by hearing what their doctors said about them? In the initial analysis, the research team expressed surprise to find that these patients were just as enthusiastic about the process as more educated patients who were healthier [10].

A later study, focusing specifically on three groups, less educated patients, non-white patients, and sicker patients, highlighted the importance of open notes and transparency in building the bridge to partnership we have been looking for [12].

There was likely to have been substantial overlap in these groups, though that was not addressed in the account of the study. Of the patients responding to the survey, 74% of patients with a high school degree or less education, 71% of African American patients, 70% of Hispanic/Latino patients, and 66% of patients with the poorest self-reported health said that access to their doctors' notes was extremely important in helping them to be informed about their care and to understand their doctor's thought processes. These patients had significantly higher rates of placing the highest value on open notes compared to their more advantaged counterparts in the study. Patients with low education levels were nearly three times as likely as better educated patients to rate open notes as extremely important to help them engage in care. Nonwhite patients were twice as likely as whites to rate open notes as extremely important. Patients with the poorest self-reported health were as or more likely than healthier patients to pick the "extremely important" rating [12].

When we discussed the multiply-disadvantaged patients (Chap. 5), those sometimes identified as complex, sometimes as having lower socioeconomic status and low education, and sometimes as having endured traumatic experiences, we found that many reported experiences with healthcare services that they found to be demeaning or to have endured shoddy care which they attributed to their low social status. We found that doctors sometimes give these patients less patient-centered care because they doubt the patients' abilities to understand the complexity of full descriptions of their conditions and treatments. Doctors may take the lower rates of adherence by these patients to be indications of their difficulties in understanding their health problems and of their need for a more directive rather than a partnering approach. We found that multiply-disadvantaged patients often are focused on the asymmetry of education, income, and power in their relationships with doctors. Trust is very difficult. Any move on the part of the doctor to be personable, to show caring, or to address difficulties that come up in the relationship is likely to be noticed and appreciated. It appears that when a doctor offers open notes, it is taken as just such a move.

The highlighted patients in this study [12] used open notes to help understand their care. They could go back to the notes multiple times and could involve the people in their lives whom they trusted to read them as well. They could be reminded about how to care for their conditions without needing to be directed. They could understand their doctors' thought processes, creating understanding of why their doctors asked the questions or made the suggestions that they did. They reported improved trust and improved adherence as a result.

The researchers ultimately suggested that access to the doctor's notes in itself may strengthen the doctor-patient relationship for these patients. They go on to suggest that doctors and other health professionals should be aware of the value of open notes for improving communication and trust. They offer recommendations for how health professionals can consciously use this tool to build engagement. They suggest that professionals authoring notes try to use clear language. In addition to improving patients' understanding of their conditions and treatments, that would allow clinicians to clearly articulate their understanding of the patient's concerns and values. Of course, to do that clinicians would need to be conscious of clearly ascertaining what the patient's concerns and values are. If clinicians take this advice, the fact of open notes could be impacting both sides of the relationship positively. Finally, they suggest that doctors should avoid using judgmental language in their notes.

7.5   Evolving the Role of the EHR

The current stage of open notes is one development in a longer series of attempts to manage the impact of record-keeping technology on the relationships of patients to their health professionals. The electronic health record (EHR) has been both a boon and a bane for doctors and patients. The role of the EHR in the transparency of doctor and patient communication up to this time has been largely a bane. Using an EHR has tended to structure the doctor's interaction in the direction of protocols and lists rather than in the direction of taking in the patient's story, contributing to the "parallel play" description of the medical interview (citation and chapter). The EHR has tended to absorb greater percentage of the doctor's attention than did paper charts [13], interrupting eye contact with the patient. This important element of nonverbal communication which conveys the HP's interest in the patient has been reduced. Multiply-disadvantaged patients, those most likely to be influenced in their self-management of their chronic illnesses by their perception of their doctors caring about them, are likely to be the most sensitive to the loss of the doctor's attention, interpreting it as relating to their relative importance to the doctor. Less eye contact and direct facing of the patient by the doctor have been correlated with less patient disclosure [14]. Should these patients believe that the doctor pays more attention to the computer during their visits compared to visits with more advantaged patients, they are not alone. One survey found that patients who were Asian, Latino, and non-English speaking or who had not graduated from high school were more likely than other patients to report that their doctor spent more than half of their visits looking at the computer screen [15].

It is probably fair to say that the period in which the EHR has functioned as a boon in the HP-patient relationship is in its infancy. The first step in transparency in relation to the EHR has involved attempts to allow the patient to see the same screen that the HP is looking at in an encounter. This has been attempted by rearranging exam rooms so that the patient and the doctor sit closer side by side, adding a second screen that can be faced toward the patient, or projecting the record on one large screen that is easily viewed by everyone in the room [16]. The introduction of a new person to manage data entry and data access from the EHR has allowed doctors to break their tether to the computer screen altogether. Each of these adaptations has been generally well received by patients who are glad for almost any step in the movement toward having more access to their own data [17].

7.6   Changing Language and Content to Build Partnership

Using open notes as a regular communication channel with patients by including information which, whether stated in the visit or not, is designed to improve the relationship between the patient and members of their healthcare team could be revolutionary. To make open notes a pathway to partnership, the early innovators are recommending three changes in how information is captured and displayed: first, a reconsideration of the way information is organized is needed to make current lists and test values more accessible; second, a regular place for information supplied by patients about their experiences of their illness and their values and preferences for their care; and finally, the usual language used by health professionals in describing their patients needs to evolve from a "neutral" recounting to a language that is experienced by the patient as coming from the commitment to them. The early innovators face the following question: if we are trying patient-centered care as a pathway to partnership by eliciting the patient's concerns and preferences, by hearing the patient's story of the reason for the visit without offering early interruptions, by addressing the emotional content and significance of what the patient is saying, or by expressing empathy or support for the patient's struggles, should not that information be as much a part of the record of the visit as the history of the present illness, the review of systems, the assessment of the doctor, and the plan?

The organization of information in most EHRs becomes a greater problem for communication when patients can view their records. EHRs are particularly good at capturing medical data for minor acute medical problems. For more complex problems such as multiple or chronic complaints, the common ways they organize information are of less help [18]. Patients often have test results presented with the normal range for each test shown, but the purpose for each test or the way a test that is out of the normal range is linked to their current treatment plan is not as clear.

As patients' preferences in relation to their care become a usual part of their record, one that is available to all health professionals using the record, standard categories reflecting these preferences need to become added to each record or to the records of some designated populations of patients. Chap. 10 goes into this issue in much more detail. It would seem sensible that a rethinking of the categories of information in the standard medical note would be undertaken by a practice or a health system that was implementing open notes. After open notes had been implemented for a while, it would be possible to assemble a group of patients from the practice to help with that redesign.

Gerard et al. [12] point out that open notes seems to add more value to the care of multiply-disadvantaged patients than it does to the care of healthier and more advantaged patients. To keep the language of the note from being an impediment, they advise clinicians not to use judgmental language in their notes. This might be a beginning, though advising doctors not to use judgmental language probably is not the best place to start. In 20 years of reading doctors' notes about patients that I shared with them, I cannot remember a single note that struck me as overtly judgmental. They were written in the ostensibly neutral terms of professional medical language. That language is full of terms such as "non-compliant," "obese," "drug user," "low cognitive ability," and "personality disorder" that are acceptable professional descriptions. While a patient reading that language might very well experience the note as judgmental, I believe that telling the doctor not to use judgmental language would seem an unnecessary instruction to almost all. They were writing in a way they were taught, a way that was designed to be free of any judgments other than medical ones. Why would professional language seem judgmental to patients if it is not meant that way by clinicians? Consider what we have said about the elements of a doctor-patient relationship that multiply-disadvantaged patients report to be helpful to them: the doctor is personable, the doctor seems to care, and the doctor tries to recognize and address times when the patient is withdrawn or alienated. Professional language, in contrast, is purposefully impersonal, leaves out the emotional experience of the author, and, if it comments on the relationship at all, focuses on patient's behavior in the visit rather than trying to report the patient's experience of the visit. OpenNotes.org, a great source of suggestions for implementation guidance for open notes, suggests that clinicians modify their note writing:

- **Difficult conversations**: If it's important enough to put in the note, it's important enough to talk about. Knowing that "you're on the same page" can improve trust and the relationship.
- **Avoid jargon, acronym, and abbreviations**: Avoid jargon and abbreviations, especially those that might easily be misinterpreted by your patients (e.g., "SOB" or "patient denies"). Briefly define or simplify medical terms (short of breath, rather than dyspneic).
- **Provide a balanced perspective**: For mental health issues in particular, describe the patient's strengths and achievements along with documenting clinical problems. This can help the patient gain a broader context within which to consider illness and tackle difficult behavioral changes (OpenNotes.org, downloaded 1/22/19).

Changing any language in the note that documents a visit, even if it will help engage the patient, has to be done very carefully. Medical notes serve multiple purposes for multiple constituencies. The note must remind the clinician and other team members in the practice of what is known about the patient and what has been done in their care so far. It must briefly give new clinicians or team members enough information to provide safe and effective care if they have to take over some aspect of the patient's treatment. It must be a true record of what was done for the sake of quality monitoring, whether that monitoring is by the practice itself or by outside regulators or payers. The purpose of documenting the visit for the information of the patient and for enhancing the clinician-patient relationship cannot undercut any of the other purposes which the note now serves.

With these requirements in mind, we can begin the process of making the note more communicative and engaging for patients. The first step is to make the note acknowledge a relationship. People in a relationship call each other by their names. Whether the patient, Mary Smith, is called "Mary," "Ms. Smith," or "Mrs. Smith," using her name is a start. (Asking a patient what they would want their doctor or team members to call them should be part of the initial information collected in any practice.) The note would document the information the patient brought to the visit using narrative conventions, not by being longer, but by being more personal. Instead of saying "patient reported ...," the note might say "Mary told me ..." or "John described ..." or "Mrs. Gonzalez explained." "Pt denied current ETOH use" can become "John says he no longer drinks alcohol." "MS, 47 yo F., with DM, obesity, and depression," becomes "Mary Smith is a 47-year-old woman who came today for help in coping with her diabetes, her weight (BMI 32), and her depression." The notes are equally communicative to other health professionals in their reworded forms and significantly more comfortably communicative with the patient that way.

Consider the way that professional language sometimes implicitly describes patients as passive receivers of both illnesses and treatments rather than as agents in their own lives. Look at any problem list for an example of this phenomenon. The characterization of patients as people who make decisions in their own lives can be helpful as we move into areas that can seem more challenging to document. Suppose the patient let the doctor know that he had not taken the medication that the doctor prescribed. A note that was not intended as a communication to the patient might say, "patient reported that he has not been compliant with his long-term asthma control medication." That phrasing connotes a person who is not doing as they were instructed to do, a person who is not cooperating with the treatment the clinician is providing to them. A note that characterized the patient as an agent in his own health might say, "John let me know that at this time, he has decided against taking his long-term asthma control medication." In a relationship, people don't always agree. In a successful relationship, disagreeing does not imply an end to working together. Phrasing the note in the second way leaves open the space for better understanding of what was behind each member's point of view, both by being clearer about why the doctor recommended a long-term asthma control medication and by clarifying why the patient would choose not to follow that advice. Clarification of the patient's perspective can open up chances for improved care by helping isolate the information that is missing from the discussion. It also highlights the patient's autonomy in making decisions about their health. Honoring the patient's autonomy is a core element of the Quality Chasm report and of the spirit of motivational interviewing, the evidence-based approach to helping patients make and keep good decisions about their health [19] discussed in Chap. 4.

Focusing on the patient as an agent in their own health tends to emphasize what they are doing for their health, rather than what they are not doing. Instead of noticing that the patient did not do the entire activity that was recommended, it tends to bring out the parts of the activity that they did accomplish. Imagine that a patient, John, has been prescribed a medication to be taken three times a day. If he is consistently missing his mid-day dose, the note might say that so far he has been able to take it two times a day. If the patient is late for an appointment, one way to describe that would be, "the visit was shortened today because the patient arrived late." Another way to describe it would be, "Mary was determined not to miss the visit today and came even though she was running behind schedule." Documenting the

Table 7.1 Change your
language to engage and
activate your patient

Negative/passive words	Positive/active words
Suffers from	Struggles with, copes with
Refused to take	Decided against
Didn't keep the apt	Was unable to be here
Was non-compliant with	Had not seen value of
Arrived late	Was determined not to miss
Work together to extend the list	

patient as an agent in their own health and noting what they are doing rather than what they are not doing is new to most people who write medical notes. When members of a healthcare team try creating similar examples of a different way of writing (while still making sure that the facts that might be needed later are not obscured), it often elicits smiles. It can become like a game. See Table 7.1.

The practice above is often called "reframing" and sometimes called "recontextualizing." It means that a description, observation, or idea is put within a different contextual background or "frame" and therefore changes meaning. This can involve changing the pattern in which an act is portrayed. "She is always resistant and now she has told me she doesn't want to follow my suggestions again" is one way of characterizing a person's pattern of behavior. Another is "she is always clear about what she is going and not going to do, unlike many of my patients who agree and then don't follow through. I appreciate her honesty." Sometimes people who are just learning to use reframing experience it as dishonest. "If I feel she is resistant, isn't it lying to say that she is honest?" The transitional step for those people is to consider what is most effective. It is, after all, our most fundamental duty to help the patient, rather than to express what we feel at the time. The Centers for Disease Control and Prevention recommends reframing when it recommends that instructions about the dangers of unsafe sexual practices that are given to HIV-positive patients be framed as being for the protection of their own health, even though the protection of their potential sexual partners is extremely important to health professionals as well. Framing the advice as protecting the patient's health, which is also factually true, has been shown to be more likely to influence patients toward safer sexual practices than a focus on the partner [20]. Health professionals tend to get more comfortable with using reframing when they see the positive impact on their relationships with their patients and when they see the effectiveness that is fostered by this better relationship.

Using clear language, making the note more personal by using patients' names, describing patients as agents in their healthcare rather than passive recipients, and highlighting what a patient is doing rather than what they are not doing for their health can create a note that is designed to improve partnership with multiply-disadvantaged patients and probably would improve the relationship with most patients. None of this means, however, that the medical content of the note should be watered down or changed. Some medical terms can be replaced by terms used by laymen, but many cannot. Medical language is more specific. To convey the same specificity of description of a particular condition in layman's language in many cases requires many more words than in medical terminology. The changes in language that highlight the patients' agency and strengths are likely more important than translating all of the medical language and abbreviations into a laymen's vocabulary. If the studies we have cited are credible, it seems that many patients are willing to make the effort to do some translating.

Behavioral health notes raise special issues in the open notes conversation, because of the history of special status for mental health and substance abuse notes and the culture of protecting notes in mental health settings. The practice of sharing notes with the patient whose care they document is a different issue than the practice of sharing notes among professionals. Sharing notes among professionals is a long discussion in itself. Suffice it to say that where behavioral healthcare is part of primary care or another medical setting, behavioral health progress notes in the medical record can and should be shared with the healthcare team, and any psychotherapy notes that cannot be shared should not be part of the medical or billing record (www. hhs.gov, Health Information Privacy).

Since 2006, all patients have had the right to a copy of their medical records if they ask for them, though some health settings have made the process inconvenient. The fact that so few have exercised that right in the past means that while all people who document in the medical record should have been told to write as if the patient was going to read it, few have had this as a consideration as they were charting. I think that if team members were a part of a workshop on reframing in chart notes, they might or might not be interested in practicing this different way of writing, but nothing in their routine would make it necessary. The skills would fade over time rather than improve. Because many medical practices will not have open notes for some time, I suggest that everyone who meets regularly with patients and then writes in the chart about the meeting tries a practice I have found to be the most helpful clinical routine I have ever used: reading back the notes of the last meeting at the beginning of the next.

Reading the note from the last visit takes very little time at the beginning of a new visit, especially for follow-ups of any sort, whether medical, behavioral health, care management, or coaching, which are not occurring because of a new complaint or concern. It focuses both the HP and the patient on the topics and brief content of their previous conversation. I found this helpful in follow-up visits because the patient often had lost the thread of our work together since the last time we talked. Instead of asking people whether they remembered what we talked about last time, the reading of the note became part of the routine of the visit. This means that the reframes or emphases that I thought would be useful at the end of the last visit are immediately made available to the patient, with the invitation in every case that they correct whatever I got wrong. This almost never happened. One of my favorite moments in my work in primary care behavioral health was the time when patients came for their second meeting with me. My reading of the note, as if that were a sensible routine practice, in almost every case was positively received by the patient. I usually remarked that I wanted them to correct any mistakes in the notes because that is the information that was shared with colleagues on the team. Patient's rarely asked for changes and then only for factual details (I have three brothers, not two) rather than in interpretations or emphases. Patient's often said that they wished other people who provided care did the same.

It is something of an aside here, but I am aware that my behavioral health colleagues may well be protesting that writing a brief note including positive reframing of the patient as an agent in their own healthcare that will be read to the patient is all well and good, but what about the requirements that mental health billing regulations have for documentation to support a fee-for-service bill for the interaction? While I would like to answer by appealing to the day when payment transformation puts all payment, formerly medical and formerly mental health, into one payment stream and pays a set price for the full care of the patient to the primary care practice and the health system within which it resides, that day may be a long way off for many of us. In the meantime, I offer the note format that I found made the practice of writing as well as reading the note simple yet defensible to auditors. (I cannot guarantee that this note format fits billing requirements in every location, so it should be vetted locally by anyone who is considering adopting it.) Together with the compliance office[1] of our health system, I created a form designed to meet billing documentation requirements and to be easy to read back to patients. I would read the text back to the patient, the same text that would be read by my colleagues, about my work with the patient. The form (see Appendix) included information delivered using check boxes substantiating the billing. I was able to fill out the form in a Word document in about 5 minutes and copy and paste it into the EHR.

From the mental health world has come an innovation in note sharing that may at some point be applied commonly in some medical settings, collaborative documentation [21]. This is a practice in which the clinician and the patient co-construct the record in the process of the conversation that the record documents. It has been developed in the treatment of people with serious mental illness whose engagement in care is often hard to sustain. The vast majority also have multiple chronic illnesses and can reasonably be called "complex." The rate of trauma histories for these patients is very high. The issues of stigma, power differentials, the need for peer support, and the need for the patient to be in the lead are central to creating successful treatment environments. In collaborative documentation the creation of the record becomes a cooperative project that involves patients and professionals discussing what will be written in the record at the end of each visit. This practice has led to increased rates of patients keeping appointments and adhering to medication [21]. Similar involvement of patients in creation of their records is done by some individual medical providers, but currently I don't find evidence that there is any broad push for adding this process into the hustle and bustle of primary care practices. Other team members, such as BHCs, care managers, navigators, or health

---

[1] Hospital systems commonly have a compliance office made up of staff members, some of whom are lawyers, who do internal monitoring of records and practices so that when external reviewers or auditors arrive, the institution will not have to give back payments that are judged to have been inappropriately obtained because the existing documentation doesn't support them.

coaches, might well consider it. Creating the time for the conversation is an important barrier, though in the evolution of alternative team routines and scheduling schemes (see Chap. 2; [22]), it may become possible. At that point the record becomes a true record of a relationship created by the relationship.

7.7 Speaking As Well as Writing

There are two ways that health professionals use their language to describe patients, writing and speaking. Just as the medical record has been a domain to which patients have had little or no access in the past, the conversations about patients, particularly among members of the healthcare team, is an arena from which patients are usually excluded. When the healthcare team is organized like a squad (see Chap. 2), i.e., staff members supporting the work of the doctor, who is the main source of expertise in the treatment, the conversation in the hall about the patient is usually fairly mundane. It consists of brief exchanges designed to coordinate the various tasks that go into making up a patient visit. Telling a patient who feels particularly vulnerable in medical visits that most conversations are brief and instrumental, rather than evaluating or judging the patient, probably would not be comforting. Observing conversations in the hall, especially if there is any exchange of smiles or if someone laughs, can increase the patients' concern that people are talking about them in less than complementary ways.

When the healthcare team expands to include a new expertise set, such as when a behavioral health clinician joins the team, the conversations in the hall tend to become longer and more detailed. One of the most common ways that a behavioral health clinician can be added to the treatment team for a particular patient is through a process called a "warm handoff." The doctor introduces the behavioral health clinician to the patient during the patient's medical visit. The behavioral health clinician can speak to the patient long enough to begin to understand the patient's view of the concern that the doctor identified and to attempt to make an engagement with the patient to work on the concern. Sometimes the BHC offers brief interventions as part of the warm handoff process. A warm handoff, with its face-to-face introduction, is much more effective at building engagement between the BHC and the patient than a simple referral by the doctor to a BHC whom the patient has never met. In an informal study in one health center, the new BHC kept a record of all his scheduled first appointments and whether or not the appointment was kept. He found that if he had been introduced to the patient by the doctor previously to the scheduled appointment (warm handoff), the chance that the patient kept the first scheduled appointment was almost double the chance that the appointment would be kept if the doctor had simply requested that the appointment for the patient be scheduled with the BHC without an in-person introduction [23].

The warm handoff is much more effective for engagement, but it can be time-consuming for doctors, particularly if they have to have a conversation with the behavioral health clinician about the medical and behavioral situation of the patient in the hall before the introduction. That tends to make the in-person introduction to the patient in the exam room feel redundant to the professionals who just spoke in the hall. On the other hand, if the introduction is done in the exam room with the patient with no orientation of the BHC to the patient's situation, it can make the conversation with the patient after the exit of the physician awkward. When the introduction and orientation of the BHC and patient is too brief, it leaves the purpose of their conversation unclear and makes their engagement more difficult. The patient may be left not sure what the new team member knows about his/her situation and uneasy about where to start. The BHC doesn't know how much of the information that the doctor shared in the hall is understood or accepted by the patient.

The more efficient solution is to have both conversations, the orientation of the BHC to the patient's situation and the introduction of the BHC and the patient, in the exam room with the patient. This is transparency in the conversation about the patient. The same skills that were discussed above for writing engaging medical notes are useful in creating engaging conversations with and about the patient. Using the patient's name, sharing the difficulty he or she is facing, and highlighting what the doctor and patient have already done can set the task for the next team member. Rephrasing descriptions to characterize a patient as an agent in his or her own health rather than as a passive receiver of illnesses or treatments forms the basis of the change. As with writing, the more one speaks with other team members in front of the patient, the easier and more natural it becomes.

7.8 Passing the Relationship

One of the challenges of a healthcare team is the inevitability that the patient will have a different sort of relationship with different members of the team, depending on their role and on how well they relate to the patient in that role. In most cases, the patient's relationship with the doctor will be the most important to the patient. It is the doctor's expertise that brings the patient for care. Occasionally a patient's relationship will be stronger with the team member who spends significantly more time with them, such as a care manager. And sometimes a patient will form the closest bond with a team member whom the patient finds most approachable, for reasons such as being of similar genders, cultures, language skills, age, or personality. If the team is going to function efficiently, it helps to have a method for leveraging the positive connection of one team member to quickly build a trusting relationship with the patient for another.

Speaking in the presences of the patient can be the basis for a thoughtful routine for the introduction of a team member who is new to the patient, made by the team member who has the closest connection. This is most effectively done by combining the conversation that orients the new team member to working with the patient and the conversation that orients the patient to working with the new team member. It is a conversation between the patient (and family members or others who are part of the patient's care), the current team member, and the new team member. When done well, this process is built on the foundational skills of talking in front of the patient that are described above. We will call this "open clinical discussion" in primary care.

Open clinical discussion as we are using the team was created originally to help doctors add the BHC to the team, though it can be used for other relationships as well. It is not meant to be the only way of passing of the relationship, but it is an example of elements that can make the process more efficient. When passing the relationship, consider using the mnemonic of SSRI[2] to organize the introduction. It is designed to help doctors, or the team member with the current relationship with the patient, conduct this process smoothly and efficiently once they and the patient have agreed that something additional in the care could be needed.

The first **S**. is for **Situation**. The doctor (or team member with the closest relationship) says to the patient and the BH clinician (or newly involved team member) what *situation* in the patient's current care makes him or her want to recommend adding the BH clinician to the treatment team. The process starts with the patient's need that the new team member will address. The current team member can try to be aware of the patient's understanding of their need and to use the patient's terminology, as well as the team member's terminology to describe it.

The second **S**. is **Skill Set**. The doctor describes to the patient the *skill set* (as opposed to the discipline) of the BH clinician that makes him or her the person that the doctor wants to add to the treatment team. Whatever the skill set of the new team member, it should be phrased to be a fit for the patient's need that was mentioned in the Situation statement.

The **R**. stands for **Relationship**. At this point the doctor says what *relationship* the work between the BH clinician and the patient will have to the overall treatment that he or she and the patient have been conducting. Remember, this isn't a new treatment; it is a new aspect of the patient's current care. In any situation, the new team member is augmenting the existing care. The "relationship" part of the statement helps a patient to know how this fits together.

The final **I**. is for **Indicators**. The doctor says to the BH clinician and the patient what would *indicate* that the addition of the BH clinician's expertise and intervention had been successful. If the care, including the efforts by the patient, that this new team member can offer does what we hope, what improvements will the patient and the team start to see occurring?

---

[2] The ideas about passing the relationship were first published in Blount, A. (2018). It takes a team. S. Gold and L. Green (Eds.) *Your Patients are Waiting: Integrating Behavioral Health for the Primary Care Physician*. Springer Publishing, New York.

Below is an example of the elements of the SSRI designed to add a BH clinician to the care of a patient in a way that allows the patient and BH clinician to begin working quickly and smoothly to address the goal(s) identified by the doctor and the patient. Notice that the doctor doesn't specify what sort of intervention the BH clinician will use nor how many contacts between the BH clinician and the patient will be involved. Those are dependent on the expertise of the BH clinician and the connection that develops between clinician and patient.

On paper this may seem like a complex process. Try reading the examples out loud. You get a complete statement that would require less time than is usually taken for either the hall discussion or the in-room introduction.

S: Bob Lawrence (patient), this is Joseph Gonzalez (BHC). Bob reports he is experiencing the early stages of a recurrence of his depression. One way in the past that he has shown that he was having a recurrence was he stopped taking his diabetes medication. Bob let me know today that he has gotten a little unreliable at taking the medicine lately and that he thinks about stopping it fairly often.

S: Mr. Gonzalez has a lot of experience helping people keep minor recurrences of depression from developing into major episodes and helping them keep the parts of their lives that they worked hard to achieve from sliding backward.

R: Bob, I am hoping that while working with Mr. Gonzalez, you can get back on track fairly quickly. I would like to get an update from the two of you in 3 weeks so that we can restart antidepressant medication if that is indicated.

I: Bob and I have discussed his situation, and we agree that if he is able to get through a mild recurrence of his depression without losing traction in his health, his work, or his social life, meaning his diabetes stays managed and doesn't cause him to miss work, it will mean that the progress he has made is getting more reliable. I think that could give him confidence about planning for his future, something that up to now he hasn't quite been able to do.

Notice that the aspect of the BH clinician's skill set that is most relevant to the patient's situation is what the doctor stresses. In the case above, Mr. Gonzalez is a skilled BH generalist, experienced at working with the mental health, substance abuse, and health behavior needs of adults and children. But it is not his skills with substance abuse care, or health behavior change that make him someone that Bob Lawrence would want to work with, it is his skill at helping a patient manage the impact of a depression recurrence. That is the skill set that is highlighted. In the early stages of their work together, Mr. Gonzales will tell the patient his discipline that he is a licensed clinical social worker, but that will be as part of the further introduction of himself and the process.

When it is possible with schedules, it is also effective to have a "report back" to the doctor by the BH clinician and the patient as their work draws to a close. It orients the doctor briefly to the specifics of what was useful in their work together. It allows the BH clinician to say complimentary things about the patient and sometimes vice versa. It passes the role of clinician regarding behavioral aspects of the patient's care back to the doctor and enfranchises him or her to remind the patient of the skills that they learned in working with the BH clinician when those skills could be useful in the future. This is most easily done if the BHC "looks in" on one of the patient's regular visits with his doctor.

Sometimes passing the relationship requires an aspect of the current relationship to be spelled out a bit so the need for the involvement of the next team member is clear. It helps to say a sentence or two about the work that has been going on in the current relationship and then to say a sentence or two about the challenge that has come up and why the challenge needs to be addressed. (Below, the doctor is introducing a care manager.)

S: Mary Smith (patient), this is Octavia Melendez (care manager). Octavia, Mary and I have been working to try to keep her diabetes under control. Since her last visit, the friend she was staying with has had to ask her and her son to leave because the landlord won't allow extra people. They are staying in a shelter, and everything is so much harder now. She has a hard time getting her medicine. She tries to keep her mood up, but she has so little privacy that anybody would find it hard. It is easy to feel hopeless. There are a lot of folks in the shelter who are using drugs, so she is worried about her sobriety.

S: Octavia is our team member who is best at solving problems, like helping people find a place to live or helping them get the additional services they need.

R: The last time Mary had secure housing, her son was doing well in school, she felt healthier, she was getting some exercise, and she was taking her medication. She was more confident in her sobriety, and she was able to go to the vocational train-ing program at the community center.

I: With Mary's connections to her family and friends, and with Octavia's knowl-edge of resources, I am hoping that fairly quickly Mary will begin to feel some hope about finding stable housing and that in not too long a time the two of you can find a stable place for Mary to stay.

Here the doctor is introducing a medical assistant who will teach the patient to use a spacer with her asthma inhaler.

S: Elena Medina (patient), this is Louis Wallace (medical assistant).
Elena has been having trouble with her breathing lately, even though she is tak-ing her asthma medication on time. She has had to go to the emergency room twice because she got so worried that she couldn't get her breath. I think that having a spacer with her inhaler could make a big difference for her in how much the medication helps her.

S: Elena, Louis is one of our team members who is very good at teaching people to use their health equipment, like an inhaler. Learning to use a spacer can take a bit of practice. Louis is skilled at teaching how it is done.

R: So, Louis, please take the time you need until Elena is confident she knows how to use the space correctly.

I: I think that if Elena was more confident that her spacer and her medicine were going to help her every time she needs help, she could feel less anxious about how her day was going to go, and that might even save her a few times of needing to use her inhaler.

The SSRI conversation can start the practice of discussing patients' situations between team members with the patient participating on a broader basis. It allows for other members of the team to see examples of what such a conversation looks like. It is much easier to have conversations about the care of patients in their presence than most team members imagine.

No one needs to change the facts that are discussed, though it helps to have a change in some of the types of language in which the facts are couched (Table 7.1).

7.9 Implementation

I suggest that if team members are uncomfortable with the idea of open clinical discussions, they be given the option of having conversations about the patient separately but that some of the weekly team meeting time be given to discussing how the same information could be passed in open clinical discussion. As a way to build the skills of team members in having conversations in front of patients, the team can practice adding to the list in Table 7.1. At first, they are likely to experience the process as humorous and forced. It is not what they "really think" about the patients. If they imagine or role play using these terms in clinical practice, the impact begins to become clear. When the experience of the patient is factored into the exercise, and the difference in the behavior that the patient is likely to exhibit begins to become apparent, people begin to see this as an exercise designed to make their work lives much easier. They begin to feel the descriptions take on more authenticity.

As team members get more comfortable in having conversations in the presence of patients, as their characterizations become more active and positive than they have used in the past, they tend to develop greater comfort and skill at speaking with patients generally. This is not something to force, but it is something worth cultivating and nurturing.

7.10 Summary

We are building a scaffold with the practices of transparency. Open notes, reading notes from the previous visit, and open clinical discussions underlie and support the other elements involved in making partnership work, in making the routines of primary care practice with multiply-disadvantaged patients empowering, activating, and mutual. We will go back through the ways of using the note, ways of speaking in front of the patient, and ways of constructing core documents and practices of care mutually with the patient, and each time we do it, it should make the processes more resonant for both patients and team members. This multiple-pass approach to describing the method mirrors a realistic approach to learning the method. Each pass adds a new layer of new techniques on top of an existing structure.

Transparency creates a novel situation for most team members. Openness to new learning is enhanced when people perceive their situation as one that is new to them, yet one in which they want to function successfully. Open notes and open clinical discussions comprise such an example. In a new situation, new rules can be learned without implying that what people did in the old situation was a problem. As people experience multiple iterations of successful actions in the new context, the situation becomes more familiar. It takes less energy for attending to being successful in the contingencies of the new environment, and people have attention freed up for observing less dramatic details. They can learn new small changes that can make a big difference, once they are oriented to the environment as a whole. Transparency is the core structure, the scaffold, of the new environment as a whole.

Next, we can add details of conversations and actions that are designed to foster empowerment of patients. From there, we begin helping patients activate themselves, to generate new behavior or to strengthen old behavior for their own health, as a refinement rather than a major change in approach, attitude, or routine. Finally, initiating and conducting the core assessment and treatment plan, the treatment plan that will be used by every member of the larger health system, in full partnership with the patient and their close network of supporters, is an affirmation of the partnership with the patient.

The preparation for and the implementation of open notes and open clinical discussion can be the first step toward the goal of caring effectively for multiply-disadvantaged patients after the team is in place. This approach to transparency requires new ways of speaking and writing for everyone. The behavioral health clinicians are no more likely than the medical clinicians or other team members to have experience communicating this way. The process of implementing open notes and open clinical discussion, because they are new to everyone and not based on an expertise that is part of the training of any particular discipline, means that learning transparent speaking and writing can be a leveling process for the team. In Chap. 2 we described a process for building the routines of the team that required the doctor to have a conception of the growth of team members and to actively foster that growth. Moving to open notes and open clinical discussion may give team members with more training, such as the doctor, opportunities to learn from and to compliment the skill of other team members in this mutual endeavor. The impact to transparency with patients ultimately can positively impact the working relationships and the transparency within the team delivering the care.

Appendix

Ambulatory Service Record:

Name, DOB, MRN, Date

Diagnosis	Code	Descriptive Statement
Primary		
Secondary		
Tertiary		

☐ Individ Psychothrpy: _____ mins(20–30)
☐ Individ Psychothrpy: _____ mins (45–50)
☐ Family Therapy w pt _____ mins
☐ Family Therapy w/o pt _____ mins
☐ Init MH Assess & Intrv

☐ Init. Hlth & Behav Assess (96150) _____ mins
☐ Subseq Hlth & Behav Assess (96151) _____ mins
☐ Indiv Hlth & Behav Intrv (96152) _____ mins
☐ Grp 2+ pts Hth & Behav Intrv (96153) _____ mins
☐ Fam Hlth & Behav Intrv w/pt (96154) _____ mins
☐ Fam Hlth & Behav Intrv wo/pt (96155) _____ mins

Problems from Treatment Plan:
Problem #1: _____
Current Status ☐ No Change ☐ Improved _____ ☐ Worse _____
Problem 2: _____
Current Status ☐ No Change ☐ Improved _____ ☐ Worse _____
Problem 3: _____
Current Status ☐ No Change ☐ Improved _____ ☐ Worse _____
☐ Medical and social history documented in medical chart and reviewed before first meeting. ☐ Reviewed limits of confidentiality.
Other Problems Discussed, Assessment / Additional Comments: (narrative portion of note)

Topics covered in visit relating to: ☐ Problem 1 ☐ Problem 2 ☐ Problem 3

Evaluation & Discussion of Problem(s):	Cognitive – Behavioral Interventions:
☐ Frequency / Severity / Other Details	☐ Self-monitoring: _____
☐ Factor Contributing to Problem, Triggers	☐ Stimulus Control: _____
☐ Factors Maintaining Problem, Barriers to Change	☐ Relaxation Training
☐ Past Coping Efforts	☐ Mindfulness / Awareness Skills
☐ Other:_____	☐ Identification of Dysfunctional Thoughts / Beliefs
Treatment Planning, Pt. Education:	☐ Cognitive Restructuring
☐ Psycho-education re: Problem & Treatment	☐ Development of Hierarchy of Treatment Targets
☐ Discussion of Treatment Plan & Goals	☐ Systematic Desensitization
Strengths, Foundation for Future Growth:	☐ Relapse Prevention
☐ Determination to Feel Better	☐ Application of Skills to Problem Situation / Symptoms
☐ Past Coping Success: _____	☐ Other: _____
☐ New Behavior Began: _____	Additional Treatment Recourses Discussed:
☐ Other:_____	☐ Psychiatric Medications: _____

Life Style Modification:	Risk Assessment:	☐ Medical Provider: _____
☐ Eating Behavior		☐ Nutritionist: _____
☐ Sleep Hygiene	HI/SI ☐Y ☐N	☐ Couples Therapy
☐ Management of Stressors	Plans ☐Y ☐N	☐ Group Therapy
☐ Physical Activity	Means ☐Y ☐N	☐ Reading Material
☐ Smoking	Active ☐Y ☐N	☐ Internet Recourses
☐ Pleasurble Activs, Self-Care	SA ☐Y ☐N	☐ Self-help (AA, NA, DA)
☐ Social Support	Agitation ☐Y ☐N	☐ Other: _____
☐ Positive Life Goals	History ☐Y ☐N	☐ Other: _____
☐ Other:_____		☐ Other: _____

References

1. Institute of Medicine. Crossing the quality chasm: a new health system for the 21st century. Washington, DC: National Academy Press; 2001.
2. Mautner DB, Pang H, Brenner JC, Shea JA, Gross KS, Frasso R, Cannuscio CC. Generating hypotheses about care needs of high utilizers: lessons from patient interviews. Popul Health Manag. 2013;16:S26–33.
3. Pollack KI, Alexander SC, Grambow SC, Sulsky JA. Oncologist patient-centered communication with patient with advanced cancer: exploring whether race and socioeconomic status matter. Palliat Med. 2010;24:96–8.
4. Willems S, De Maesschalck S, Deveugele M, Derese A, De Maeseneer J. Socioeconomic status of the patient and doctor-patient communication: does it make a difference? Patient Educ Couns. 2005;56:139–46.
5. Shenkin BN, Warner DC. Sounding board: giving the patient his medical record: a proposal to improve the system. N Engl J Med. 1973;289:688–92.
6. Tollast O. Transparency and medical records. Salzburg Global Seminar. March 12, 2017. https://www.salzburgglobal.org//calendar/2010-2019/2017/session-553.html
7. Delbanco T, Berwick DM, Boufford JI, et al. Healthcare in the land called PeoplePower: nothing about me without me. Health Expect. 2001;4:144–50.
8. Delbanco T, Walker J, Darer J, et al. Open notes: doctors and patients signing up. Ann Intern Med. 2010;153:121–5.
9. Walker J, Leveille SG, Ngo L, et al. Inviting patients to read their doctors' notes: patients and doctors look ahead: patient and physician surveys. Ann Intern Med. 2011;155:811–9.
10. Delbanco T, Walker J, Bell SK, et al. Inviting patients to read their doctors' notes: a quasi-experimental study and look ahead. Ann Intern Med. 2012;157:461–70.
11. Walker J, Meltsner M, Delbanco T. US experience with doctors and patients sharing clinical notes. BMJ. 2015;350:g7785.
12. Gerard M, Chimowitz H, Fossa A, Bourgeois F, Fernandez L, Bell S. The importance of visit notes on patient portals for engaging less educated or nonwhite patients: survey study. J Med Internet Res. 2018;20:e191.
13. Rathert C, Porter TH, Mittler JN, Fleig-Palmer M. Seven years after meaningful use: Physicians' and nurses' experiences with electronic health records. Health Care Manag Rev. 2017:1–11.
14. Makoul G, Curry R, Tang P. The use of electronic medical records. J Am Med Inform Assoc. 2001;8:610–5.
15. Ratanawongsa N, Barton JL, Schillinger D, et al. Ethnically diverse patients' perceptions of clinician computer use in a safety-net clinic. J Health Care Poor Underserved. 2013;24:1542–51.
16. Schutzbank A. V.P. of Iora Health. Personal communication, 29 Sep 2018.
17. deBronkhart, D. Let patients help. Richard Davies deBronkhart Jr.;2013.
18. Ventres W, Kooienga S, Vuckovic N, et al. Physicians, patients and the electronic health record: an ethnographic analysis. Ann Fam Med. 2006;4:124–31.
19. Rollnick S, Miller WR, Butler CC. Motivational interviewing in health care. New York: Guilford Press; 2008.
20. Gerbert B, Danley DW, Herzig K, Clanon K, Ciccarone D, Gilbert P, Allerton M. Reframing "prevention with positives": incorporating counseling techniques that improve the health of HIV-positive patients. AIDS Patient Care STDs. 2006;20:19–29.
21. Stanhope V, Ingoglia C, Schmelter B, Marcus SC. Impact of person-centered planning and collaborative documentation on treatment adherence. Psychiatr Serv. 2013;64:76–9.
22. Jain N, Okanlawon T, Meisinger K, Feeley TW. Leveraging IPU principles in primary care. NEJM Catalyst. June 27, 2018.
23. Apostoleris NH, DeGirolamo S, McConarty P, Mazyk B. Overcoming barriers to mental health utilization: examining the referral process in a community health center-based family medicine residency. Presented at the Annual Conference of the Society of Teachers of Family Medicine. 2005.

Chapter 8
"E" Is for Empowering

8.1 Getting to Empowerment

Empowerment of patients is a crucial element of an approach to primary care that improves outcomes for patients and lowers cost for payers [1, 2]. Patients who experience themselves as empowered, as partners in their relationships with their doctors, are generally the same patients who feel empowered in relation to their own health [3]. They are more likely to take the actions that maintain or improve their health. These are patients, on average, whose healthcare will cost significantly less in the long run than those who do not feel able to influence their healthcare or impact their health.

"Empowered" patients should not be confused with patients that health professionals sometimes call "enfranchised" because they seem inappropriately demanding of their healthcare teams. Empowered patients are able to participate in a partnership, to share in planning their care, and able to act autonomously to maintain their health. Enfranchised patients generally are not experiencing a partnership with health professionals; rather they tend to see health professionals as controlling their access to tests or treatments that they think they need. When a genuine partnership can be developed with these patients, one that involves an agreement on the goals and the methods for reaching the goals and that honors the expertise of the professionals as well as the desires of the patients, both patients and clinicians experience themselves as more empowered.

In Chap. 5, we looked at a group of patients who have particular trouble forming partnerships with their doctors and healthcare teams. These are patients who are described in different ways in different literatures. They are a subgroup of "complex" patients, those who are high utilizers of healthcare resources, who have multiple chronic illnesses, often including behavioral health disorders. Many are people of low socioeconomic status, whose low levels of educational attainment make participating in the complexities of healthcare difficult for them and for their clinicians. Many cope with language barriers and/or with societal discrimination. Many have

© Springer Nature Switzerland AG 2019
A. Blount, *Patient-Centered Primary Care*,
https://doi.org/10.1007/978-3-030-17645-7_8

histories that include experiences of trauma that have affected their coping abilities and their health. Studying these extremely high-cost individuals, Mautner et al. [4] found that besides their histories of trauma, a great many had histories of what they experienced as inadequate, dismissive, or demeaning interactions with the health-care system. Doctors commonly are less likely to take a patient-centered approach to these patients, believing instead that they need a more directive approach because of their challenges in understanding and in adherence [5, 6]. These are people for whom an offer of empowerment, in its more political sense, i.e., an invitation to share a partnership with health professionals in planning their care, is not likely to have the desired effect. Building trust and the experience of self-efficacy has to precede the invitation to partnership.

In working with multiply-disadvantaged patients, the meaning of "empowerment" that is most immediately relevant is the meaning used by practitioners of trauma-informed care (TIC) [7]. In the TIC approach, "empowerment" means that wherever possible, the patient's strengths and successes are used as a basis for building toward their better health and functioning. In addition, hierarchical relationships between health professionals and the patient are likely to be a reminder to the patient of unsafe times in the past, when they did not have power to avert one or many traumatic experiences. TIC becomes an organizational commitment that flattens hierarchy among team members as well as between team members and patients [8].

To a person in any of the helping professions who has been trained to ease suffering by solving or alleviating problems, either physical, emotional, or social, the idea of starting by focusing on what the patient does well, or where they have been successful in the past, can appear to be inefficient at minimum or even misguided. In simple situations, this might be true. Studying the functioning and health of the arm that isn't broken rather than treating the arm that is broken is certainly not the best use of the time of the health professional or the patient. However, in situations in which the patient's understanding or definition of their own situation, and the future actions they take based on that understanding, will make a difference in their physical, emotional, or social outcome, focusing them on what has worked in the past and how that can relate to the future can be the most efficient use of time and energy.

The precepts of trauma-informed care (TIC) provide conceptual guidance for implementing the "the patient as the source of control" of their healthcare, but in general they do not specify in detail what actions can be taken or what words can be used to accomplish the purpose outlined. There is a proven methodology for enacting this sort of empowerment. In Chap. 11, we describe one version of this methodology, the version targeted at developing collaboration within groups of co-workers and teams in organizations, when we talk about "appreciative inquiry" for building the healthcare team [9]. We highlight how working from staff members' strengths helps build the empowerment for them to take on more complex and more autonomous roles.

In a clinical situation the same general methodology is called "solution-focused interviewing" (SFI) [10]. SFI consists of questions designed to highlight strengths, successes, and solutions in a way that is oriented toward helping a person make further progress. The method is a distillation of some of the techniques developed in the 1960s and is called systems-oriented (or "systemic") brief therapy [11]. SFI resulted from research that attempted to rigorously correlate behaviors by a clinician in systemic brief therapy sessions with a patient's subsequent report of improvement [12]. The researchers, studying videotapes of visits, sought to isolate the behaviors by therapists that correlated most strongly with improvement and achievement of patient goals. They used a method called "sequential analysis" [13] for reliably designating specific categories of therapist behaviors. This naming of categories of behaviors allowed for mathematical correlations of therapist actions with later behaviors of patients to be done. The findings were striking. They determined that the more the therapist talked about problems, analyzed problems, looked at sequences in which the problems occurred, and talked about causes of problems, the less likely positive change was to be reported by patients. The more the therapist *elicited* descriptions of change or of exceptions in the problem patterns, or *amplified* the patient's description of change, or *initiated* descriptions of change by reframing a problem or by suggesting new behavior, the more the patient was likely to report a positive outcome and the achievement of therapeutic goals [12]. Therapists interviewed for solutions by asking: What would the solution look like? How would you recognize the beginnings of a solution as it developed? What previous examples of similar solutions had occurred? What exceptions to the problem patterns had occurred? What had the patient said or done that seemed to help toward those solutions?

The insights of the study of solutions in brief therapy and the focused approach to interviewing that it engendered are useful and effective outside of a psychotherapy setting. While "solution-focused therapy" describes an approach to creating change in a brief psychotherapy, "solution-focused interviewing" describes a general way of approaching communication in a helping relationship that tends to lead to improvement by focusing on strengths, on what works, and on a patient's history of exceptions to problem patterns.

Solution-focused questions are not contrived to lead patients to certain conclusions or realizations; they are ways one person tries to understand the strengths or determination or creativity or values of another. In the process, the other person is likely to become more aware of their own strengths, determination, creativity, or values. As the patient experiences themselves as more likely to achieve positive results or solutions, their hope for success and their willingness to try are likely to be strengthened.

The findings of the Gingerich et al. study [12] correspond with more mainstream science of brain function and memory. Recent neuroscience [14] helps to explain a phenomenon that I have observed in my clinical experience of using SFI for over 30 years. I found that early in a visit if a patient was asked about times when they did better than in their current problem situation, times when they were successful to some degree in the problem area, the answer was often, "Never." They could not think of a single time in which there was an exception to the current pattern of problems or pains. After a conversation that featured some of the solution-focused questions discussed below, their report of their history often had changed. They could remember actions that worked, how they had helped to create instances that were an improvement on their current problem situations. When people experienced themselves as currently unable to find a solution, they often experienced their history as characterized by a continuous sequence of failures. When they experienced themselves as having been able in some instances to effect better outcomes, they remembered a pattern of events that supported that picture. This change in their experience of one part of their history tended to correspond with a small change in their current sense of themselves which connected to a small change in their understanding of the possibilities for the future. "If I made it work in the past, possibly I can make it work in the future." A small change in a person's expectations of the possibilities for the future can make an important difference in their commitment to action toward improving their situation, such as working for better health.

Hasselmo [14] reminds us of the difference between "semantic memory," the memory of facts and knowledge of the world; "procedural memory," the memory of how to do something; and "episodic memory," the memory of an episode of experience in space and time. He points out that one memory can cue access to other memories that have similar elements, based on the salient details of the first memory as determined at the time of access. He uses the concept of "reciprocal richness" to describe the way in which, when one memory of an episode cues access to a similar memory, the richness of a detail in the first memory can mean that the second memory is accessed with a richness of detail borrowed from other elements in memory, enhancing the newly recalled memory with a vividness it may not have had at the time it was created. Our current purpose or emotional state helps determine what memories are accessed, and the details of those memories that we experience as important are enhanced in richness. Research on memory and the brain supports the observation about SFI above [14, 15]. Garry and Polaschek [16] express it clearly in their summary for a popular audience:

> The "autobiographical (episodic) memories" that tell the story of our lives are always undergoing revision precisely because our sense of self is too. We are continually extracting new information from old experiences and filling in gaps in ways the serve some current demand. Consciously or not, we use imagination to reinvent our past, and with it, our present and our future. (p. 66)

Put another way, our personal history is the story we remember and unconsciously create to explain our current experience of ourselves and our situation. When our current experience of ourselves and our situation changes, a somewhat different history is likely to become available in memory. Helping people experience themselves as able to create solutions makes different episodes in their lives come to mind, episodes that logically lead to their being able to continue in their more adaptive path. In the process, the interviewer's experience of the patient, about the strengths and potential of the patient, changes as well. New hope and energy are infectious. New hope and energy, the experience of being effective, correlate with lower burnout for health professionals.

Coping is a daily challenge for multiply-disadvantaged patients. For many people, asking about what works or about their strengths will not be an approach that engages them. Feelings of frustration or vulnerability tend to be primary when they think about their experience. Accounts of successes or of taking steps to make their lives better may be hard to elicit. Solution-focused interviewing can also include coping questions that ask not about patients' successes but about how they have kept their currents situations from being worse. Sharing information that the patient experiences as characterizing their coping and their determination can begin to build engagement between the patient and the team. As people feel more confident in the importance of their knowledge about their lives and their functioning, and as they are surer of the respect with which they are regarded by their care team, they are likely to become more open in sharing their thoughts and to ask for the specific information that will help them.

Using solution-focused interviewing may seem to team members to add too much time to the little time they have for their interaction with the patient on a given day. In the cases of many patients, that could be true, and good care through partnership can be achieved without the addition of solution talk for those patients. In the case of multiply-disadvantaged patients, however, the likelihood of their taking up a lot of time is very high, perhaps not in one visit, but in the many visits required by their care in the health system. Any extra time that is given to helping them engage more effectively in their care and to experience themselves as more empowered in relation to their care team will be likely to save time later. Teams that become proficient at solution talk will find that they use it throughout their day. Over time, it is likely to become not an extra approach added on but a way of working with everyone.

8.2 Solution-Focused Questions[1]

Questions that tend to help discover solutions can be grouped into several categories. The following are common, but there can be many more [17]: pre-visit change, coping questions, questions about what you would keep, exception questions, scaling questions, and questions about what the solution would look like. Each of these questions can be the beginning of a period of "solution talk" [18]. Solution talk, as opposed the "problem talk" that is usual in healthcare settings, tends to focus on the future rather than the past, to notice resources rather than problems or failures, to highlight the agency of the patient rather than their being a victim, and to build partnership between the interviewer and the patient. Noticing when the conversation is in solution talk can help the interviewer in assessing the interaction. While

---

[1] The descriptions of SFI and the questions offered here were influenced by a number of sources, both by the pioneers (de Shazer, Berg, Furman) and by my students, particularly the family medicine residents that I taught over the years. I do not claim, however, that any of them would endorse my formulation of the method.

problem talk is inevitable, the more the interaction can be conducted in solution talk, the more the patient is likely to experience their past, their current situation, and their future as empowering and energizing toward partnership on their health-care team.

Pre-visit Change Questions   help a patient notice any slight improvement that has occurred since they made the decision to come for a visit about a particular problem or symptom. These questions are particularly applicable in the first visit about the problem or symptom. The question can be phrased, "Sometimes when people make a decision to get help in addressing a problem or symptom, they notice that there is a slight easing of its intensity for a time before the visit occurs. Is that something that you noticed in your situation?" If the patient says everything stayed the same or got worse, the questioner can move on to another topic. If the patient says that things did get slightly better for a time, the next questions can be phrased to have them describe very briefly how they experienced things during that slightly easier time and if they did anything that seemed to correspond with that slight improvement. Whenever there is a report of things easing or getting slightly better, there is an opportunity to ask if the patient did anything that might have contributed to the improvement, however temporary. If they can identify something they did, the interviewer has helped to identify in the patient's mind an instance in which the patient had some effect on their situation or created the beginnings of a solution. If the patient can't identify anything that they did, the topic of their potentially being someone who makes a difference in their own problems or symptoms still has been broached. This introduces the topic of self-efficacy which will be useful to the interviewer and the patient in the future.

Note the incremental language: "slight improvement," "ease up a bit," "for a brief time." When people have struggled with physical, emotional, and/or social problems for a significant period of time, the changes and improvements that they can notice are likely to be small. Helping them begin to notice and to look for these small changes can make it easier for them to notice future improvements.

Coping Questions are helpful in the many situations in which patients cannot remember instances when things had been better or easier. At such a point in the conversation, the next question can be about how they have managed cope as well as they have. Another way to ask about coping is to enquire about how they have kept their situation from getting worse than it is. The question might be worded something like the following: "You have been facing this terrible difficulty for a long time. How have you managed to keep it from affecting your life (pick whatever fits — your work, your relationships, your family, your sobriety, your coping with your symptoms, etc.) even more than it has?" When the person can't think of anything that counts as coping, sometimes a question that can get a brief time of solution talk going is to say: "You know I work with a number of people with similar levels of struggles to the ones you face. I have to tell you that many of them, if they felt like you do today, would not have made it in for this visit. They would not have made it out of bed, much less have kept their appointment here. What was it that helped you make it to this visit in the face of the difficulties (or symptoms or pain) you have?"

Often the answer to the question about keeping the appointment is something that allows a second question that highlights the personality or values of the patient. If they say they made it to the appoint because they try to keep their commitments, the interviewer can ask if that determination to live up to their commitments is typical of them. If they say that they had to try to get some relief, the interviewer can observe that they seem to be determined to find some solution or improvement. Is that determination typical of their approach to troubles generally?

The word "determined" in the follow-up questions begins to create a characterization of the patient as showing self-efficacy, even in a very difficult situation in which they have not seen any relief to date.

What Would You Keep? When the patient's situation seems overwhelming, to the patient and to the interviewer, the "what would you keep?" question can be a way of changing into a conversation about what is working or is valuable in their lives. This is sometimes used as a part of creating an agenda for a visit or meeting. The interviewer has gone over the problem list and has heard of new problems that the patient brought on that day. They are preparing to focus on what can be addressed in the meeting time that is available. The question can be phrased in the following way: "You are facing so many difficulties, no one could blame you for wishing there was a way to get a life where your list of troubles was much shorter. Suppose you were able to make a lot of things change for yourself, what part of your current life, your current activities, your current relationships would you want to keep in any future time?"

Whatever elements the patient identifies are likely to be things that they identify as valued or as working. Those elements can then be the focus for a brief discussion in solution talk. How has the patient kept those elements going amid all their difficulties? How have those elements of their life helped or sustained them when they faced other challenges? Are there things that they learned in maintaining or growing those elements in their lives that they will use today as a help as they work with the current team member to address the challenges to be addressed in the current visit? Setting an agenda for work is more likely to be experienced as a partnership and as likely to be productive by the patient if they start the visit in solution talk.

If the conversation about what they would keep has already occurred, the visit can be started by asking about the life elements identified in the what-would-you-keep conversation earlier. The health professional might say, "I still remember when we talked before about how you would want to keep your relationship with your daughter as important, no matter how your life changed in other ways. Have you been able to do anything to maintain that relationship or to enjoy time with her since we talked?" To be able to keep this continuity of solution talk, it has to be documented. The health professional should include enough information in a note about what the patient would keep to remind both of them of the conversation next time. The note can also be helpful to other team members who know the significance of the question. Another team member who was meeting with the patient might say, "I can see in Dr. Peterson's note that no matter what we do, we want to be sure to support your relationship with your daughter. That is very helpful. So I can understand what works for you, maybe you can say a little about how you have been able to keep that relationship alive and valuable in the past."

Exception Questions are used to study times when things work better, even when the vast majority of the conversation is about problem times. Exception questions look for times when the problem did not happen, or happened with less intensity, or happened as usual but had a slightly less powerful impact on the patient or their functioning. To start a conversation about exceptions in a medical setting can usually be done by asking if the problem or symptom is worse on some days. Does the patient have bad days and good (or not as bad) days? In the majority of cases, the answer is yes. While the patient may expect the next question to be about the worse days, the interviewer focuses on the better days. What makes a better day? What happens or doesn't happen that lets the patient know it is going to be a better day? Is there any point on the day before the better day at which the patient could predict that the next day would be a better day? Is there anything that the patient does or that someone else does that seems to contribute to increasing the chances of a better day? For any of these questions, if the answer indicates some pattern to the exception, it can be investigated for another question or two.

Another way to identify an exception is to count instances of the problem. In a medical setting, it is common to ask patients to keep a pain diary, or a record of the intensity of their anxiety, or a record of some health behavior that they are trying to improve. When reviewing the diary at a subsequent visit, the interviewer who is looking for exceptions focuses on the days when things were less problematic or painful. Because the patient has kept the record of the better day, the study of the patterns on that day is experienced by patients as a reasonable focus of their care, not a failure to stay on target in looking at the problem.

Even when no day is identified as having an absence or less intensity of the problem, the interviewer can look for days on which the patient was able to maintain their functioning in some area slightly better than on other days with similar levels of the problem. The exception and the consequent solution talk in these situations are about the maintenance of function rather than about the lessening of the problem.

When patients do not have any idea of what they did to influence the exception that has been identified, it is possible to stay in solution talk by looking "downstream" from the exception. The patient can be asked what they are able to do or able to enjoy on the days when things are slightly better that they are not able to do or enjoy on the worst days. Any answer can be discussed for another question or two.

Interviewer: "It sounds like the days of lower pain come pretty much without warning. You can't see anything that you do or anything that you don't do that helps you have a less painful day. What can you do or what can you enjoy on one of your lower pain days that you can't do on a bad pain day?"

Patient: "I can sometimes go for a brief walk, just around the block or up to the corner store."

Interviewer: "What do you particularly enjoy about these walks, when you can take them?"

Patient: "I just like to get out. Sometimes I get to chat with my neighbor for a little while."

Interviewer: "Sounds like you have made some important relationships that you try to keep up when you can. Can you say a little more about that?"

Even if a patient cannot think of anything they do to influence the exception, if they can report the things they do when the exception occurs, they create a brief time to discuss their self-efficacy in those moments. Conversations about their self-efficacy, in whatever context, help patients build a sense of themselves as effective in some area of their lives. The dynamics of memory increase the likelihood of their remembering times of self-efficacy in other areas of their lives. The last question above, in which the interviewer tries out the idea that the patient has built a network of relationships based on the report of her chatting with a neighbor, is an example of looking for a pattern of efficacy when offered an exception to a problem pattern. Sometimes the patient doesn't agree that there is such a pattern and the topic can be dropped. Sometimes the patient agrees, and that pattern of self-efficacy can continue as a topic in future conversations.

The pattern of the exception, like any answer that describes a possible solution, should be documented with a sentence in the note of the visit. It is captured and made part of the information that informs future conversations and treatment. It becomes available for follow-up by other team members in their conversations with the patient. Solution talk can be a greater part of the interaction of the patient with the team when solution examples are documented and shared. All of the members of the team can present themselves as interested in solutions and as adding to their documentation when another example comes up in conversation. None of the other tasks that team members need to do in their interactions with the patient have to be dropped or curtailed because of added solution talk, unless those tasks become unnecessary because of solution talk. It is always easy to get back to the problems that need to be addressed in a visit by saying, "Maybe you and I can keep this (exception example) in mind as we try to get you more of your better days in the future."

Scaling Questions are ways of orienting the conversation to observing small changes, rather than looking for larger changes or resolutions that are unlikely at the time. Having people rate the difficulties of their symptoms on a scale, such as the 1–10 scale of pain, can help to discover exceptions in the problem or in the impact of the problem that otherwise would be unnoticed. Asking a patient "How was your week?" invites an answer that will be too general to bring a story of better days or better functioning to the patient's memory. Asking patients to rate the level of the symptom or of their functioning or to count instances of the occurrence of the problem every day gives access to the patient's memories about the exceptions that otherwise are not available. (For a way of helping patients keep records that can be the basis of solution-focused conversations, see the discussion of Tracking in the Appendix of Chap. 12).

"What-Might-It-Look-Like" Questions invite the patient to imagine specifically what their experience would be if the change that is a goal should come about. The more vividly the patient can experience in imagination the various aspects of life in the future they would like to achieve, the more they can have access to pieces of those experiences in the present. What-might-it-look-like questions can help in designating short-term goals, long-term goals, and treatment pathways as part of informal conversations with patients who otherwise might be uncomfortable with a "goal setting" meeting. Short-term goals are elicited by asking what event or observation would be the first sign of a solution developing. A long-term goal can be a formulated by asking the "miracle" question. A description of a treatment pathway sometimes emerges from a "how-did-it-heal" question.

An idea of the short-term solution can be elicited by asking about how the solution, or the improvement, would first be noticeable. The patient is asked, "If this problem were starting to improve, what would tip you off that an improvement that wasn't just temporary had begun?" The answer then can be examined further. Has that first indicator of an improvement happened before? Did you or someone else do anything that helped it happen? Has any part of it occurred recently? What will you begin to be able to do if that small change occurs? If the first answer is a bit general or seems to be an unrealistically large step toward a solution, a question that asks about the first element of that change can help define a more reachable goal.

Sometimes when a problem that has had recurrent cycles of being better and worse, the question can be phrased as, "What have you noticed in the past that let you know that the worst part of a bad period was past and you were starting to come out of a bad time and go into one of your better periods?" Simply studying all of the elements of the evolution from a bad period to a good period can make those elements more vivid and more accessible to the patient. The search for a more permanent solution can then be phrased, "What would happen in a better period that would let you know that this better time was going to last longer or be even better than the good periods in previous cycles?" In this situation, the elements that signal improvement can become a short-term goal, and the elements that would indicate a changing for the better of the overall pattern become the long-term goal.

Whenever a patient can articulate what would happen that would indicate that the beginning of a solution was starting, it can be helpful to follow with an exception question. If we know just what would indicate to the patient that things were just starting to improve, we can ask if that event has occurred recently. Often it has happened. That gives an example of a solution pattern to examine in more detail, more solution talk.

Interviewer: "If you were starting to get a handle on your diabetes, I don't mean get everything managed completely, but just the first step, what would you be likely to see happening?"

Patient:	"I guess I would start to take my medication more regularly. I often forget and sometimes I just don't feel like taking another pill."
Interviewer:	"How many doses in a row would you have to take for you to notice that you were starting to do slightly better at keeping on your schedule?"
Patient:	"I guess if I took it morning and night three days in a row, that would be different enough for me to think I was starting to be more regular."
Interviewer:	(Clear answer to a what-might-it-look-like question creates an opportunity for an exception question). "Has there been a time in the last few months that you can think of when you took your medication twice a day for three days in a row?"
Patient:	"I guess I did when I was at my sister's house. I did four days in a row then."
Interviewer:	"What was it about being at your sister's house that made it possible for you to be able to take care of your diabetes a bit better?"

Sometimes when a conversation like the one above is possible, the event that was going to be designated as a short-term goal turns out to have already occurred. Then the focus can be changed from having one occurrence of the event as the short-term goal to looking for multiple occurrences.

The "miracle" question is a way of helping a patient imagine their life in a world in which the current problem has resolved or lost its impact. De Shazer articulated the question in 1988, and it has continued to be used in essentially the same form since:

> Now I want to ask you a strange question. Suppose that while you are sleeping tonight and the entire house is quiet, a miracle happens. The miracle is that the problem which brought you here is solved. However, because you are sleeping, you don't know that the miracle has happened. So, when you wake up tomorrow morning, what will be different that will tell you that a miracle has happened and the problem which brought you here is solved? (de Shazer [19], p. 5)

The term "problem which brought you here" is a place holder for whatever problem is under discussion. Phrasing that problem in a way that makes it possibly solvable can be helpful and grounding in the process. Instead of saying "your diabetes was gone," saying "your difficulties managing your diabetes were gone" might be more possible for the patient to imagine. Instead of saying "your trauma never happened," saying "the power that your traumatic experiences have over your life was completely gone" would make the goal more accessible.

It is important that the question focus the patient experientially on what they would see or hear or think or notice as they went through their day and discovered the miracle. What would or would not occur that would indicate that the problem was resolved. This is different from asking at the start for a list of all the changes that would have occurred. The miracle question should focus on one problem area in the lives of multiply-disadvantaged patients with complex health issues, rather than on a resolution of all problems. The follow-up discussion between the health professional and the patient about the patient's imagined experience after the focus problem was miraculously resolved can then look at what the impact of that resolution would be on other problem areas. This conveys a picture of the way that, for most people, any significant improvement in one problem area is likely to have positive impacts on other problem areas. That means that as the patient improves in one area, their hope and experience of self-efficacy can be improving to at least a small degree in others.

An example:

Interviewer: Now I want to ask you a strange question. Suppose while you are sleeping tonight and all the house is quiet, a miracle happens. The miracle is that your depression is over. However, because you are sleeping, you don't know that the miracle has happened. So when you wake up in the morning, what will tell you that a miracle has happened and the depression that you have been coping with for so long has gone.

Patient: I guess if my depression was really gone, I would want to get out of bed and go make breakfast for me and my grandson.

Interviewer: What else might you notice as you get further into the day?

Patient: I guess I would be more interested in what my grandson was going to do at school when we talked at breakfast and I would clean up the dishes when I got back from walking him to the bus.

Interviewer: Anything else?

Patient: I probably would go for a walk or maybe call and talk to my sister.

Interviewer: So if you had a morning where you wanted to get out of bed, you liked making breakfast for you and your grandson, you were interested in what he was going to do that day at school, you cleaned up the kitchen when you got back from walking him to the bus and you felt like going for a walk or calling your sister, what would you be telling yourself about how your day was going and about your depression?

Patient: I guess I would notice that I was having a really good day.

Interviewer: What would happen sooner or later that would let you know that your depression was really not coming back, not just that you were having a good day?

Patient: I guess if my grandson had a problem at school, if he didn't do his homework or if he got in trouble and it didn't make me really sad or angry and make me go back to hating to get up in the morning, that would let me know that things were really changed.

Interviewer: Suppose you were doing so much better, how would that help you with your diabetes?

Patient: Well, for one thing, I would feel like getting more exercise because I would like walking. I guess I would feel like it was worth it to do all the stuff I am supposed to do for my diabetes because I would feel like I had more good times to look forward to.

Interviewer: How do you think the disappearance of your depression would affect your grandson?

Patient: I guess he would worry about me less and maybe do better in school.

It is possible for this kind of conversation, exploring the impact of the miracle, to go in multiple directions and to be continued as part of multiple visits. In the process of the conversation, the elements that would be involved in achieving the long-term goal can be enumerated. For the patient in the example, getting up quickly, talking to her grandson at breakfast, getting exercise, being in contact with other family members, and doing a targeted amount of cleaning can be isolated as things to be tracked. To keep the process from seeming impossible, at any point in which a long-term goal needs to be articulated, the term "resolved" could give way to "significant progress." Tracking any or all of these elements can mean to the patient that they watch themselves approach an element of the long-term goal. Always be sure, when reviewing any tracking form or diary that the patient keeps to ask how the patient was able to do as many of the elements of the goal as they were able to do, rather than why they didn't do more.

How-did-it-heal questions are useful after a patient has begun to make progress on a problem. In situations in which there is a good relationship between the interviewer and the patient, sometimes it is possible to help the patient imagine the solution or visualize achieving the goal in a way that helps them imagine the entire pathway to achieving that goal. I have often been surprised at the clarity and specificity of the steps to the goal that a patient has produced in response to this question. When the question works, the steps that they imagine can be incorporated into the treatment plan as the patient's expectation of the course of treatment.

To ask a how-did-it-heal question, the interviewer invites the patient to imagine a time in the future when the problem is resolved and then to imagine telling the story of the journey to the resolution to the interviewer as part of a chance meeting on the street. In the future scene, the patient is characterized as managing their life without professional help in the problem area.

An example:

Interviewer: I know you've been struggling with this problem for a good while and you are just beginning to feel like you are getting a handle on it, but let me ask you to imagine a time in the future after your current efforts have had time to really pay off. Let's imagine that you are able to reach your goal in terms of this problem. You don't have to be working on it anymore. Keeping on track is much easier. You haven't been seeing me or anyone else about this problem for a good while. How long in the future do you think we are talking about?

Patient: I don't know, maybe five years?

Interviewer: So, let's imagine it's five years from now. You reached your goal in this area and you are focusing on other areas of your life. And let's say you and I run into each other on the street or in Walmart or someplace, and we say hello, and I say that I am glad to see you looking so well. And I say, "I haven't seen you in years, you look like you are really thriving, what's working for you?" and you say, "you know that problem we were working on? I pretty much put that behind me a while ago and now I am on to another part of my life" and I say "so what did you do to make this work, to get to where you are?" What would you tell me? What would be your story of how you got yourself to where you are?

Patient: Well, I guess I would say that first I kept sober finally. That was real important. Then maybe I went back to the job training program and I did the whole thing. And after that I got a job and got my own place … got my own place, and from there I started to be able to visit with my kids regularly.

As the patient is telling the story, the interviewer can help make the details richer by commenting on the emotional experience that would likely go with any of the success experiences the patient describes. Comments such as "that must have made you pretty proud" or "I'll bet your kids were happy about that" help the patient experience each step more vividly and thereby be more specific with the steps that they create.

The conversation can be capped with a statement by the interviewer that it seems that the patient, consciously or unconsciously, has a plan for their future that they have been working on. The interviewer can suggest that maybe it will be possible to talk in the future about how they could use help for some of the parts of their plan and how they are likely to handle some aspects of their plan on their own.

8.3 Solution-Focused Questions and Different Team Roles

Each member of the team can use solution-focused questions in ways that fit the tasks that are part of their role. There is no question that needs to be the sole province of one role or of a particular license. Questions are not inherently medical or mental health in character. Different teams are made up of members with different roles. Teams working with multiply-disadvantaged patients might have more members than teams for patients presenting less complexity. Team members will have varying levels of engagement with different patients and be able to ask different sorts of questions depending on their level of engagement with each. Patients will present widely varying sorts of problems and illnesses, for which different questions will be a fit. The examples below are just to suggest some common possibilities, not to assign types of questions to particular roles.

A medical assistant doing vitals for a patient with hypertension who notices a lower blood pressure than the last visit can ask if the patient had been doing anything to try to help with their BP. If the answer is yes, the MA can say that she will make a note that the patient has been working on blood pressure because the doctor will want to hear more about it. If there is an open conversation (see Chap. 7) between the MA and the doctor in the exam room with the patient, the fact that the patient was making efforts on her blood pressure would be mentioned. If there is no overlap, the doctor can mention the MA's note before asking about what the patient had been doing for her blood pressure. Passing solution talk from one role to another as part of the patient's visit sets a tone of respect and engagement that makes the team a positive reality for the patient.

The doctor might use an exception question as part of discussing the pattern of the occurrence of a symptom. Asking about times when a symptom occurred can give hints into what might be causing or triggering the symptom. If the symptom is happening regularly, asking about times when the symptom does not occur might give hints into what tends to prevent or alleviate the symptom. A quick question about whether the patient can identify anything that they or anyone else did that might have helped create the symptom free (or symptom reduced) period can lead to a quick characterization of the patient as already having some success in dealing with symptoms. This highlights the patient's efficacy in the situation and can help support future partnership of the patient.

The behavioral health clinician can use coping questions in engaging patients, exceptions questions in supporting a developing process of change, and what-might-it-look-like questions when they have time to talk in depth about a problem pattern with which a patient is struggling. In fact, most BHCs can spend a good part of their day in solution talk, working on depression, anxiety, substance use, and health behavior change and consulting to other team members.

Care enhancers will probably use coping questions quite a lot. They will be the team members most likely to see the specific ways that the social determinants of health are affecting their patients' lives. That knowledge lets them ask questions about how people have coped with, for example, homelessness, trauma, challenges of the dominant culture, challenges of the culture of the medical system, personal loss, unemployment, or trying to keep a job. In the case of any of these examples of coping, the care enhancer can share a sentence or two with coping story they obtain from the patient with the other team members. Through the brief notes of the CE, the whole team gets more knowledgeable about the patient's strengths and successes in their situation.

8.4 Summary

The methodology of solution-focused interviewing provides a way to start the process of empowering multiply-disadvantaged patients by helping them experience their self-efficacy in relation to their health, a basic step that can help them participate as partners with their doctors and health teams. As members of the healthcare team ask questions that focus patients on their own abilities to find solutions, the perception of these patients about themselves and the perception of them by the members of their health teams tend to evolve. Both sides experience the patient as more capable and tend to experience the team as more perceptive. This lays and important foundation for motivational interviewing and shared decision-making. The transparency of information about the patient in a practice seen in the use of open notes and open clinical conversations creates an important vehicle for sharing the solutions envisioned and achieved by the patient. In the next chapter, we will explore the way in which a solution-focused information exchange creates an environment in which multiply-disadvantaged patients can become activated for improving their health.

References

1. Berwick D. What 'patient-centered' should mean: confessions of an extremist. Health Aff. 2009;28:w555–65.
2. Delbanco T, Berwick DM, Boufford JI, et al. Healthcare in the land called PeoplePower: nothing about me without me. Health Expect. 2001;4:144–50.
3. Bodenheimer T, Lorig K, Holman H, Grumbach K. Patient self-management of chronic disease in primary care. JAMA. 2002;288:2469–75.
4. Mautner DB, Pang H, Brenner JC, Shea JA, Gross KS, Frasso R, Cannuscio CC. Generating hypotheses about care needs of high utilizers: lessons from patient interviews. Popul Health Manag. 2013;16:S26–33.
5. Agency for Healthcare Research and Quality (AHRQ). National healthcare quality and disparities report. Rockville: Agency for Healthcare Research and Quality (AHRQ); 2016. July 2017. AHRQ Pub. No. 17-0001.
6. Willems S, De Maesschalck S, Deveugele M, Derese A, De Maeseneer J. Socio-economic status of the patient and doctor-patient communication: does it make a difference? Patient Educ Couns. 2005;56:139–46.
7. Harris M, Fallot R, editors. Using trauma theory to design service systems. San Francisco: Jossey-Bass; 2001.
8. Krause DJ, Green SA, Koury SP, Hales TW. Solution-focused trauma-informed care (SF-TIC): an integration of models. J Publ Child Welfare. 2018;12:117–35.
9. Cooperrider DL, Whitney D. A positive revolution in change: appreciative inquiry. Oakland: Berrett-Koehler; 2005.
10. De Jong P, Berg IK. Interviewing for solutions. 4th ed. Belmont: Brooks/Cole; 2013.
11. Watzlawick P, Weakland J, Fisch R. Change: principles of problem formulation and problem resolution. New York: W. W. Norton; 1974.
12. Gingerich WJ, de Shazer S, Weiner-Davis M. Constructing change: a research view of interviewing. In: Lipchik E, editor. Interviewing. Rockville: Aspen; 1988.
13. Gottman JM. Marital interaction. New York: Academic Press; 1979.
14. Hasselmo ME. How we remember: brain mechanisms of episodic memory. Cambridge: MIT Press; 2013.
15. Cappas NM, Andres-Hyman R, Davidson L. What psychotherapists can begin to learn from neuroscience: seven principles of brain-based psychotherapy. Psychother Theory Res Pract Train. 2005;42:374–83.
16. Garry M, Polaschek D. Reinventing yourself: who you are is limited only by your imagination. Psychol Today. 1999;32:65–9.
17. Bannink F. 1001 solution-focused questions. New York: W. W. Norton; 2010.
18. Furman B, Ahola T. Solution talk: hosting therapeutic conversations. New York: W. W. Norton; 1992.
19. De Shazer S. Clues: investigating solutions in brief therapy. New York: W. W. Norton; 1988.

Resources

Solution-Focused Interviewing

Furman, B., and Ahola, T. (1992). Solution talk: Hosting therapeutic conversations. New York: W. W. Norton. A classic book in the field that can be borrowed at no cost with examples of SFI conversations from a broad range of settings and with many types of problems and symptoms. https://archive.org/details/solutiontalkhost00furm

Chapter 9
"A" Is for Activating

9.1 Patient Activation: The Concept and the Practices

There are a number of concepts used in medical literature to reflect the understanding that despite advances in medical treatments, the largest factor in how well patients with chronic diseases do in the long run is a product of how well they take care of their own health. Whether or not they take their medicine, get exercise, avoid tobacco or too much alcohol, eat a healthy diet, and do other actions to control their particular chronic illness will make a major difference in how well they are able to function and in how long they live. Where the standard of care was once focused largely on proper prescribing and other actions taken by health professionals, now the standard of care is becoming focused on ways of influencing patients to do their part in their own care.

In the case of chronic illness care, the patient is the most important member of the team, whether health professionals or patients like it or not. Concepts such as stages of change in health behaviors [1], health locus of control [2], self-efficacy in self-management [3], self-determination theory [4], and patient engagement [5, 6] reflect the array of efforts at understanding what makes patients more likely to take the actions that only they can take to improve or maintain their health. Each of these concepts is now supported by a metric to locate a patient's functioning with regard to an ideal. Some of these concepts have spawned broad adoption efforts involving training of professionals to use the methods shown to move patients along the metric of the concept.

The concept of "patient activation" is one in this line of research, one that has rapidly growing acceptance currently. The concept measures an amalgam of the will, the knowledge, the skills, and the confidence that the patient has, to predict the likelihood that they will take the actions necessary to manage their illnesses and to stay healthy. It has had broad acceptance in part because of the elegance of an instrument for measuring patient activation that embodies a rigorous definition to the concept. The Patient Activation Measure (PAM) [7] is good at distinguishing

© Springer Nature Switzerland AG 2019   147
A. Blount, *Patient-Centered Primary Care*,
https://doi.org/10.1007/978-3-030-17645-7_9

which patients are likely, and which are not likely, to be active in self-care for their chronic illnesses. Because of its success as a prediction of health behavior, it can be used as an intermediate outcome to measure interventions that would take too long to show the changes in patients' health status that good self-care eventually brings [8]. The ability of the PAM to sort patients hierarchically into groups that are more and less likely to do successful self-care means it can be used to target specific interventions to patients based on their answers to the questions of the measure.

The Patient Activation Measure was constructed through a multistep process involving many experts and patients that isolated a consensus list of the core elements of "activation" in healthcare [7]. The measure is based on self-report of the patient about their beliefs and abilities. The original form of the PAM had 22 items, but a reliable short form with 13 items was developed shortly after the introduction of the first form [9]. The 13-question short form and a subsequent 10-question version are both currently in wide use. Subsequent testing has shown that people whose responses are higher on the PAM tend to behave in more activated ways in relation to their health. The beliefs and self-descriptions measured by PAM do predict people's health behaviors well. It sorts patients into groups that can be studied further.

The PAM is built on a developmental model of activation, meaning that it assumes that patients go through the PAM's four levels of activation in sequence. A patient with low activation is likely to first need to believe that they have an important role to play in maintaining their health and then to gain elementary knowledge about their condition and their treatments. Those who achieve that step will then need to develop skills and confidence so that they practice self-care for their specific illness burden. Finally, in their development toward higher levels of activation, they need to learn to maintain their health gains in the face of stress.

One shortcoming of the PAM is that its concept of activation tends to be patient focused rather than patient-in-context focused. It measures the patient's ability to maintain gains in relation to context factors (stress) only for the highest stage of activation. The impact of stress on patients' confidence in their importance as part of their healthcare team, or in their ability to take the actions that are needed for self-management, for example, is not measured.

The role of context, however, is very important in understanding which patients are identified as being at different levels of activation. While there have not been any nationally representative samples done, multiple smaller studies have found that demographics are powerful correlates of activation [10–12]. In a study by Smith and his colleagues [12] of 3400 patients, higher patient activation was shown to be associated with higher income ($p < 0.001$), higher levels of education ($p < 0.01$), better self-rated health ($p < 0.001$), and having fewer chronic conditions ($p < 0.05$). Wealthier, better educated patients who have fewer illnesses and feel that they are healthy are the people who show up as most activated on the PAM. The converse wasn't stressed, but the data said that patients with lower incomes and lower education levels, who experience themselves to be in poorer health, are the patients that the PAM shows to have lower levels of activation. The more a patient might be classified as "complex" in other literature, or as fitting the "multiply-disadvantaged" term we have used in previous chapters, the lower their initial activation score is likely to be. Demographics are not destiny, however, in that patients with low activation scores can make the most gains when interventions to improve activation are offered [13].

Patients with lower activation scores tend to have different ideas of what constitutes good self-care than patients with higher scores based on their having different understandings of what constitutes an ideal relationship between a patient and their doctor [14]. This study involved in-depth interviews with patients whose scores represented every level of activation. At lower levels of activation, patients identified compliance with the directions of the doctor as constituting better self-management of their condition. They believed that patients who do what they are told to do by their doctor are doing their part of the physician-patient relationship. At higher levels of activation, patients identified partnership with the doctor as the best physician-patient relationship for successful self-management.

Given the finding about patients' different conceptions of the doctor-patient relationship, it makes sense that less activated patients have been found to be less likely to perceive shared decision-making with their doctor as a value. As patients' level of activation rises, they report interest in sharing decision-making with their doctors on more types of medical decisions. The most activated patients want to participate in shared decisions relating to lifestyle, preventive screening, choosing treatments, choosing between medications, and deciding the necessity of a diagnostic test [12]. Patients with low levels of activation, complex patients, cannot be assumed to want to participate in shared decision-making despite the literature that promotes shared decision-making as the fix for building partnership for complex patients [15].

Another difference between patients with low and high activation scores was identified by Aung and her colleagues [16] when they added a measure of patients' experience of the quality of care that they receive to the assessment of their level of activation. All of the patients in the study had type 2 diabetes. The outcome measure was the level of glycemic control patients maintained. For patients with high levels of activation, the quality of care had little effect on their glycemic control. They tended to have good control, whether or not they thought they were getting the best care. It was for patients with low activation that the quality of care made a significant difference in how well they controlled their blood sugar. Patients tended to interpret their perceptions of the quality of care they got as reflecting their health professionals' judgment of the care they deserved. Whether or not they are seen by their health professionals as deserving the best care was important to the patients we have called "multiply-disadvantaged" and made an important difference in their levels of adherence.

While some approaches emphasize patients' lack of knowledge about their chronic condition as a central explanation for poor self-management [17], in the study by Dixon et al. [14], lack of knowledge was identified by only a small number of low activation patients as a barrier. As patients gain activation, their own searching for information increases [18]. In fact, patients at low levels of activation had learned strategies for self-care from professionals and from trial and error, just as patients with high activation had done. The difference was that patients with high activation were applying that knowledge consistently. Patients with low activation levels tended to see their low self-confidence about making requests of their physicians, their perceptions of their physicians' lack of respect for them, and their lack of ability to successfully carry out self-care actions as much more significant barriers.

Patients with low activation scores get significant benefit from both interventions designed to improve their skills at self-care and from interventions designed to improve their self-assertion in interacting with their physicians. This improvement in activation is particularly true of patients whose low activation is combined with passive relational styles in their interactions with their doctors [13]. This group showed the highest increase in activation when they were taught how to formulate questions to ask in their visits with their physicians. In the intervention, interviewers helped patients become aware of common health-related decisions in several domains and brainstormed questions that might help them make the decisions from that list that were relevant to them. Patients practiced prioritizing information and developing questions with the help of the interviewer, and, perhaps most importantly, they were reminded that the questioning they were learning was expected by their doctors and is associated with better health outcomes. In some team-based care settings, one team member is explicitly assigned to help patients formulate questions, and sometimes even role play asking them, before their visits with their doctors [19].

Measuring activation does not distinguish which patients will struggle with certain barriers to self-care [14]. Patients at all levels of activation perceived the symptoms of their illness, such as pain, as barriers to self-care. Many listed multiple drug combinations and the potential side effects as a barrier. Perhaps the most telling agreement about barriers among patients across levels of activation was the report that feelings of stress and depression were significant in impeding their being able to manage their conditions. This finding supports the routine assessment of the "footprint" of the disease and its treatments in patients' lives as part of deciding what care and what self-care to recommend [20]. It also supports a routine (more than once a year) screening for depression and anxiety for all patients with chronic illness, whether they are highly activated or not.

The authors of the studies of patients with different levels of activation make certain limited recommendations about what can be done to help patients with low activation scores improve the likelihood of their achieving successful self-care. At the same time, they tend to be much less confident about their recommendations for interventions than they are about their research findings. Smith and his colleagues [12] endorse programs that teach these patients to ask better questions and feel more confident in their medical visits [13], but they stress that multifaceted approaches are likely to be necessary to help patients with low activation achieve partnership in decisions with their doctors. Aung and her team [16] offer a recommendation: "The benefits of good quality chronic care can be best seen in patients at low levels of activation, and health care providers should ensure that these patients receive the full range of chronic care including self-management support, follow-up, and care coordination. On the other hand, improving activation in patients may serve as a safety net when care is deficient" (p. 123). Dixon et al. [14], stressing the importance of building self-confidence, suggest that reminding patients of their past experiences of success in managing their health is likely to be a useful strategy in instilling self-efficacy for new self-management actions in the future (p. 264). It is a strategy that fits nicely with a solution-focused approach to building confidence.

As I look at the research on patient activation and particularly descriptions of patients with the lowest levels of activation, I am drawn back to the picture of the chasm between some patients and their doctors that is the theme of Chap. 5. Activated patients tend to have higher income, be better educated, and have images of themselves as being healthy people. They see partnership with their doctors as a desirable element in their managing any illness and in maintaining their health. They appreciate high-quality care and are likely to act in ways that elicit good care and partnership [18, 21]. On the other hand, they don't need best practices in order to stay healthy. The picture of patients with very low activation is similar to the picture of complex patients or multiply-disadvantaged patients in Chap. 5. They tend to have low income with lower education levels. Whether they have more chronic illnesses, they experience themselves as less healthy. They are not confident in their dealings with their doctors, and they are very sensitive to whether or not they are being given good care. If they experience their care as of lower quality, they are less likely to take the actions necessary for managing their conditions. They are more likely to experience the asymmetries of power and social status in their relationships with their doctors and to feel that they are treated unfairly by their doctors [18].

Patients designated as complex, or as deprived, or as trauma victims (to a great degree the same group of patients; see Chap. 5) have high rates of depression. Patients found to have the lowest activation meet the same description. Magnezi and her colleagues [22] studied the relationship of patient activation to depression for 278 patients. The participants were recruited from all the adults who visited two participating doctors at each of two primary care clinics during the same 53-day span of time. Patients were given the PAM plus a measure of depression (PHQ-9) and a measure of perceived quality of life (SF-12). The scores on the PAM correlated negatively with the PHQ-9, i.e., the more activated, the less depressed ($p = 0.0001$), and correlated positively with the SF-12, i.e., the more activated, the higher the reported quality of life ($p = 0.0001$). Of the patients who scored at the lowest level of activation, the majority of patients (58%) scored at or above the PHQ-9 threshold of 10, the point at which patients can be expected to meet criteria for a diagnosis of depression [23]. Symptoms of depression can be part of a picture that is also called low activation. Patients who are depressed are less likely to be actively involved in self-care [22]. A group of patients at all of the levels of activation were positive on their depression screen.

The PAM is not a stand-in for depression screening. However, for patients displaying lower activation levels, the possible role of depression treatment should be considered as one way of facilitating activation. Effective activation efforts can also have an impact on lowering depression scores [22]. In this study, of the patients who were identified as depressed by the PHQ-9, 93% said they would like to have treatment or follow-up for depression in primary care by their family doctor. Depression treatment in primary care by a behavioral health clinician who is part of the same team as their doctor is acceptable to most patients, with or without their doctor prescribing medication treatment (see Chap. 3). This can be a good plan because brief treatments for depression in primary care such as solution-focused therapy [24], cognitive behavioral therapy [25], or acceptance and commitment therapy [26] can all be effective in helping patients become more successful at coping with chronic illness and improving self-care.

The suggestions for interventions with patients identified as having low activation are in line with the emphases so far on empowerment and transparency. Recommendations advise that these patients receive the full array of best practices: care coordination, coaching in how to formulate and ask questions about their healthcare, and efforts to build their self-confidence in relation to their own self-care as well as in relation to their health professionals. These patients need to feel that when they are asking questions or expressing their concerns in the process of their care, they are doing the "right" thing and that their participation is expected and valued. In the rest of this chapter, we will discuss ways of adapting the empowerment approaches described in the last chapter specifically to building the skills and confidence of patients in their roles as patients, as partners with their health professionals, and as self-managers of their health conditions.

9.2 Building Expectations for Activation

The tools of empowerment described in Chap. 8 that can be so effective in building engagement and partnership can be targeted with very minor adaptations toward building patient activation. Adaptation or targeting requires only looking for exceptions, or successful coping, or a vision of a successful future, which are the elements of empowerment, in the specific areas that have been identified as comprising successful activation. Where solution-focused questions look for strengths in any area relevant to the complex problems that multiply-disadvantaged patients face, activation focuses the same techniques on the specific elements that are necessary to successfully manage one's chronic illnesses in partnership with one's health professionals.

Interventions targeting the activation level of patients, whatever else they may impact in the way of knowledge or skills or confidence, also involve trying to change expectations. These interventions must change the expectations of patients about themselves and about their health professionals as well as change the expectations of health professionals about the patients. In this case, I am using "expectations" to mean what a person consciously or unconsciously predicts will happen in a situation or relationship, rather than in the sense of "standards" that a person should meet to achieve a goal.

The power of expectations to influence events in relationships has received a great deal of attention in psychology. One of the most famous studies of the power of expectations was led by Robert Rosenthal [27]. His study tried to assess the impact of elementary school teachers' expectations (predictions) about their students on how well they would learn. The study involved manipulating the expectations of teachers in a way that would not be acceptable in research today. All of the students in an elementary school south of San Francisco were given an IQ test. The teachers were told that it was a special test designed to identify students with previously unrecognized learning potential. A list was given to each teacher of the likely "growth spurters" in their class. The core deception was that this list contained randomly generated names, rather than being based on any results of the test. Their potential "spurters" were just randomly selected kids.

When the IQ test was administered again at the end of the year, the randomly selected students on the list had made nonrandom gains in their IQ scores. The most dramatic gains ("spurters," +27 points; controls, +12 points) were made by students in the first grade. The second grade also showed significant results. In the higher grades, the differences were much smaller or nonexistent. The finding later confirmed in numerous other studies [28] was that enhanced expectations on the part of teachers or therapists or researchers can make significant and sometimes dramatic differences in the performance of students, patients, or research subjects. In the elementary school study, Rosenthal and Jacobson speculated that these expectations were enacted in subtle ways, ways of which teachers tended not to be conscious, and that these subtle changes had very real impacts on students. A change of tone of voice, an expression of optimism that the child could learn a concept or complete a task successfully, a moment of particularly positive focus on a child's success, and likely many other even more subtle manifestations all worked together to influence the child's perception of themselves and to create mutually increased confidence in the child's learning abilities.

The effect of expectations was conceptualized as circular. Others' beliefs about us cause others' actions toward us which reinforce our beliefs about ourselves which influence our actions toward others which impact others' beliefs about us. Rosenthal called this cycle of changing expectations leading to changing behavior leading to changing expectations the Pygmalion effect.

As Rosenthal and others attempted to reproduce the Pygmalion effect, they found that it only worked when the authority was unconscious of having their expectations affected [29]. When teachers or other authorities "acted as if" they had higher expectations, the results were not nearly so positive. The authority had to believe the evidence for the new expectations.

The attenuating of the Pygmalion effect in the upper grades speaks to the difficulty of changing expectations for people who have a history of functioning in a given way. The longer students had been in school, the more time they and their teachers had had to observe their functioning and to form expectations (predictions) about their functioning in the future. A longer history of functioning has more power to keep future expectations constant, though new information, if it is believed, still can make a measurable difference.

In considering how expectations might be relevant for patients with low activation who have complex and expensive health burdens, who are multiply-disadvantaged, who have long histories of coping with chronic illnesses, and who face behavioral health challenges and other challenges in the area of the social determinants of health, the concept of the impact of attributions can be an important addition. "Attribution" is another way of naming what Rosenthal calls "our beliefs about ourselves," "others' beliefs about us," and "our beliefs about others."

If I believe that I am a healthy person and that I have a history that shows I can manage my health effectively, I am likely to expect or predict that I will manage my next health challenge effectively. None of this necessarily will be conscious or spoken overtly. It is an assumption about what sort of person I am. It might be what we could call an "implicit attribution" about myself. If my doctor says to me, "I know that this is a challenge for you, but you have always done so well in the past in managing health issues that I expect you will do well this time also," we might call that an "explicit attribution." An explicit attribution will be helpful in strengthening my own expectations of my functioning – if I believe it. There, as Hamlet would say, is the rub. If, instead, I think of myself as a sickly person who has difficulty managing health challenges, particularly if I have a long history of struggling with health challenges, and I hear my doctor or other health professional say that they are sure I will do well with the new challenge I am facing, I am likely to find their explicit attribution unconvincing and even alienating. I am likely to experience the positive attribution from the expert who should be helping me as being out of touch with my situation. In addition, if my doctor is expressing expectations (predictions) about how I will do that I believe are unrealistic, it means that either my doctor is poorly informed or is not being truthful with me. Either contributes to my experience of alienation.

We know that in the case of patients with complex health burdens, multiply-disadvantaged patients who are likely to show low activation, doctors tend to change their approach to care, becoming more directive and less partnership oriented [30, 31]. The implicit attribution drawn by patients from such a relationship is that they do not have the knowledge or skills or confidence to manage their conditions. The behavior of their health team implicitly indicates what others think of them. We talked in Chap. 5 about the reciprocal process set up between multiply-disadvantaged patients and their clinicians. These patients who are less healthy are also less likely to engage actively in a visit. They are more likely to internalize stigma about themselves from the implicit attributions they perceive in the care they are given. They need more experiences of support and positive relating than more advantaged, more activated patients to receive the intended benefit from their care. Yet they commonly receive more directive and less supportive care from providers. Health professionals mistakenly assume that these patients are less active in visits because they want less information or care less about their health than more activated patients, making a more directive, less patient-centered approach seem to be best for them. The concept of low activation which fits these patients can become both a cause and an effect in the reciprocal cycle. This is not to suggest that health professionals should act as if they expect patients with low activation to successfully understand and manage their health conditions and their treatments. To do that would be to ask them to be disingenuous with their patients which is unreasonable and possibly unethical.

How can we help the doctor and the health team on one hand and the less acti-vated patient on the other to move beyond this impasse? Let's go back to the discus-sion about solution-focused interviewing and the neuroscience of memory in Chap. 8. We saw that when a person makes a generalization or an attribution about them-selves, based on the episodes they remember, that attribution tends to influence what other episodes can be remembered. People remember events that fit with their cur-rent attributions about themselves. When solution-focused questions help the per-son to notice or discover exceptions to their generalization about themselves, they are often able to remember other events that fit the new pattern, leading to a new implicit attribution that fits the new discovery. This provides new data to modify the expectations of both the patient and the interviewer. Memories of exceptions to problem patterns which provide clear examples of the patient managing better than they or their clinician might have expected offer the possibility of new explicit attri-butions. The new attributions can be a way of solidifying the impact of the discovery for both patient and interviewer.

Sometimes the new explicit attribution can come from the patient:

Interviewer: When you remember a time like the one you just mentioned, when you handled things well, how does that impact how you think of yourself in this situation?

Patient: I guess I can be more effective than I usually give myself credit for.

Sometimes the attributions can come from the interviewer:

Interviewer: When you remember an incident like this, where you handled things so well, I start to get the impression that you have more ability to handle this problem than you give yourself credit for. Does that sound sensible to you?

Explicit attributions made by the clinician need to be offered tentatively. If a clinician says confidently that the patient has skills or abilities in relation to their health that they have not been aware of, even after a clear exception to the problem pattern has been found through solution-focused interviewing, the statement creates the implicit attribution that the interviewer knows more about the patient than the patient knows about him or herself. This is not a message, no matter how positive it is, that fosters partnership. By offering explicit attributions about a person's commitment, knowledge, or self-confidence in a way that is tentative, the implicit attribution is that the patient is the final arbiter of whether an explicit attribution about them is valid. The interviewer is modeling the same relationship that they would like to encourage, that the patient will be the final decider about their health and healthcare.

The interviewer as well as the patient needs to believe a new attribution when an exception based on solution-focused questioning is uncovered. This is possible when the initial articulation of the attribution is tentative, a trial balloon, for the interviewer as well. When the attribution is thought of as trying out an idea to see if it fits, the tentative formulation is genuine, and, when the patient accepts an explicit attribution based on actual events, both the interviewer and the patient tend to expe-rience that attribution as valid to some degree.

Offering an explicit attribution tentatively requires that the interviewer accepts the patient's judgment about the validity of the attribution without question or argument. The patient is the best authority about themselves, their actions, and their potential. Offering an explicit attribution can be effective even if the attribution is not accepted at the time. Often, in my experience, a patient denies a positive attribution when it is offered, only to report later that they kept thinking about it and found it useful. Sometimes offering an explicit attribution can start the interviewer thinking differently, even when it is not accepted by the patient. In those situations, the interviewer can maintain an impression, even after agreeing with the patient that it is probably wrong:

Interviewer: When you described how you quit smoking on your own after 15 years of resisting your family's pressure to quit, I got the impression that you have a determination about you that is powerful. Whether you are determined to do something or not to do it, you make your health actions follow your determination. Does that sound right to you?

Patient: You give me too much credit. I think I just don't have any will power.

Interviewer: Well, you know yourself better than anyone. I will try to believe that you just don't have will power, but I can't promise that I'll succeed in believing it.

Solution-focused questions and explicit attributions make good pairs. A solution-focused exception question would ask about the times when a patient took specific actions that helped manage their health:

Interviewer: I see that it is very hard for you to get exercise in the face of all the other demands on your time, yet on Tuesday and Friday you somehow managed to take the walk you were hoping to take every day. What was it about those days that made it possible for you to get your walk in, even though I am sure it wasn't easy?

Patient: I got things cleaned up from breakfast earlier those days, so I had time before I had to go to work.

The patient's answer then can open an opportunity for an attribution that is a generalization about the patient's commitment to their health:

Interviewer: When we talk about how you tried to put things together to be able to get in your walk, I get the sense that you have a growing determination to find a way to manage your diabetes better. Does that sound right to you?

Patient: I guess I am thinking about it more these days.

One way of making attributions that are on target for supporting activation is to target the elements of activated functioning in those attributions. Because the concept of activation is based on a hierarchy of beliefs and actions, it provides a pathway for matching solution-focused questions and attributions with the current state of activation that a patient expresses [7]. At the lowest level, questions or attributions would look for instances in which a patient's statements or actions indicated that they believed in the importance of their role in managing their illness, rather than simply following their health professional's instructions. This would be discovering that a patient was moving from the lowest level of activation to the second level. In another instance a health professional might highlight an exception or an example of coping that demonstrated the patient's determination to get the information they needed to do their part in managing their illness. A patient could be observed looking for information on their own, or using information supplied by their health team, or asking more questions and sharing their concerns with their doctor. This would be an example of a patient who was moving from the second to the third level of activation. Finally, a patient might be observed either by what they said or what they did, to be using information that they had gathered, or to be using the habits of self-care they had developed, or to be using their partnership with their health professionals, to maintain their successful management of their illness in the face is particularly challenging life stresses. This would be a transition from level three to level four in the patient activation hierarchy.

While using the levels of activation as a template has been shown to be useful for clinicians, teaching the levels of activation to patients is not likely to be useful. Doing this tends to set up the levels as steps patients are expected to climb, or the level of a patient can become an explicit attribution about them that can tend to fix the patient where they are.

Sometimes attributions are made on the basis of behavior that occurs as part of the relationship with the patient rather than based on solution-focused questioning. These explicit attributions can be a way of defining the patient's behavior differently than the patient expects their behavior to be defined. They can redefine the motivation or the impact of the behavior. These explicit attributions are a way of putting into practice the redefinitions that were part of writing open notes that we described in Chap. 7:

Doctor: Were you able to take the medication that I prescribed last month?

Patient: I picked it up, and I took it a couple of times. I quit because it didn't make me feel any better and I don't like taking more pills.

Doctor: I really appreciate your honesty. When patients are that honest, it makes it so much easier to work together successfully. I also respect your having high standards for your healthcare. Clearly, if something doesn't make a significant difference for you, you are not going to do it just because I recommended it. I agree, you are the one who should be the final decider about your health. Would you like me to go over why I recommended that you take this medicine, or should we drop that subject for a while?

In the list of changes of definition of a patient's behavior for open notes, we suggested that where a health professional might write "failed to take" the medicine, that instead they write "decided against" the medicine (Chap. 7). Here the same change is part of a conversation. The explicit attribution, based on the patient's behavior, is that the patient is actively engaged in their healthcare rather than being uncooperative. In a usual situation in which the patient doesn't take the prescribed medication, the implicit attribution is that the patient is not cooperating and may not care about their health. They have low activation. The explicit attribution above changes the definition of the relationship to one in which the patient is making decisions about their healthcare and cooperating with their doctor by being honest. They are more activated.

9.3   Reasons for Activation

The reasons for patients making health-related changes, i.e., acting in activated ways, are many. Health professionals often expect that managing their illness, maintaining health or functioning, reducing discomfort, or living a longer life are the most important reasons for a patient acting in an activated way. For many patients, these outcomes are valuable mainly as means to other ends. Eliciting the particular reasons that motivate each patient toward self-care can be important so that all team members can use language targeted to what motivates each patient. When asked what makes them work to manage their illness and to stay healthy, many patients report reasons that are about family or values. "I want to be able to spend more time with my grandchildren." "I want to live to walk my daughter down the aisle." "I want to take care of this body that God has entrusted to me." Focusing only on the elements of activation in the PAM can keep a healthcare team from a richer understanding of their patients' motivations and from discussing considerations that can be especially compelling to each patient.

In order to be sure that some member of the team asks about the particular reasons for managing illness and staying healthy for each patient who shows low activation, it makes sense for the team member in a specific role to have that question assigned. It could be the team member, perhaps care manager, doctor, or behavioral health clinician, who is in a role likely to have substantial contact and to develop a comparatively strong relationship with the patient. The patient's answers would be shared with other team members. We will discuss this step in more detail in the next chapter.

9.4   An Attribution Generator

Offering explicit attributions is unfamiliar to many health professionals. Their training may well have discouraged attributions. While some psychotherapies suggest using compliments toward the patient [32], explicit attributions can be uncomfortable for those trained not to offer judgments about patients. The exercise outlined below is the one I have used for teaching attributions to all the members of a team. It is somewhat tongue in cheek. Probably no one has the "Attribution Generator" on their wall. The elements are not a prescribed list. The practice, however, is to give health professionals experience in constructing explicit attributions targeted to a specific patient using a tentative formulation, invoking the patient's reasons for being healthy, and a generalization about their approach to their health that fits with the concept of activation (Table 9.1).

The questions on the PAM can provide ways of formulating the phrases in "C" that are even more precisely targeted to activation.

Table 9.1 Activation script generator: 1 phrase from "A," then 1 phrase from "B," then 1 phrase from "C"

A	B	C
It looks to me like…	…you are determined to…	…work on goals to make yourself healthier
I suspect that…	…you are learning to…	…prevent health problems down the road
I may be wrong, but I am thinking…	…your values are helping you to…	…be sure you get the information you need to maintain your health
I get the impression that…	…you are getting more confident that you can…	…follow through on treatments on your own
	…for your sake and for your family, you are going to…	…maintain the lifestyle changes you have made
	…you are getting back on track to…	…get your life back from the effects of your (illness)

9.5   The Team's Role in Changing Expectations

The focus on finding exceptions, redefining patient behavior, and creating accept-able attributions in the service of increasing patient activation could give the impres-sion that I am recommending that all members of the team add a new segment to the work they already would be doing with a multiply-disadvantaged patient. That is not the case. If the questions and attributions that I am recommending take up sig-nificantly more time, they will be impossible to maintain in the long run. No one on the team has time to spare. I can imagine that the patient, as well, would start to wonder about their care if most of their time with their doctor or other team mem-bers was taken up with solution-focused questions and attributions.

Team members will use opportunities that come up in the course of their contact with the patient to look for an exception in a pattern of problems or failure. They may articulate a possible new attribution about a patient's movement toward greater activation and better health. Different team members spend different amounts of time with the patient and have different opportunities for these sorts of questions and observations. Team members will vary in their facility at using this approach. It would be very difficult to characterize a question or an attribution that would be used only by one team member or one role. It is important, however, that as the expectations of the patient begin to evolve through their relationship with one team member, that all team members have access to that information in the medical record as well as in team discussions.

Positive attributions about patients fit well into the practice of open notes and open clinical conversation. Recording an attribution that was accepted to some degree by the patient in a note gives it a bit more reality and likely a bit more impact for patients who read their notes later on. It is in the medical record, in black and white. Such a positive attribution impacts patients' experience of themselves and their experience of the support and perceptivity of their health professionals. This kind of documentation does not need to be long or detailed:

Note entry: Mr. Jones reports his alcohol intake is down significantly on more
                than half the days. He agreed with my suspicion that his efforts at
                improving his health are starting to show results.

This brief note documents an exception that was noted by the patient and his
clinician during the visit and briefly refers to the attribution that the clinician offered.
This sort of entry might appear in the documentation of the doctor, the behavioral
health clinician, or the care enhancer. When other team members mention the attribution that appears in the note to the patient, the reality of team care is brought
home to the patient. Changes in expectations of the patient's potential that emerge
from one relationship become reflected in their relationships with other team members. The more a new attribution is discussed and confirmed, the more impactful
new expectations are likely to be. Rosenthal's experiment worked only on the
expectations of the authority. Unlike Rosenthal who tried to secretly manipulate the
expectations of teachers about students, in patient-centered care in the course of a
team working with a patient, the expectations for the patient's success in managing
their health on the part of team members and on the part of the patient can reciprocally evolve.

9.6 Summary

The concept of patient activation is one of an array of concepts designed to help
professionals encourage patients, particularly patients with chronic illnesses to be
active in caring for themselves. The Patient Activation Measure has proved to do an
excellent job as distinguishing which patients are most likely to be successful at
self-care. The PAM helps to target specific steps for each patient to help them
become more active so they can achieve better health. While the PAM helps identify
a group of patients as having low activation, it is a mistake to think of these patients
only in terms of their levels of activation. In general, these are the same patients
designated as complex and as needing care management [33], as disadvantaged and
as needing information targeted to their level of health literacy [34], and as patients
with a high likelihood with traumatic experiences as measured on the ACEs screen
and needing trauma-informed care [35]. We have used the term "multiply-disadvantaged" to describe this group. Studying the effective approaches in the literature for
each group gives options for expanding approaches for patients with low activation.
In Chap. 8, we described the elements of trauma-informed care that have been
shown to be empowering to these patients. Focusing on strengths and what they do
well, called "empowerment" in the TIC literature, can be enacted using the methodology of solution-focused interviewing. In this chapter we have described the way
in which a solution-focused approach can be adapted to fostering patient activation.
We used the evidence on the impact of changing expectations from Rosenthal's
work on the Pygmalion effect to support an approach that uses mutually acceptable
explicit attributions about patients to change the expectation of the patients' success
at self-management on the part of both health professionals and the patients

themselves. In the next chapter, we will focus on ways of using a patient-centered care plan to structure a path to partnership and to better health for multiply-disadvantaged patients.

References

1. DiClemente CC, Prochaska JO, Fairhurst SK, Velicer WF, Velasquez MM, Rossi JS. The process of smoking cessation: an analysis of precontemplation, contemplation and preparation stages of change. J Consult Clin Psychol. 1991;59:295–304.
2. Wallston KA, Stein MJ, Smith CA. Form C of the MHLC scales: a condition specific measure of locus of control. J Pers Assess. 1994;63:534–53.
3. Lorig KR, Sobel S, Steward AL, et al. Evidence suggesting that a chronic disease self-management program can improve health status while reducing hospitalization: a randomized Trial. Med Care. 1999;37:5–14.
4. Williams GC, McGregor HA, Zeldman A, Freedman ZR, Deci EL. Testing a self-determination theory process model for promoting glycemic control through diabetes self-management. Health Psychol. 2004;23:58–66.
5. Graffigna G, Barello S, Bonanomi A, Lozza E. Measuring patient engagement: development and psychometric properties of the Patient Health Engagement (PHE) scale. Front Psychol. 2015;6(274):1–10.
6. McCormack L, Thomas V, Lewis MA, Rudd R. Improving low health literacy and patient engagement: a social ecological approach. Patient Educ Couns. 2017;100:8–13.
7. Hibbard JH, Stockard J, Mahoney ER, Tusler M. Development of the Patient Activation Measure (PAM): conceptualizing and measuring activation in patients and consumers. Health Serv Res. 2004;39:1005–26.
8. Hibbard JH, Greene J. What the evidence shows about patient activation: better health outcomes and care experiences: fewer data on costs. Health Aff. 2013;32:207–14.
9. Hibbard JH. Development and testing of a short form of the patient activation measure. Health Serv Res. 2005;40(6 p1):1918–30.
10. Greene J, Hibbard JH. Why does patient activation matter? An examination of the relationship between patient activation and health related outcomes. J Gen Intern Med. 2012;27:520–6.
11. Hibbard JH, Cunningham PJ. How engaged are consumers in their health and healthcare, and why does it matter? Res Briefs. 2008;8:1–9.
12. Smith SG, Pandit A, Rush SR, Wolf MS, Simon CJ. The role of patient activation in preferences for shared decision making: results from a national survey of U. S. adults. J Health Commun. 2016;21:67–75.
13. Deen D, Lu WH, Rothstein D, Santana L, Gold MR. Asking questions: the effect of a brief intervention in the community health centers on patient activation. Patient Educ Couns. 2011;84:257–60.
14. Dixon A, Hibbard J, Tusler M. How do people with different levels of activation self-manage their chronic conditions? Patient. 2009;2:257–68.
15. Bodenheimer T, Lorig K, Holman H, Grumbach K. Patient self-management of chronic disease in primary care. JAMA. 2002;288:2469–75.
16. Aung E, Donald M, Williams GM, Coll JR, Suhail AR. Joint influence of patient assessed chronic illness care and patient activation on glycemic control in type 2 diabetes. Int J Qual Health Care. 2015;27:117–24.
17. Lorig KR, Sobel DS, Ritter PL, Laurent D, Hobbs M. Effect of a self-management program on patients with chronic disease. JAMA. 1996;276:1473–9.
18. Alexander JA, Hearld LR, Nittler JN, Harvey J. Patient-physician role relationship and patient activation among individuals with chronic illness. Health Serv Res. 2012;47:1201–23.

19. Schutzbank, A. (2018). V.P. of Iora Health. Personal communication, 29 Sep 2018.
20. Leppin AL, Montori VM, Gionfriddo MR. Minimally disruptive medicine: a pragmatically comprehensive model for delivering care to patients with multiple chronic conditions. Healthcare. 2015;3:50–63.
21. Kaplan SH, Greenfield S, Ware JE. Assessing the effects of physician-patient interactions on the outcomes of chronic disease. Med Care. 1989;27:S110–27.
22. Magnezi R, Glasser S, Shalev H, Sheiber A, Reuveni H. Patient activation, depression and quality of life. Patient Educ Couns. 2014;94:432–7.
23. Manea L, Gilbody S, McMillan D. Optimal cut-off score for diagnosing depression with the Patient Health Questionnaire (PHQ-9): a meta-analysis. CMAJ. 2012;184:E191–6.
24. Katon W, Robinson P, Von Korff M, Lin E, Bush T, Ludman E, Simon G, Walker E. Arch Gen Psychiatry. 1996;53:942–32.
25. Freedy JR, Carek PJ, Diaz VA, Thiedke CC. Integrating cognitive behavioral therapy into the management of depression. Am Fam Physician. 2012;85:686–7.
26. Glover NG, Sylvers PG, Shearer EM, et al. The efficacy of focused acceptance and commitment therapy in VA primary care. Psychol Serv. 2016;13:156–61.
27. Rosenthal R, Jacobson L. Pygmalion in the classroom. Urban Rev. 1968;3:16–20.
28. Rosenthal R. Interpersonal expectancy effects: a 30-year perspective. Curr Dir Psychol Sci. 1994;3:176–9.
29. Ellison K. Great expectations: being honest about the Pygmalion effect. Discover. December, 2015Issue. http://discovermagazine.com/2015/dec
30. Agency for Healthcare Research and Quality (AHRQ). National healthcare quality and disparities report. Rockville; 2016. July 2017. AHRQ Pub. No. 17-0001.
31. Willems S, De Maesschalck S, Deveugele M, Derese A, De Maeseneer J. Socio-economic status of the patient and doctor-patient communication: does it make a difference? Patient Educ Couns. 2005;56:139–46.
32. De Jong P, Berg IK. Interviewing for solutions. 4th ed. Belmont: Brooks/Cole; 2013.
33. Bodenheimer, T., Berry-Millett, R. 2009. Care management of patient with complex health care needs. Robert Wood Johnson Foundation. https://www.rwjf.org/en/library/research/2009/12/care-management-of-patients-with-complex-health-care-needs.html
34. Bernheim SM, Ross JS, Krumholz HM, Bradley EH. Influence of patients' socioeconomic status on clinical management decisions: a qualitative study. Ann Fam Med. 2008;6(1):53–9.
35. Purkey E, Patel R, Phillips SP. Trauma-informed care: better care for everyone. Can Fam Physician. 2018;64:170–2.

Resources

https://health.ubc.ca/pcpe/projectsactivities/past-projects/talk-your-doc-ttyd is the address for the listed reference

Patient Activation Measure

Questions of the PAM Short From
Permission to Use the PAM

Coaching Patients to Talk to Doctors

"Talking With Your Doctor... and other Healthcare Professionals" by Donald Cegala, MD.
P.A.C.E Manual for Facilitators, a manual for facilitators for a workshop called "Talking with Your Doctor" for patient groups.
More resources: https://pcpe.health.ubc.ca/ourwork/ttyd/community; https://health.ubc.ca/pcpe/projectsactivities/past-projects/talk-your-doc-ttyd

Chapter 10
"M" Is for Mutual

10.1 A Tool for Mutuality

Primary care is a highly organized process, always struggling to balance the need to serve a large number of patients with the need to allow time for the relationships on which successful care is built. For primary care settings to successfully care for patients with chronic illnesses, the patients have to take an active part in the effort. The effort to make patients meaningful members of their own healthcare teams, however, presents a challenge to whatever balance between speed and relating time a particular primary care setting has already achieved. Wherever there is an opportunity to include patients in the standard processes of their healthcare, it makes sense to employ those processes as vehicles for partnership.

The use of open notes is a good example of a standard process in medical care that can promote the patient's participation on the team. It undoes an often-unnoticed outcome of the usual way of keeping medical notes that every member of the team has access to the notes except the patient. The patient is excluded. Notes are going to be kept on every interaction, and, with some very minor reconsiderations of wording, they can become an important way for patients, particularly multiply-disadvantaged patients, to become better informed about their illnesses and their care and to build trust in their healthcare team (see Chap. 7).

In the first pilot of open notes, the patients who, up to that time had never been exposed to the possibility of reading their doctors notes, were excited by the new option. Once this new channel of communication was opened, patients quickly envisioned what might be considered the next logical step: two-way communication [1]. Sixty percent said that they would like the ability to add comments about the doctors' notes. In this one area, the doctors, all of whom had volunteered for the program, overwhelmingly disagreed with the patients. They did not want patients' comments on their notes recorded as part of the medical record, though they were willing to have patients offer ideas or comments to them by secure email. It is impossible to be sure of the specific concerns behind this opinion

© Springer Nature Switzerland AG 2019
A. Blount, *Patient-Centered Primary Care*,
https://doi.org/10.1007/978-3-030-17645-7_10

because they were not elicited in the survey [1], but we only have to consider the time and energy that might be required of doctors if they had to read and react to new questions relating to their patients' notes, coming at any point between visits and appearing in the EHR, to understand why the doctors thought this was untenable.

What can we learn from the fact that patients so clearly wanted to be involved in two-way communication about notes? I suspect that the notes, as a core element of the official medical record, have a special status to patients, especially multiply-disadvantaged patients who are likely to experience the providers of medical care as authorities. It is great, as a patient, to be able to see what is being said about you, but it can still feel like you are in a vulnerable or lower position if you have no opportunity to respond to what is said (see Chap. 5). It doesn't seem to be a partnership.

So far in this volume, we have been working to lay out an approach to serving patients in primary care who have been particularly challenging to engage and help, even for the team-based patient-centered primary care as it is currently practiced. We have described this population of patients for whom these approaches tend not to be fully adequate and sometimes are quite unsuccessful. The population we are describing are patients that are often described as "complex" or high utilizing. A good deal of work has been done to find ways to provide care that improves their health and lowers their cost. These patients are known in other literature as "disadvantaged" patients because they are generally of low socioeconomic status because of their incomes or because of discrimination against their racial group. They are often discussed in literature on equity in healthcare. As Mautner and his colleagues [2] showed, a large percentage of them have histories of trauma and are appropriate for trauma-informed care. We have been using the term "multiply-disadvantaged" to describe this group and the many aspects of their challenges in relation to their health and healthcare.

The patient-centered care plan (PCCP) can be a vehicle for engaging these patients in the creation of a document in their medical record that is a central guide to their own care. Using the PCCP gives the patient a role on their healthcare team and at the same time gives doctors and the health team a way of focusing this important contribution by the patient to a particular time and structured process, a process that can make the patient's activation toward self-management more likely.

Anyone first encountering the topic of patient involvement in care plans would be justified in being confused by the terms they encounter. The terms "patient-centered care plan" or "person-centered care plan" or "shared care plan" or "collaborative care plan," any one of which could be designating the kind of document and relational process we are describing in this chapter, are also used in other places to designate other relationships and processes. It is important to distinguish their meaning in each context of their use. Sometimes "patient (or person)-centered care plan" is used to indicate the shift from care plans focused on a particular disease, e.g., a diabetes care plan, to a care plan focused on the array of needs of one patient, particularly when more complete information about their life circumstances or preferences are included. There may be no implication that the patient was involved in the creation of the plan except as a source of information and did not see or approve the final product. A "shared care plan" can mean that multiple providers are working together to share care of a patient, rather than having each provider operating in a silo. In this use, the term implies that there is a common record of medical history, problem list, medication list, allergies, and so forth and a plan for care to which all providers have access. The same sometimes applies to the use of "collaborative care plan" in which the entities collaborating may be providers in the same health system or a collaboration between medical, mental health, and social service agencies. In these cases, as well, the participation of the patient in the creation of the plan may not be implied. In this chapter we will be focusing solely upon care plans that give the patient a substantive role in creating the plan and regular access to the completed product.

10.2   Role of the Care Plan

The care plan has a long history as a document in inpatient care. It is usually a plan for the nursing care of a patient, sometimes employing subsections of standardized nursing plans for the patient's individual illnesses or wounds. The Medical Dictionary for the Health Professions and Nursing [3] defines care plan as:

> A carefully prepared outline of nursing care showing all of the patient's needs and the ways of meeting them; a dynamic document initiated at admission and subject to continuous reassessment and change by the nursing staff caring for the patient; typically includes nursing diagnoses, nursing interventions, and outcomes; ensures consistency of care; may be standardized or preprinted.

By this definition, the care plan is a guide for the many nurses and other professionals who will care for a patient during the course of a day and of an inpatient stay. It insures consistency of care by guiding the actions of each health professional.

The care plan was adopted by the American Academy of Pediatrics for its medical home approach for children with complex medical conditions [4]. In this use, it is meant to be a single synthesis of all the relevant information about medical situation and the care of a child. These children are often cared for by several specialists and even several agencies. Having one place, in the primary care pediatrician's office, where each provider or agency can go to obtain an overall picture of the child's situation supports coordinated care and spares parents the task of having to be responsible for orienting each new care provider. In this use of a care plan, the expertise of each user is assumed. It is access to the information that improves and coordinates care.

The belief in care plans as ways of informing and guiding practice for high-utilizing patients seems to be growing, particularly in large corporate approaches to care improvement. The demand for plans developed by "experts" has created a growing business. In my research, I found a company that will provide its report on the use of "coordinated care plans," including a list of potential vendors of plans for different clinical settings, for $2000. I was not able to learn the cost of the individual plans from the different vendors.

The PCCP adds a new function to the informing and guiding functions that have characterized care plans, that of engaging patients in their care. It creates a process that requires health team members and the patient to discuss the patient's preferences and values and record them for use by all. It allows the patient to describe themselves and their social situation in ways that can offer information which team members and other providers can use to guide important decisions in the process of care.

If the discussion of patient values and preferences is framed as a way of helping the healthcare team to understand the patient better, it is particularly engaging for multiply-disadvantaged patients, those with low levels of trust, empowerment, and activation. For a brief time in the process of care, the patient is a consultant to the team about themselves. In my experience, and in the experience of others (Valeras, 2018), this part of the PCCP process gives an opportunity for the team, represented by the member explaining the PCCP to the patient, to express humility in relation to knowledge about the patient and their life. Implying that the team has things they need to learn about the patient in order to do their part of the care better often fits the patient's experience of what has been a poor fit between themselves and their team up to that point. The information elicited about the patient is aimed at giving the team access to the context for the problem lists that usually are the core information about patients. This gives team members new insights to help them improve their side of the fit. Just the fact that the team wants to obtain the information tends to enhance the patient's trust and optimism about working with the team. Some of the most noticeable immediate impacts of creating a PCCP can be the improvement of the working relationship between the team and some of their patients who were particularly hard for them to engage.

Team members who might be skeptical about the need for this sort of brief reversal of roles tend to be willing to participate when they observe that the conversation with the patient about their preferences and values can transition seamlessly into a conversation about health goals. Empowerment improves activation (see Chap. 9). Patients who are more activated take care of themselves better, and that makes providing care for them more rewarding.

Adding the engagement function to the care plan through the PCCP inevitably impacts its other functions. The care plan continues to be important in the role of informing health team members and external providers, but it also informs the patient as well. This requires a change in the assumptions about the expertise of those reading the plan. The information in the care plan will need to provide some guidance for team members and other providers on caring for the patient, and it will also be guiding to the patient as a member of the team.

The informing and guiding functions will need to be engaging to team members as well as to the patient. The engagement of the health professionals needs attention, because they may be as untrusting of new efforts that impact their work routines as multiply-disadvantaged patients are untrusting of authorities who want to manage their lives. In order for the PCCP to be engaging to team members, the use of the care plan needs to fit as seamlessly as possible into their clinical practice routines.

Helping with all three functions is, at best, a complex balance that takes determination and creativity for successful implementation. Determination is needed to enlist team members in what will certainly be an inconvenient process at its beginning [5]. Determination is also required to keep the PCCP from being driven out of balance by forces in the health system that want to emphasize guidance of team members in caring for the patient or guidance of the patient in self-management, or increasing the care plan's role as a repository of clinical information about the patient. As we look at implementations of the PCCP, the requirement for the balance between the three functions (informing, guiding, and engaging) will help to understand the lack of durability of some these implementations.

10.3 A Brief History of PCCP Trials

10.3.1 The Shared Care Plan

The Pursuing Perfection program was a grant program of the Robert Wood Johnson Foundation, with consultation from the Institute for Healthcare Improvement that ran from 2001 to 2008. One of the first grantees was a group from Whatcom County, Washington. Their program strove to make patient-centered care an attribute of the entire county health system, rather than a characteristic of a few healthcare sites. The central tool they developed to help in this effort was the shared care plan (SCP). The SCP was an attempt to involve patients in the creation of a care plan that would inform any medical provider about their medical history, their needs, their social situation, their religion or spirituality, their life goals, and their health goals. When the program was designed, it was expected that any physician would be able to access the care plan electronically at the time of a visit with the patient. The plan template was designed through a process that involved physicians, staff, and patients working with the technical staff of the project. It had tables for capturing complex medical information including the list of medications and instructions for taking each. It listed life goals and short-term goals and had forms for tracking actions for health improvement by the patient in very detailed ways [6].

The design of the program was to help patients in obtaining the information needed to complete the form and in setting health goals. The help came from a "clinical care specialist" who was a nurse or social worker serving as the patient's health coach and advocate. Then the patient would keep their SCP updated so that any new clinician could be oriented about the patient's care and the patient's own health efforts. The original goal was that 70% of patients would have an up-to-date SCP in place at any one time. Ultimately, at the height of the implementation, the percentage of patients with SCPs in place got to just over 40%. Today the program is no longer active, and the website through which patients created and accessed their SCPs has been taken down.

Dr. Bertha Safford is a family physician in Whatcom County who was centrally involved in the creation and implementation of the SCP. She has pointed to several factors that led to the lack of durability of the program [7]. One factor was the inconvenience of the plan for providers. At the time (2001) there was no interoperability between EHRs in the county. Many practices were still using paper records. A provider who was using a computer in a visit would have to log out of the EHR, log into the internet to be able to access a patient's SCP, and then log back into the EHR. The process could interrupt the flow of the visit and add a few minutes to the total time needed. The lack of interoperability meant that the hope that there could be a cue to the provider in any electronic record about the existence of an SCP for a patient could not be realized. In the end, SCP was reliably available to providers only if the patient brought a printed copy to the visit.

Dr. Safford believes that the patients on the committee that created a SCP were some of the most activated in the county. Their passion for patient participation was not necessarily shared by the majority of their patient colleagues. They created a form that required extensive information gathering in order for it to be completed accurately. A good deal of ongoing maintenance was required of the patient as they interacted with the health system. When the plan was implemented, the more activated patients who were sick had "too much on their plates" to keep up their SCPs, and the less activated patients, the ones the health system most wanted to reach, never became engaged in the process. The fact that patients were not reliably updating their SCPs meant that a provider who was presented with a copy by a patient had no idea how current the information in the plan was.

The fate of the shared care plan of Whatcom County provides confirmation of the necessity for balancing the informing, guiding, and engaging function of a PCCP. The SCP was created by physicians and patients together and expressed the belief in the power of partnership of both groups, but it was out of balance in that it was not convenient or reliable for providers, and it was not convenient or engaging enough for patients.

In 2012, during my tenure as editor of the journal, *Families, Systems, & Health,* we received two inspiring reports on pilot implementations of patient-centered care plans in primary care settings, one in New Hampshire and one in Seattle. In both cases these implementations were led by clinicians with a commitment to improving the ability of their practices to provide truly patient-centered care. The two programs were similar in many ways, particularly in vision of the potential role of the care plan in patient-centered care. They were different in ways that are instructive about the options and approaches for patient-centered care plans.

10.3.2 Concord, NH

The PCCP in Concord, NH, was developed in a family medicine residency practice serving both rural and urban patients [8]. A significant percentage of patients in the practice would be seen in a federally qualified health center in most cities. The research team consisted of a physician with research experience, a behavioral health clinician with qualitative research experience, two physicians with quality improvement experience, and an outside researcher from a medical school with a national reputation as a center for primary care and behavioral health research. This group designed the PCCP used in the program. The research team in the Concord project was aware of the shared care plan effort in Whatcom County.

The implementation of the PCCP was done by one out of the four healthcare teams in the practice. The team included faculty and resident physicians, medical assistants and nurses, nurse practitioners and physician assistants, and behavioral health clinicians. The care plan had three sections: a medical summary, a "patient snapshot," and a "goal directed action plan" [8]. The medical summary included a brief medical synopsis or "sign-out," a problem list with suggested actions, information on the current continuum of care for the patient, and an emergency plan of action for the patient. The "patient snapshot" included what the patient wanted the care team members to know about them, what the primary care team wanted to communicate about the patient, and information on the patient's assets, supports, and strengths. The "goal directed action plan" included the patient's goals and the negotiated action plan with the person responsible for each action. Note that the action plan details steps to be taken by the team members as well as the patient. This was one of the many efforts to create a plan all users would experience as a team agreement rather than as patient instructions. See Fig. 10.1.

Part 1: Medical Summary

Name: Cynthia Brown _____ Nickname ____ Cindy __ DOB 1/1/1967

Address: 11 Pleasant Lane, Apt 3C, Pleasant Town, NH

Phone # (preferred) _603-111-1111_ (Blocked? Y x N) Best time to reach: 5–7 in the evening.

How do you prefer to be contacted: Phone, but I never answer. I'm the one who checks my voicemail, so you can leave messages

E-mail n/a _____ Alt.Phone_n/a_____

Emergency Contact ___Lucy Brown__ Phone 603-545-4545 Relationship mother

Health Insurance/Plan Medicare _____ ID# VX00111

Emergency Plan? Y   Advance Directives? N

Allergies/reaction:

• Lisinopril – angioedema

• Bees – hives

Medications/dose/purpose:

• Ibuprofen 600 mg four times a day for arthritis

• Amlodipine 5 mg at bedtime for blood pressure and migraine prevention

PCP_____ Dr. Sally Sunshine____   **Phone** 603-777-7777 **Fax**____ **E-Mail**_____

Care Manager Carol Park_____   **Phone** _603-888-8888 **Fax**____ **E-Mail**_____ F

Team RN Jamie Bosana_____   **Phone** 603-888-8989

Medical Synopsis/Sign-out:

Cindy has rheumatoid arthritis, s/p hip replacement. She does not drive and was dismissed from her rheumatology practice for no-shows, but they are willing to answer questions about her care from our office.

Who else is involved in your care? (specialists, nurses, outside agencies)

#1 Name	Clinic/Hospital	Phone	Other (fax, e-mail, etc.):
Dr. Gupta	Rheumatology	603-999-9999	Release? Y
#2 Name	Clinic/Hospital	Phone	Other (fax, e-mail, etc.):

Fig. 10.1 Patient Centered Care Plan (Concord) (Council et al. [8])

Jay Upton	NH P.T.	603-222-2222	Release? N
#3 Name	Clinic/Hospital	Phone	Other (fax, e-mail, etc.):
Dr. Lee	Orthopedics	603-333-3333	Release? Y

Who are the most important people in your life? (family members, a partner, friends, coworkers, people you live with)	• My son, but he is in jail. I miss him. I haven't seen him in 19 months. • My daughter doesn't speak to me. • My best friend is Bonnie. She goes to AA with me. • I also talk to Robert, my minister, every Sunday after church.

Who can we talk to about your care?

#1 Name	Relation	Phone	Other (fax, e-mail, etc.):
Robert Jones	Minister	603-555-5555	Release? Y
#2 Name	Relation	Phone	Other (fax, e-mail, etc.):
Lucy Brown	mother	603-444-4444	Release? Y

Part 2: Snapshot

Snapshot: What do you want your healthcare team to know about you? (This can include your most important medical and/or emotional concerns. You can also include information about what you like to do in your free time, what you do for work, what your spiritual or religious affiliations are, what your financial situation is, what your unique talents or hobbies are, and what makes you happy.)	• I play the guitar. I taught myself. Music is important to me. • I attend church every Sunday. I like going to church, but I'm not religious. • I don't eat meat. • I never have transportation when I need it. I need at least 3 weeks advance notice to arrange a ride, and I don't always know if my transportation is going to show up. • I am quick-tempered, but I don't mean to be.
My provider wants my care team to know:	Because Cindy is in active recovery, potentially addictive medications need to be prescribed with a specific plan as to how to take them (e.g., take at 8 am and 3 pm). Always let her know if a medication could be sedating because this makes her anxious.
Urgent Plan of Care: *Do you have any recommendations for how your healthcare team should respond if you are in a crisis?*	• If I'm angry, tell me, "Everything is going to be okay." Don't put me on hold. • When I'm in pain, I want to kill myself. When I feel like this, I need a plan. I don't want to be told that you'll call me back. Reassure me the pain is not life-threatening, and ask me if I'm thinking about hurting myself. If I am, help me get in touch with Robert. He always knows what to say.

Fig. 10.1 (continued)

Part 3: Action Plan

Patient goals		Provider goals	
Short-term			
• To be able to move like I could before my hip replacement • To stay sober • To be able to visit my son in jail		• Fully participate in physical therapy rehab to achieve maximum mobility post-hip-replacement • Use medications appropriately	
Long-term			
• To become a sponsor in AA		• To decrease use of NSAID medications	
Negotiated Goal	**Action Plan**	**Person Responsible**	**Time Frame**
1. Do physical therapy exercises at home	Cindy will put pictures of her exercises on her fridge door and do them twice a day	Cindy	Now
2. Re-establish care with a rheumatologist	Care manager will call rheumatology office to see if they will conditionally re-establish care	Carol Park	Within 1 week
3. Attend PT sessions	Ensure transportation to PT appointments	Cindy will reschedule appointments to be before AA meetings, Bonnie will drive to PT appointments and then meetings	Now

Fig. 10.1 (continued)

The Concord PCCP included the patient in defining what information went into it in a way that was a good deal more inclusive of the patient's perspective than the shared care plan. Unlike some other plans that offer space for only one answer to important patient descriptions, the Concord plan assumes that the patient and their care team might have different perspectives and offers space for both. That frees the patient to answer certain questions from their perspective without requiring that their answer be shaped through a negotiation with a health team member. The result can seem particularly personal, while still reflecting what the patient wants to communicate. It invites a more personal response from any new provider in the patient's care.

Fully completing the PCCP requires a care management role, whether that is played by a team member designated as a care manager or by another team member. Releases of information, which up to that point had not been needed, have to be obtained. Often multiply-disadvantaged patients are unclear about the details of their care in other settings, who they see and how to contact that person, and the team member in the care manager role makes contacts to clarify. These contacts can include conversations that improve the team's communication with the patient's personal or care networks, a helpful step that also would not have occurred without the PCCP process.

The process of negotiating a PCCP that is as complete at the Concord document takes too much time to be offered to all patients. Usually, a practice would start with a fairly small group until the team is experienced and efficient at their part of the process. Then an expansion of the target group can be considered. In Concord patients to be offered participation in the PCCP were selected at each clinic session in a huddle among the team before the session began. They tended to select patients with complex health pictures who were already requiring significant time and energy from the team and from other parts of the health system such as the emergency department. These were likely to be patients with whom the team did not feel well engaged.

The reports from team members about the impact of the PCCP were very positive. In a residency practice where physicians come and go regularly, they reported improved continuity of care. Physicians reported that this continuity commonly saved doctors who were covering for the patient's PCP or new residents who were taking over the role of the PCP from ordering unnecessary tests. They judged that the way the plan reflected the patient's perspective and life circumstances was helpful in establishing rapport and in lowering team frustration when patients did not do what was expected of them. The program was engaging to team members as it developed, because they found that the initial investment of extra time in creating the plan led to less time spent overall on the patients with PCCPs. Nurses who were members of the team reported that the PCCP made it much easier to address patient calls or to respond to a contact from the ED about a patient. Multiple team members described increased job satisfaction as the program progressed.

In several cases, both health team members and patients noticed a lowering of tension or conflict. Patients reported that they felt known by their team and were more willing to work with team members who were not their doctor after the PCCP process. Many said that when they met a new doctor or other team member, they could tell whether the new person had read their PCCP by how they acted. Some patients were proud of the results of the work they had put into their PCCP. They felt new team members should be accountable to have read their plans and told them so.

The PCCP was excellent at building partnership, but it did not impact the ED use of certain patients as much as hoped. Over time, the practice undertook a QI project to further improve the impact on ED utilization for its high-utilizing patients [9]. The unique aspect of the QI project for the PCCP was that every patient who was in the top 5% of ED utilization in the previous year was invited to participate in designing the QI plan. While the group that agreed to participate was small, the impact was substantial. The group met monthly for 6 months. Working with representatives of the QI team, they came up with an addition to the PCCP that specified what both patient and HPs should do when the patient perceived an urgent need for care. The addition in its most recent form [10] was the answers to the questions below (Table 10.1):

Table 10.1 Patient Centered Care Plan (Concord) Urgent Plan of Care

1. Symptoms
(a) What are the symptoms that typically lead to ED visits or frequent calls for perceived urgent healthcare needs?
(b) Why are these symptoms important or worrisome to you?
(c) What has worked for you in the past to address these concerns?
2. Who is on your team?
(a) Who knows you best at the health center?
(b) Who has been most helpful in addressing your concerns?
(c) Who outside of the health center has been most helpful in meeting your urgent needs?
3. Detailed executable plan
(a) What do you want to happen when you have an urgent care need?
(b) How do you want the plan relayed to you (by phone, in person, by whom)?
(c) When would be a good time to check in with you after addressing your urgent need?

During its implementation, there was a significant reduction in ED utilization for the 127 patients originally identified as the high utilizers, both in number of uses and as a percentage of total usage. These patients tended to "rotate off" the high utilizer list and others came on, for whom the urgent plan of care was then offered. Team members tended to exhibit more understanding and tolerance for the patients in the program, which the patients noticed and commented upon. The patients, for their part, were more activated in handling the problems they had previously taken to the ED.

10.3.3 Seattle, WA

At about the same time as the Concord effort, a pilot program was developed in the Seattle area [5] built on the work begun in Whatcom County, WA, in the shared care plan. It took a problem-solving approach [11] that focused on helping patients articulate and achieve goals for their health [12]. The designers of the program were particularly aware of the time pressures that face primary care doctors [13] and that negotiating goals might not be part of the training of many doctors [14]. To overcome these barriers, they chose to enhance the role of the nurse/medical assistant using the "teamlet" model of Bodenheimer and Laing [15]. In this model, the medical assistant role is expanded beyond basic collection of information for the doctor, to activities that might be said to "tee up" the content of the patient and doctor visit. Besides taking vitals, the MA in the Seattle program begins the agenda setting for the visit, orients the patient to a discussion about health goals, and often goes through the initial process of setting goals with the patient.

The teamlet approach was chosen so that, as far as possible, the process of creating and the monitoring of the patient's care plan would be embedded within the routine flow of a clinical visit in primary care. Discussions that in other programs are located in the relationship between the patient and a care manager, or a behavioral health clinician, were streamlined and kept in the patient's relationship with their MA and their doctor.

The design team met with selected patients and reviewed the literature at the time, and after a great deal of discussion, they settled on a structure for the PCCP that had three sections: "About Me," "My Goals," and "My Progress." As in other PCCPs, the description of the patient that is part of the care plan is from the perspective of the patient (see Figure 10.2, Section A).

Patient-Centered Care Plan
"About Me" (Patient Preferences, Needs, and Values)

Figure 10.2, Section A

A. I prefer to be called:
B. I speak (language) as my main language.
C. I sometimes need help understanding written information about my health (yes/no).
D. I live with:
E. I believe the following person(s) in my life are supportive of my healthcare goals:
F. Religion/spirituality may impact my healthcare in the following way:
G. My healthcare team and I agree it is important for the people working with me to know the following information (consider working with your MA and provider to fill out this section):
H. In addition to my healthcare team at family medicine, others important to my care are (e.g., cardiologist, mental health provider, naturopath, or any provider you see regularly):

Name Discipline/specialty Location

1.
2.
3.

This section of the care plan was filled out by the patient on paper before the visit with help, when necessary, from the MA. The copy of the paper document went with the patient into the visit with the doctor and was entered into the EHR later by the MA.

The section called "My Goals" attempts to help the patient define personal healthcare goals in ways that lead to specific actions that can be monitored by the patient and their health team. This PCCP has the process of goal setting built into it in more detail than others. In most cases this process of identifying goals would be started by the MA before the patient met with the doctor. She would orient the patient to the idea of health goals and, using a structured stepwise approach, work with the patient to define at least one goal and actions that the patient could take to begin to move toward the goal. The ideas generated in the meeting with the MA and the patient could be reviewed and endorsed or modified in the patients' visit with the doctor. In general, the process of finding an overarching goal and breaking it into activities and then specific actions took about 5 minutes for the patient and the MA to accomplish, once the MA had the experience of a few iterations [16] (Figure 10.2, Section B).

"My Goals" (Personal Healthcare Goals)

Figure 10.2, Section B

These healthcare goals represent what you want to do to live a healthy life as well as the areas of your health that you want to monitor and manage.

1. My healthcare goal #1: (Describe your healthcare goal as specifically as possible as well as why this goal is important to you.)
2. Healthcare goals are most often accomplished by breaking them down into small, specific steps.

   My ongoing health activities: What areas do you need help with in order to reach your healthcare goal?

   (a) _____
   (b) _____
   (c) _____

3. There are often several steps to reaching a goal. Consider the options, and choose one of the above areas on which you would like to work.

   My ongoing action steps

   (a) What I will do: _____
   (b) How often? _____
   (c) When? _____
   (d) Potential barriers? _____

4. On a scale of 1 (*low*) to 10 (*high*), my confidence in reaching this goal:
5. What can help increase my confidence? _____

The use of the confidence rating comes from motivational interviewing. In some cases, the action which could give the patient more confidence that they would be able to follow through on their ongoing action steps could become an ongoing action step in itself. In cases of a patient having low confidence about achieving the goal, the rating focused the conversation on barriers and kept the conversation from spending time on goals the patient didn't think were possible.

The "My Progress" section is the monitoring part of this PCCP. Compared to some others plans and to the goals section of this plan, this section is comparatively less elaborated. It offers the opportunity to revise goals as care progresses but doesn't prescribe the way in with information about the patient's efforts is collected (Figure 10.2, Section C).

"My Progress" (My Health care Goal Successes and Challenges)

Figure 10.2, Section C

My Healthcare Goal:

Date:

Successes:

Challenges:

Does the goal need to be revised? (Y/N):

The PCCP was offered to patients who had at least one chronic illness that required regular monitoring and who had already established care with the team. The team was made up of four family medicine residents and three faculty, all with part-time clinical practices. The team was supported by one MA, who usually had two doctors seeing patients on any given half day session. All of the doctors and the MA received the same 2 hour training experience in the PCCP process and patient-centered behavior change and viewed a video on negotiating goals. Doctors were given 40 minute visit times with patients who were part of the program and 1:1 support from the MA for the first few visits only. Then they had their usual visit time and the MA supported two doctors.

The program ran for a year. Evaluations at the end identified some consistent experiences among team members. Team members found that allowing time for training and practice was important and that ongoing conversations about the program and about possible refinements were very useful. Training as a team (or teamlet) was very important. While the training they received allowed both members of the teamlet to start using the PCCP, they would have liked more. The process was a new way of interacting with patients, and both doctors and the MA would have appreciated some ongoing reassurance. Both doctors and the MA appreciated the greatly enhanced role of the MA. The PCCP increased continuity of care for the patient among providers within the team. It became a training and a clinical problem-solving intervention for providers and the MA as they gained practice in its use.

Patients tended to report that they felt better known as a person through the PCCP process. They trusted their doctor and the team more and appreciated their doctors taking the time to talk about their health goals. They all were comfortable with the MA talking to them about health goals.

In this implementation, there was a group of patients with low activation (such as multiply-disadvantaged patients) for whom the idea of health goals was difficult. They thought that doing what they were told to do was what was required to manage their chronic illnesses. This confirms the findings cited in Chap. 9 that more activated patients tend to see partnership with their doctor as a value and as part of their managing their health needs, while patients described as at a low level of activation tend to see doing what they are told to do by their doctor as fulling the patient's role in self-management [17]. The emphasis on defining goals and taking the actions needed to achieve them tipped the balance for these patients toward feeling guided rather than engaged by the process. For those people, the engagement function of the PCCP, as it was implemented in the Seattle program, was not adequately realized. This finding highlights the risk of a "health goals" approach rather than a T.E.A.M. Way approach for the multiply-disadvantaged patients.

Ultimately, in both the Seattle and the Concord programs, the accessibility for providers envisioned by the designers of the programs was never achieved. Instead of being immediately available when any provider opened a patient's record, the PCCP was delegated to the status of "additional documentation" in the EHR. After opening a patient's record, the PCCP was two or three extra clicks away, and a new user could not always tell that there was a PCCP in place without checking for it. That meant that the plan tended not to be reviewed before each patient visit.

If the PCCP has no utility for the doctor in a patient's visits, over time it gradually loses the organizing and engaging impact that it had when it was being created by the team and the patient. Patients notice the difference, and it can feel like an attrition in the team's interest in their health. It is the PCCP that to them represents their views and suggestions in their medical record. For multiply-disadvantaged patients, that can correlate in an attrition in their efforts toward partnership and self-management that they began to develop during the process of creating their PCCP. The benefits of the creation of the plan, as seen in the increased understanding between challenging patients and their care team and in somewhat lower ED use, then follow the pattern of regression to the mean that happens after the excitement at the beginning of many promising programs.

Perhaps the greatest challenge in trying to achieve a smooth implementation in both the Concord and Seattle programs was the EHR. The EHR was controlled centrally in each health system, as it is in most health systems. The technicians and managers who control these large and extremely complex pieces of software have to address system-wide issues and problems. Because many EHRs are set up primarily to manage types of information needed for billing and for retaining medical data, incorporating a form that was not imagined in the design of the system can require a lot of time and energy, even if the software is able to be adapted to include the new information. Without support and direction from the top levels of the organization, IT departments are unlikely to share the urgency or enthusiasm of the clinical developers for the changes that are required for the PCCP implementation. It is clear that administrative and IT support personnel need to be at the table in the initial development of the project. These people need the time and experience in the project enough to share the enthusiasm and the commitment that tend to grow in the clinicians and patients involved.

In other settings the PCCP has been broadly implemented and is still used. Legacy Health, a large health system serving the metropolitan and suburban areas around Portland, OR, and Vancouver, WA, uses a PCCP for patients who have the services of a care manager [18, 19]. Iora Health is an innovative health system with practices in several areas of the USA. It serves patients on contract to large Medicare health plans. Iora uses a PCCP that doubles as a face sheet for a patient when it is opened by any health team member [20]. These settings have not offered the same level of detail as the Whatcom County, Concord, and Seattle programs partly because they believe that the tools they have developed give them a competitive advantage in the markets they serve.

The patient-centered care plan needs to be a living and evolving record of the evolving relationship between the patient and their healthcare team. We have discussed the impact the PCCP can have on the engagement between the healthcare team and the patient and on healing rifts that may have developed. The increase in continuity of care that has been noted by multiple authors as a result of the PCCP is one element in that improved engagement. The effect of the continuity of relationship, when the health team is using the techniques of empowerment and activation described in Chaps. 8 and 9, usually leads to a changing picture of the patient on the part of the team members. The evolving image of the patient as they become better connected as part of their team should be reflected for the patient and for the larger health system in the PCCP.

10.4 Suggestions for Implementation

The implementations of PCCPs described and evaluated in the current literature cannot be described as more than pilots. The findings, however, when placed in the context of a much larger body of evidence, such as described in the early chapters of this work, allow us to distinguish the outlines of a comprehensive program using patient-centered care plans in primary care. For patients with chronic illness who have moderate to high levels of activation, the Seattle approach to the PCCP, using the teamlet of an MA and a doctor, could help increase their experience of partner-ship with their doctor and help them work on reasonable, doable goals. In those cases, the emphasis is away from teaching patients and toward facilitating their own decision-making and helping them structure their approach to self-management. It makes shared decision-making a regular part of care rather than a process used only in specific clinical situations. Doctors and MAs who use this approach will require training in facilitation and in goal setting, but this training does not have to be expensive in terms of time spent.

Multiply-disadvantaged patients with complex health needs will require a PCCP approach with more emphasis on engagement, even if that has to be at the cost of the focus on goal setting in the early stages. This was demonstrated by the finding that patients with low activation often do not understand the concepts involved in goals and self-management [5, 17]. For those patients, partnership in defining the treatment plan should be a central feature, so that engagement is more prominent. It is likely that this care plan will need additional staff efforts, either from the care manager or the behavioral health clinician functioning as care manager. Some larger implementations of PCCPs assume that all of the assembling of information and discussing goals with patients will be the province of a care manager on the team [20]. This is thought to lower the inconvenience for doctors and to increase their support for the PCCP process.

The role of patient goals in a patient's PCCP may evolve over time. Setting health and activity goals for the patient that are judged by the team to be the best for their health may not produce the best-chosen goals from the perspective of long-term values of the patient. We need to face the fact that the steps that a patient might choose to take to begin to be activated as part of their health team might be of negli-gible value in reducing risks. The wisdom of minimally disruptive medicine [21] is in the choice to define goals that do not add stress on top of the stress patients already experience in coping with their illness burden. Reflecting these more doable goals in the care plan can inform other specialists or services in the health system, to restrain other providers from expecting self-management actions from a patient that are not currently possible for them. The PCCP may also need to evolve because as patients become more empowered, they may learn to ask for and expect better information from their health team, information that should be reflected on the care plan and pos-sibly in new goals. Below is a synthesized example of a PCCP drawn from several of previous plans with some adaptation to fit the T.E.A.M. Way.

Figure 10.2 is an example of a PCCP that incorporates elements from other care plans and adds other elements designed to support the empowerment and activation

Example of a Patient-Centered Care Plan

About Me:

Name: _____ I want to be called: _____ DOB _____

Address: _____

Phone# _____ Best time to reach _____ Can leave a message? _ Y _ N

Email _____ Alternate phone# _____
Emergency Contact: _____ Phone: _____ Relationship _____

I speak _____ as my main language. I sometimes need help
understanding written information about my health _ Y _ N

My Care Team:

PCP_____ Phone _____ Fax _____ E-mail _____

Care Man. _____ Phone _____Fax _____ E-mail _____

RN/MA _____ Phone _____ Fax _____E-mail _____

BHC _____ Phone _____Fax _____E-mail _____

Other _____ Phone _____ Fax _____ E-mail _____

Who else is involved in your care? (specialists, nurses, outside agencies)

Name _____ Role _____ Phone _____ E-mail _____ Rls _ Y _ N

Name _____ Role _____ Phone _____ E-mail _____ Rls _ Y _ N

Name _____ Role _____ Phone _____ E-mail _____ Rls _ Y _ N

Who are the most important people in your life?

Who can we talk to about your care?

Name _____ Rel. _____ Phone _____ E-mail _____ Rls _ Y _ N

Fig. 10.2

Name _____ Rel. _____ Phone _____ E-mail _____ Rls _Y _N

Name _____ Rel. _____ Phone _____ E-mail _____ Rls _Y _N

What do you want your healthcare team to know about you?
(This can include your most important medical and/or emotional concerns.
You can also include information you would be happy to talk with people
about: what you like to do in your free time, what you do for work, what your
spiritual or religious affiliations are, what your financial situation is, what
your unique talents or hobbies are, what makes you happy)

What my provider wants my care team to know about me:

My Health:

Medical Summary/"Sign-out" by my doctor:

My Medications:

Name	Dose	When (BLDB)	Purpose.

Allergies/reaction:

Advance Directives? _Y _N HC proxy? Name _____ Phone _____

Things I do to maintain my health (e.g., try to eat a healthy diet,
try to exercise, try to take my medication as prescribed, check
myself (weight, blood sugar, feet, others), get doctor check-ups,
ask for information I need from my doctor, avoid excessive drinking,
avoid illegal drugs, spend enjoyable time with friends or family, try to
get enough sleep, build in time to relax and decompress,
use breathing techniques or mindfulness to calm my body or control pain):

Ways the care team has noticed that the patient tries to contribute to their
own health and healthcare: (e.g., tries to come to appointments on time,
calls for advice or help before a problem gets too serious, tries to be

Fig. 10.2 (continued)

honest with team members even if that makes things uncomfortable at times, tries to be supportive of health team members):

_____

_____

Barriers to doing what I want to do to maintain or improve my health (e.g., pain, other symptoms of illness, housing instability, hard to obtain food for healthy diet in my area, no place to exercise, family responsibilities or pressures, difficult to get rides to appointments):

_____

_____

Urgent Plan of Care:
1. *Symptoms*
   a. *What are the symptoms that typically lead to ED visits or frequent calls for perceived urgent healthcare needs?*
   b. *Why are these symptoms important or worrisome to you?*
   c. *What has worked for you in the past to address these concerns?*
2. *Who is on your team?*
   a. *Who knows you best at the Health Center?*
   b. *Who has been most helpful in addressing your concerns?*
   c. *Who outside of the Health Center has been most helpful in meeting your urgent needs?*
3. *Detailed Executable Plan*
   a. *What do you want to happen when you have an urgent care need?*
   b. *How do you want the plan relayed to you (by phone, in person, by whom)?*
   c. *When would be a good time to check in with you after addressing your urgent need?*

My future:

What I am able to do or enjoy at this point in my life when illness or stress doesn't get in the way. Things that I would like to be able to do more often:

_____

_____

Things I would like to be able to do in the future, for myself or for people I care about:

_____

_____

Fig. 10.2 (continued)

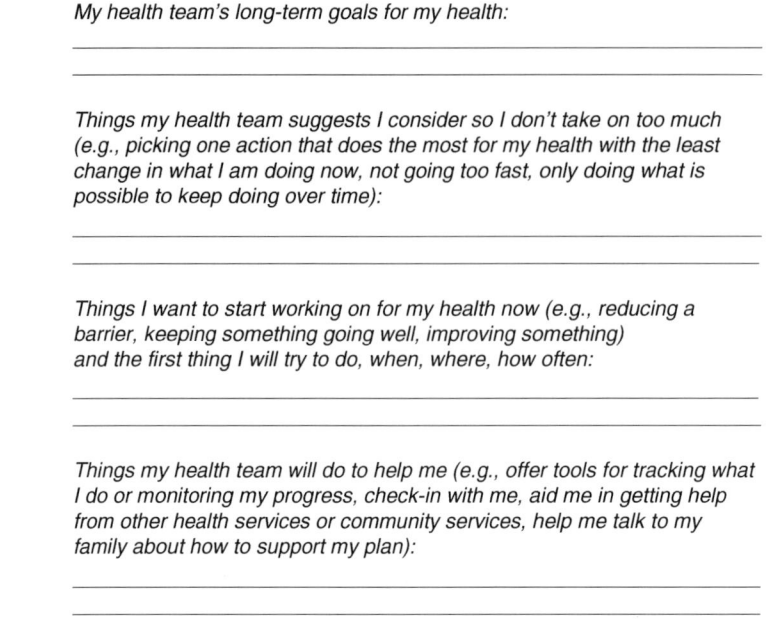

My health team's long-term goals for my health:

_____

_____

Things my health team suggests I consider so I don't take on too much
(e.g., picking one action that does the most for my health with the least
change in what I am doing now, not going too fast, only doing what is
possible to keep doing over time):

_____

_____

Things I want to start working on for my health now (e.g., reducing a
barrier, keeping something going well, improving something)
and the first thing I will try to do, when, where, how often:

_____

_____

Things my health team will do to help me (e.g., offer tools for tracking what
I do or monitoring my progress, check-in with me, aid me in getting help
from other health services or community services, help me talk to my
family about how to support my plan):

_____

_____

Fig. 10.2 (continued)

of the patient as part of the team. It elicits goals without using that terminology, and it modifies the goal orientation with considerations of what is possible for the patient to undertake due to the burden of their illnesses. It should fit comfortably with a minimally disruptive medicine orientation for serving multiply-disadvantaged patients. Each practice will choose items that fit for its approach to patient-centered care. It is longer than some others. It will require input from the patient and multiple members of the team. The process of completing it may take multiple conversations at different times. One team member should monitor its stage of completion and discuss (probably in the huddle on the day the patient comes for each visit) what parts of the plan are still to be completed and what parts might need to be reviewed and updated.

In any PCCP implementation, a practice will choose which elements of other PCCPs are best to support their approach to patient-centered care. They will format the plan in a way that is the best fit for their population of patients and to fit the contingencies of their own EHR. Some may find additional efficiencies such as having elements of the PCCP pre-populated from other parts of the record they currently collect. For all of these adaptations, a program will need the support of central leadership in their health system or an EHR that they can modify to their own purposes. The current variability in approaches to the PCCP will be likely to continue until there is a good deal more research in the area.

10.5 Summary

The four parts of the T.E.A.M. Way interact recursively to help a primary care practice implement team-based patient-centered care for high-utilizing multiply-disadvantaged patients. The transparency of open notes and open clinical conversations begins the shift of language toward strength-based descriptions of patients. Empowerment takes the shift in terms about the patient and begins a process of questioning designed to create a narrative concerning the patient's strengths and successes that begins to build the self-efficacy that patients need for participating as partners in their care. Activation uses attributions to refine and expand the narrative in a way that solidifies the identity of the patient as an active member of their healthcare team and creates mutual self-fulfilling expectations of what the team can accomplish for the patient's health. Mutuality is made official through the patient-centered care plan that is an evolving "official" record of a developing partnership.

In the next chapter, we will discuss ways that a practice might go about training a team to use the T.E.A.M. Way and how it might set up a professional development structure so that it can retain team members by allowing them to advance in their roles and their salaries without having to leave their jobs for schooling.

References

1. Delbanco T, Walker J, Bell SK, et al. Inviting patients to read their doctors' notes: a quasi-experimental study and look ahead. Ann Intern Med. 2012;157:461–70.
2. Mautner DB, Pang H, Brenner JC, Shea JA, Gross KS, Frasso R, Cannuscio CC. Generating hypotheses about care needs of high utilizers: lessons from patient interviews. Popul Health Manag. 2013;16:S26–33.
3. Medical Dictionary for the Health Professions and Nursing. 2012. Retrieved 2018, August 22 from https://medical-dictionary.thefreedictionary.com/care+plan
4. American Academy of Pediatrics. Care plan. Retrieved 2018. AAP.org
5. Chunchu K, Mauksch L, Charles C, Ross V, Pauwels J. A patient centered care plan in the EHR: improving collaboration and engagement. Fam Syst Health. 2012;30:199–209.
6. Patient Centered Primary Care Institute. The shared care plan of Whatcom County, Washington, slides 17–24; 2013. Accessed 20 Aug 2018.
7. Safford B. Conversation with Bertha Safford, MD, 8/20/18. 2018.
8. Council LS, Geffken D, Valeras AB, et al. A medical home: changing the way patients and teams relate through patient-centered care plans. Fam Syst Health. 2012;30:190–8.
9. Morse J, Valeras A, Geffken D, Eubank D, Orzano AJ, Dreffer D, DeCook A, Valeras AB. Using a team approach to address avoidable emergency department utilization and rehospitalizations as symptoms of complexity through quality improvement. In: Sturmberg JP, editor. The value of systems and complexity science for healthcare. New York: Springer; 2016.
10. Kahtri P, Gunn W, Talan M, Valeras A, Peek CJ. Beyond hotspotting: identifying complexity and solutions at the micro, meso, and macro levels. Presented at the collaborative family healthcare conference, Rochester, NY. 2018.
11. Oxman TE, Hegel MT, Hull JG, Dietrich AJ. Problem-solving and coping styles in primary care for minor depression. J Consult Clin Psychol. 2008;76:933–43.
12. Mold J, Hamm R, Scheid D. Evidence- based medicine meets goal-directed health care. Fam Med. 2003;35:360–4.

13. Østbye T, Yarnall KS, Krause KM, Pollak KI, Gradison M, Michener JL. Is there time for management of patients with chronic diseases in primary care? Ann Fam Med. 2005;3:209–14.

14. Rosal MC, Ockene JK, Luckmann R, et al. Coronary health disease multiple risk factor reduction. Providers' perspectives. Am J Prev Med. 2004;27(Suppl. 2):54–60.

15. Bodenheimer T, Laing BY. The teamlet model of primary care. Ann Fam Med. 2007;5:457–61.

16. Mauksch L. Personal communication. 2013.

17. Dixon A, Hibbard J, Tusler M. How do people with different levels of activation self-manage their chronic conditions? Patient. 2009;2:257–68.

18. Ross J. Care plans best practices for development and implementation. Patient Centered Primary Care Institute, Portland, OR, slides 33–39; 2013. Accessed 2 Aug 2018.

19. Ross J. Conversation with Jackie Ross, 8/28/18. 2018.

20. Chait S. Conversation with Sari Chait, 8/28/18. 2018.

21. Leppin AL, Montori VM, Gionfriddo MR. Minimally disruptive medicine: A pragmatically comprehensive model for delivering care to patients with multiple chronic conditions. Healthcare. 2015;3:50–63.

Resources

Developing a Care Plan for Complex Patients

Examples of Shared Care Plans – PCPCI – Patient Centered Primary Care Institute, Portland, OR https://bit.ly/2LBb3AJ.

Whatcom County Shared Care Plan – Institute for Healthcare Improvement http://www.ihi.org/resources/Pages/Tools/MySharedCarePlan.aspx.

Setting Goals

Setting Goals with People with Complex Needs: A Collaborative Approach. National Committee for Quality Assurance. https://www.ncqa.org/hedis/reports-and-research/measuring-what-matters-most-to-older-adults/.

Goals to Care: How to keep the person in "person-centered". National Committee for Quality Improvement. https://www.johnahartford.org/newsroom/view/ncqas-goals-to-care-how-to-keep-the-person-in-person-centered-now-available.

Setting Goals, Care Management, Staff Training

The COACH Model of the Camden Coalition. https://www.camdenhealth.org/the-coach-model/.

Chapter 11
Growing and Retaining an Expert Team

11.1 Team Learning

The T.E.A.M. Way is different enough from the way that most health professionals have been taught to interact with patients that it presents a substantial training challenge for successful implementation. Complex patients present so many illnesses, psychosocial problems, and difficulties in relating to their healthcare team that many of the routines and interviewing techniques that are successful for the majority of patients fail to engage them. This group is different enough to require special training for health professionals who care for them.

One example of this training is a curriculum for caring for complex patients developed as a rotation experience in a family medicine residency and evaluated by a group at the University of Washington [1]. When it was initiated, the rotation was a 4-week training experience, consisting of 33 half-day training sessions out of the 40 half-days in the 4 weeks. The training included didactics, experience visiting community agencies, observation of the residents' work by faculty with feedback, and individual study by residents. The knowledge and experience that were built into the rotation included community medicine, social determinants of health, health disparities, health literacy, violence and abuse, substance abuse, at-risk populations, mental health, provider-patient communication, health behavior change, patient self-management, cultural competency, and the development of interdisciplinary teams ([1], p. 36). The competencies that the rotation sought to foster were improving relationships and agenda setting, understanding the patient's perspective, encouraging behavior change, co-creating care plans, counseling and mental health, coordinating the carrying out of care plans, navigating complex health systems, leading teams, linking with community resources, and treating complex patients. The program used the Minnesota Complexity Assessment Method [2], which is now the Patient Complexity Assessment Method [3], as a way of identifying complex patients and as a means of assessing the types of needs that they were presenting. To organize the observation of the residents'

© Springer Nature Switzerland AG 2019
A. Blount, *Patient-Centered Primary Care*,
https://doi.org/10.1007/978-3-030-17645-7_11

interviews and feedback about what they did well and what they could improve, they used a standardized, evidence-based form, the Patient-Centered Observation Form [4].

Twenty-four residents completed the rotation over a 2-year period. They reported that the training experience resulted in significant changes in their abilities to relate to and empathize with complex patients who were part of their patient panels. They saw increases in almost all of the competencies that the rotation was designed to teach. The majority reported that despite their improvement, they did not feel fully competent in most of these skills. The authors concluded that observation and feedback, learning to work as part of a team, didactic input, and exposure to community resources were all good ways to approach training, but an intense 1-month training experience (170 hours) was not enough to develop the competencies needed to be able to offer state-of-the-art care for complex patients.

Duplicating or expanding the training program described by [1] especially if the training is given to all team members, is probably not possible in most primary care settings. That would require a practice to import didactic speakers, to offer mentors who can observe and give feedback to team members in their work with complex patients, to make time for reading and discussion about the social determinants of health, to free up team members to visit community agencies that also serve these patients, and to do this over a period longer 170 hours in a 4-week period. There would need to be additional time in role play and discussion of their mental models of care for many team members. Even then, when the team had learned the state of the art in caring for complex patients, it still would need to learn the T.E.A.M. Way.

When describing the development of the T.E.A.M. Way, I am using the term "growing" rather than "training" the team even though most people would not call "growing" an evidence-based concept. I find the idea general enough and familiar enough to convey the complexity of the process, whereas "training" has a much more limited set of associations, many of them misleading. Growing encompasses the many facets of change that are involved in successfully putting the T.E.A.M. Way into practice. There are changes in team members' understanding of patients' life situations, changes in team members' perceptions concerning patients' behavior, changes in the distinctions of what are helpful acts of patient-centered behavior, changes in culture and relationship with other team members, and ultimately changes in the way one understands the mission of healthcare in general.

A program of intensive training sufficient to create the changes above is not practical economically or pedagogically. People don't learn a set of skills as complex as these in a short time. It is an evolutionary process, involving gradual change of "mental models of care" as well as new routines and new uses of language [5]. Instead, teams will need to identify, grow, and share expertise that resides in its members as part of the routines of care for their patients.

The team learns together. Continuity of relationships with their panel of patients and the continuity of team members working with each other create an environment that fosters relationships. These relationships are the foundations for experimenting with new behaviors. A culture of continuous improvement, of Plan, Do, Study, Act [6] in the practice as a whole, fosters the type of learning needed to grow as a team. The work of improving protocols and routines requires an openness to discovery that leads toward new ways of thinking about patients, their life situations, and their care.

Team-based care in this setting is challenging because each team is made up of members with different training, different roles, and, therefore, different experiences of any one patient or group of patients. The T.E.A.M. Way presents all team members with the task of learning to enact an approach that is likely to be equally new to all of them. The team members share a learning task. And while everyone is learning together, the team tolerates and supports the variable paths of its members toward incorporating the T.E.A.M. Way in their own work with patients. It is the same tolerance and support the team offers in working with its complex patients who are on a journey to learn to be partners in their own healthcare.

Learning becomes a team task and a team process. To go more deeply into the elements that this task requires, we have to look briefly at the concept of "learning organizations." If we think about the team as a small learning organization, this literature helps to lay out the tasks and pathways forward. One of the best known and most influential authors on the phenomenon of learning organizations is Peter Senge. His book, *The Fifth Discipline* [7], was identified by the Harvard Business Review as one of the seminal management books of the past 75 years [8]. Among many aspects of his work, certain of his insights are particularly relevant for the task of growing an expert team in healthcare. He offers ways of understanding "mental models," "building a shared vision," and "team learning" that can provide a launching point for defining the process.

Senge defines "mental models" as "deeply ingrained assumptions, generalizations, or even pictures and images that influence how we understand the world and how we take action" ([7], p. 8). This definition of models is more abstract than many concepts or protocols that are also termed "models." Often "models" are general patterns of actions and role descriptions based on research findings (e.g., [9]). Senge's definition of mental models is more akin to what might be called "cognitive lenses." They are ways of organizing perceptions built on assumptions about the world, assumptions that may not be available to the consciousness of the perceiver at a given moment in time. He describes access to one's mental models as a process of increasing self-reflection and understanding that requires interaction with others, their perspectives, and their feedback.

Senge points out the need for a "shared vision of the future" among members of the learning organization as a condition for the types of conversations and mutual observations that make up the process of change in mental models. This is very different from a "vision statement" that is created somewhere in an organization and promulgated to the members. In an organization the size of a team, the shared vision arises over time through robust exchanges of information. In Senge's view of the process, "As people talk, the vision grows clearer. As it gets clearer, enthusiasm for its benefits grow." ([7], p. 227). The richness of the information exchange gradually transforms the experience of the team members. The team develops a shared vision as part of "…the process of aligning and developing the capacities of the team to create results its members truly desire" (p. 236). The learning of the team could be thought of as "organismic" in the sense that any learning organism will have multiple ways of taking in information about its environment and about its operation within that environment. These multiple sources of information are combined or synthesized to guide its continued successful operation within its context.

Successful operation in its environment over time impacts the structure of the organism. Its structure comes to reflect the patterns of "information" it has encountered to guide its successful operation in its environment. Each of the team members is a different source of information for the team about its operation in its environment. Each will have different experiences and expertise, both personal and disciplinary. The richness of team exchange of information synthesizes these differences of experience and guides the team's operation toward the shared vision of the future. This exchange occurs both within the team meeting and in the process of each enacting their roles and expertise for their shared patients. Over time the rich exchange of information impacts the informal structure of the team. For example, one MA may become the leader when discussing the care of patients with a particular type of history or from a particular culture. The BHC might lead self-care classes. Each becomes a leader, changing the expected structure of communication, within a recurring context.

There are practical ways of learning within the clinical practice and in routine meetings of the team that fit with Senge's ideas about growing a learning organization. These include mutual observation and feedback, sharing information about team members individual experience in narrative form, mutual rehearsal and discussion of new skills for speaking with patients, and problem-solving meetings with patients and sometimes with their families. These are done at the cost of additional time, though the mutual benefit can justify the added time required.

Mutual observation and feedback can be done by having one member of the team observe and offer feedback to another member of the team who is fulfilling his or her role in patient care. The feedback is offered either at the time of the observation or, more likely, at another time when feedback is more convenient. The observer is not required to be of the same discipline as the observed. In fact, having the observer from a different discipline creates opportunities for new perspectives and learning for both observer and observed. The process is done by overlapping team members' times with the patient, times that are usually sequential. In some settings one team member follows the patient through the sequence of interactions that make up a visit, observing their interactions with each team member. In other settings the team members interacting with the patient do the observation of each other. The MA might observe the interaction of the patient with the registration staff member and then be observed in their interaction with the patient by the doctor, who is then observed in their interaction with the patient by the care manager or behavioral health clinician and so on. This is a process that is done for the sake of the learning of the team with the permission of the patient. Patients tend to appreciate the process and the fact that the team is using self-observation in order to provide better care. Typically, extra time is allowed at the beginning of a morning or afternoon, and the process is done with the first patient in a session. This one person is usually the only one with whom it is possible. A team might conduct a mutual observation once a month or once every other week. Enough observations are generated in each instance for a good deal of conversation and learning, which might take place over lunch or at the end of the day.

The mutual observations and feedback can benefit from structured observation tools. An excellent example is the Patient-Centered Observation Form (PCOF) [4] for doctors' visits and a second version designed to help observe nursing or medical assistant visits. Both versions draw on extensive reviews and syntheses of literature on patient-centered interviewing. The tools introduce expertise in interviewing by the categories of behavior they cause to be observed and recorded. They help both the observing and the observed team members to distinguish behaviors that have been shown to be useful. Without the observation guidance, numerous actions that are helpful would not be identified. By helping team members distinguish desirable behaviors, the process allows for clearer and more rigorous conversation using an appreciative inquiry approach. This focuses observation on what is done well and encourages precise description of those behaviors for the person being observed. When the conversation focuses on what each observed team member did well, it is easier to appreciate their expertise because it becomes more visible to someone from another discipline as well as to the observed health professional. Listing and discussing what each person did "right" are likely to help all experience the conversation as supportive and therefore as more conducive to learning. Plus, seeing the list of other behaviors on the PCOF that would make the patient-centered part of the visit better provides additional teaching for everyone. As people get more invested in the process, they tend to push for feedback on how they might have introduced more elements rather than accepting only feedback about what they did well. The assumption that we are all learning together and that each individual effort to improve helps us all provide better care is one that should be stressed regularly. The "we are learning together" value tends to be easy to maintain because each team member will be both observer and observed over time.

Another contributor to a learning team occurs when some of the information about patients and interactions with them is exchanged in *narrative form*, rather than solely in descriptions in medical professional language. Medical professional language is designed to report events and facts in only as much detail as required, as briefly as possible. Perhaps a few readers remember Sgt. Joe Friday on the crime drama of the 1950s called *Dragnet*. Sgt. Friday caught the spirit of any professional language and how it differs from narrative language. He used to direct witnesses who were telling their narratives of their experiences of the crime, to stick to "just the facts, Ma'am." Professional language is "just the facts, Ma'am." A narrative of the crime is an account of the experience of the witness, data that Sgt. Friday did not feel the need to hear.

Medical professional language, by its nature, is likely to lead to different and very individual responses by each team member in a team meeting. When medical professional language is the only type of information exchanged in a meeting, team members of different disciplines judge the accounts offered by other members by whether or not they needed those facts in order to do their jobs better. A description in professional language of the involvement of one team member with a patient, as it gets more detailed, can make other members of the team wonder why they need to spend so much time on this. What the care manager did with the patient may be judged by the doctor, MA, or BHC as something they do not need to know about in detail to do their jobs. "Just the facts, Ma'am." That does not mean that medical professional language does not have a place in meetings. It does. There is a lot of data that needs to be exchanged efficiently. But its contribution to the process should be noticed so that a different type of exchange can be used when that would be more useful.

Narrative knowledge, exchanged in the form of a story, impacts the listener's as well as the teller's experience. Patients who want to tell the story of their experience with their illnesses often feel that the doctor doesn't know them until the doctor has heard their story. For these patients the doctor's hearing of the story increases the possibility of the patient being part of their healthcare team and pursuing self-management. In the mind of patients with complex health challenges, if the doctor is able to make a diagnosis and prescribe a treatment through processes that only the doctor knows, e.g., tests, vital signs, and the patients' brief answers to the doctor's questions, then the entire process is one in which the patients' experiences play no role. The process enacts the model of doctor-patient relationship that is expected and often resented by patients who have low levels of activation [10]. These patients believe that doing what the doctor tells them to do is their only responsibility. It is an understanding that is associated with very poor adherence and less active self-management (Chap. 9).

A narrative is not the "facts," it is the story of an experience in terms that allow a listener or a reader to have some of the experience of the event. The training curriculum on treating complex patients at the University of Washington [1] stressed the value of residents visiting community agencies that serve many of the complex patients in the practice to understand the lives of the patients better and to understand the work of agencies that might be part of the patient's larger care team. As desirable as this might be, sending all the team members to many community agencies is not likely to be possible. But what if one team member who had to go to an agency as part of their job brought back a narrative that allowed all the team members to have some of the experience of the visit? Consider the difference in how the team might experience a professional description versus a narrative account by the care manager reporting on her visit to the Vietnamese Cultural Center.

11.1.1   Just the Facts

"Our patient, Tran Pak, is currently attending the Vietnamese Cultural Center at least 3 days a week. The Vietnamese Cultural Center is located on Chestnut St. It was established in 1989 to serve the social and cultural needs of the large influx of Vietnamese people who came to our city in the early 80's. The center is supported by grants and by the United Way. It provides housing support, navigation and translation for Vietnamese people in medical and social services organizations, and offers events at the center to build the cohesion of the community."

11.1.2 A Narrative Account

"I learned that Tran Pak spends a good deal of time at the Vietnamese Cultural Center. I went to see her there so I could better understand her functioning in the community. I also hoped to make contact with an agency that serves many of our Vietnamese patients. I asked Tran how I could call and make an appointment to come. She said she didn't know a phone number and that I could come any time. The center is in a fairly simple storefront on Chestnut Street with a barber shop and a small Vietnamese grocery store on the same block. When I came in, I was surprised that the whole center was in one large room. There were different groups around the edges of the room doing different activities. In one corner there was an open kitchen and a group of women involved in a cooking class. In another corner, a group of women were taking turns reading out loud in English. In another corner a group of men were sitting at a table playing a game I didn't recognize. There were three people sitting at another table having some sort of meeting. I guessed they were the staff. As soon as she spotted me, Tran got up from the reading group and came to meet me with a smile that I don't think I had ever seen on her before. She took my arm and took me to each of the groups to introduce me. It turned out that the director of the center was the woman leading the cooking group. She is an older woman named Mai Nguyen who explained what they were cooking and insisted that after my visit with Tran, I had to stay for lunch. As Tran introduced me around the room, she translated for the few people who spoke to me in Vietnamese. People tended not to offer to shake my hand. Several seemed not to want to make eye contact, so I tried to greet them without staring at them in the eyes. When I was eating lunch with the cooking group, they wanted to know what I usually eat for lunch. I found it difficult to describe a turkey and swiss sandwich, so I went quickly out to my car and got my sandwich out of my cooler. We cut it into small squares and put it on a plate for people to try. They all said that they thought it was delicious, but I think they were just being polite. I have never seen Tran looking so relaxed and happy as in that center. Ms. Nguyen said that I could come there anytime to meet with any members of the center who are our patients. ("Members" is what they call their clients). I was surprised at how effective their limited staff seemed to be with the members. I know how depressed Tran seems at times when she is at our practice, and so I was particularly impressed with the power of the center to bring out a very different side of her."

The second description takes more time than the first. It is likely that the second description is more interesting and conveys a familiarity with the Vietnamese Cultural Center that the first one fails to impart. It gives every team member some personal experience of the center because they could imagine the visit that was described. The fact that one team member vividly conveys their experience of an agency helps build confidence for other team members to contact the agency should that become needed.

The narrative of the visit is the story of a new relationship between the team and the agency. All team members are more familiar with the center, so when Tran Pak comes back to the practice, they seem to know something about her daily experience, an important step in engagement. A second benefit comes from the fact that one positive relationship can be leveraged into a positive relationship with the center for other members. When the next team member contacts the center, there is already the beginning of a relationship on both sides. People who feel familiar to each other can establish working relationships much more quickly. The introduction for the next team member can be made by the person with the original relationship, or if that is not possible, the next team member can reference the relationship already established by the first team member. The first positive connection can open the door for professional collaboration on behalf of other patients.

11.1.3   A Brief Example

In the health center in which I practiced, as we got behavioral health clinicians more integrated into day-to-day care, there was less available time for longer-term therapy. We needed to refer more people who needed longer-term therapy to the mental health services in town. Our behavioral health clinicians were frustrated by the intake practices of these services that made achieving a successful connection for our patients difficult. The fact that our BH staff were mostly doctoral-level clinicians and well known in the field of integrated primary care added no value in dealing with the intake workers at these agencies, and letting the patients call for themselves rarely led to a successful connection. They were not used to the type of formality and the wait times they encountered. We knew we needed a more personal connection, but none of the BHCs had the time for all the meetings that would require. We decided to send out a second-year psychology graduate student who was doing a practicum placement in our health center. She was given instructions to make a personal connection with the intake worker or the clinical director at each service. We weren't as interested in the service array (though that was the ostensible reason for the meetings) as we were in her building a person-to-person relationship. Stephanie was an upbeat, curious person who was great at getting to know people quickly. She found the meetings interesting, a meaningful training experience. She ended up making friendly relationships with almost all of the people she met, knowing a bit about their lives, their kids, their hobbies, and their professional stories. After her connecting meetings, BHCs had much better luck making timely and successful referrals, as long as Stephanie made the introduction or the BHCs started their conversations with Stephanie's contact at each agency saying they were her colleagues. After she left us, we were dropping her name in our referral calls for another year or more.

The evidence for narrative accounts comes in part from neuroscience. A vividly told story, one that lets the hearer envision the setting, the characters, and the action in the narrative, imparts an experience for the hearer of having had a version of the experience described in the story. This is due to the fact that the neural substrates that are activated by envisioning an experience are the same ones activated by personally having the experience [11, 12]. The same account in professional language, just the facts, doesn't have the same impact.

> Whereas imagery techniques are already commonly used in psychological settings, these findings clarify why imagery is effective in treating conditions such as pain, fear, phobia, and anxiety. However, an understanding that imagined events differ little from actual perception also suggests that imagery techniques may yet be applied too narrowly. For example, a more creative use of imagery may be to cultivate empathy and compassion among practitioners for the experiences of their patients (i.e., to purposefully imagine being in the physical and emotional situation of the client). (Cappas et al. [13], p. 380)

Sometimes professional language is protective when an experience is upsetting to hear. Professionals, such as those who work with abused children, populations in disaster events, or traumatized veterans, who hear vivid stories of abuse or tragedy as part of their helping roles, commonly show some of the symptoms of the PTSD, depression, or anxiety of the victims they serve. In those situations, when talking with their colleagues, professional language protects others from envisioning the traumatic story, but it leaves the helping professional alone with the experience of hearing the narrative of the traumatic events. In these situations, narrative can help in a different way. First-person accounts of the professional's feelings and reactions to the story, rather than sharing the actual patients' stories, can be helpful [14]. In working with complex patients, many with traumatic histories, sharing a story of the experience of the professional with the patient, rather than the story told by the patient, allows team members to experience providing care to the patient. A story of the reframing that was helpful, of successes and solution stories that were elicited, or of attributions that seemed to enhance the patient's activation can add to the engagement options with the patient for other team members.

Narrative descriptions allow the whole team to learn from the experience of successful patient-centered care by each team member.

A crucial element in growing a learning team is *practicing the four skills* of the T.E.A.M. Way. These skills are likely to be new to all members of the team. The learning tasks involved are more equally shared than in most situations where differences in expertise tend to create a hierarchy of teachers and learners. The skills are reframing for a successful move to transparency, eliciting successes and solutions in conversations with patients, offering attributions that can help adjust the perceptions and expectations of both the patient and team member for the patient's motivation or activation, and working with patients on a patient-centered care plan to help them define achievable goals in their move toward improving their health and their lives. Each of these skills is discussed in much greater length in one of the T.E.A.M. chapters. Each is a definable skill that can be practiced in a team meeting, eliciting ideas from team members and feedback about those ideas. Through the recursive interplay between "practice" (learning and rehearsing) in the team meeting and "practice" (using skills in their work with patients) made possible by observation and feedback sessions or by narratives of providing care, team members refine the skills of reframing, solution-focused interviewing, creating attributions, or co-constructing a treatment plan.

For most members, practicing is likely to be a new sort of activity for a team meeting. The initial sessions teaching these skills may be done on an organization-wide or practice-wide basis. It is likely that no member of an individual team will already have enough expertise to teach these skills. But once the initial concepts are taught and practiced in larger groups, using team meetings for practice builds the skills in the context of discussing how to approach particular patients on the team's panel.

Some organizations will decide to use a facilitator of team meetings when learning skills is on the agenda. The facilitator of the team meeting might ask about the behavior of the patient being discussed that members found particularly challenging. Then members could be asked to offer positive reframes of that behavior, no matter how far-fetched. As the list is discussed, some reframes will start to seem potentially credible to some team members. If the team picks a reframe to introduce to the patient, the discussion can turn to how this might be done, perhaps through an open clinical conversation between team members with the patient present or as an attribution used by a team member. At other times the facilitator might ask the team to consider strengths of the patient, often by thinking about how the situation might be even worse and examining who is doing what to keep that from happening. The team might practice interviewing the patient for exceptions to the current problematic patterns in their care or their self-management. Discussing the framing of the team's portion of a patient-centered care plan is another rich opportunity for formulating descriptions in ways likely to be engaging to a patient. In each case, the practicing and learning are woven into discussions of patient care that are part of the business of a team meeting.

Patient/Family/Team Meetings   Finally, an opportunity for the team to put the four T.E.A.M. Way skills into practice is created when the team has patient/family/team meetings. The most common of these will be patient/team meetings. These will usually be brief get-togethers of team members who are actively caring for one patient when the patient comes for a routine visit. These meetings allow for a check-in that can be for clarifying an understanding of patient's symptoms or life struggles and for problem-solving, to introduce a new team member to the patient's care or to revise the care plan. The patient is treated as an enfranchised member of the team. Deciding on a patient/team meeting can be a common outcome of a discussion of a patient's situation in the team meeting which needs further information or further discussion. The meetings can be booked in one of the standard visit times. The more the team practices doing these meetings, the more the format can be streamlined, the more matter-of-fact they can be in describing the meeting to the patient, and the less intimidating it can be for patients.

Patient/family/team meetings are initiated by inviting patients, their relevant family members, and/or their most important service providers from community agencies to come to meet with the team. Such a meeting provides a way to improve engagement of the patient and the team, and to work on problems of the patient in their network. Situations in which adding the patient to the team meeting can make an important difference can be times when a patient is at odds with the team or with one member of the team, times when the patient disagrees with their family about their care plan, whether the patient supports the plan and the family disagrees or vice versa, or when there is conflict in the family or between the patient and another agency that creates a stress that impedes the patient's self-management. The idea of the meeting can be intimidating to some team members, to patients, and to family members. Framing the meeting as an opportunity to practice the skills of the T.E.A.M. Way is one possibility for reducing the uneasiness of team members. Team members can feel vulnerable in an unfamiliar setting where they can imagine feeling publicly on the spot. Making participation by team members voluntary can help. Over time, they are likely to feel more comfortable as they hear the processing after meetings by other team members. Including only team members that have a relationship with the patient can make the process less challenging for patients, family members, and representatives of community agencies. It is important to make sure people don't feel "called in front of" the team. Defining the meeting as assembling the extended version of the team involved in helping and supporting the patient's progress can be helpful. This definition makes patients and other members of the network feel that they reasonably have a place in the meeting. Steps for conducting the meeting are offered in the Appendix.

11.2 Guiding the Developing Team

Determined leadership is necessary to build engagement in the T.E.A.M. Way among team members. Particularly early in the team's development, it will feel odd to some staff to be having conversations in meetings that have never been part of previous team meetings. It will take determination to install the new practices over time.

The commitment of time to the team will be one of the demonstrations of the commitment to the new way. Andrew Schutzbank, MD, MPH, Vice President of Product and Technology, for Iora Health, makes the point that in athletics, another type of expert practice, the ratio of skill development time to performance time is about opposite of the time ratio in medicine. In medicine we expect masterful performance with almost no time to learn and refine skills. At Iora Health, a for-profit health system with primary care practices in many states across the nation, the teams meet for a 45-minute huddle at the beginning of every day and take another 3 hours per week for meeting and learning time [15].

There may be some on the team who are skeptical. I would suggest that there be no forcing of the issue in regard to their opinions. Expect the judgements of team members about the new way to be variable. Treat any open show of skepticism as a gift. Define holding on to past ways as a commitment to patients, a commitment not to embrace unproven changes unless the skeptics are convinced they will help their patients. But the skepticism doesn't change the direction of the new way. The team meetings will gradually become obviously necessary, even to the skeptics, to support successful functioning of team members. The impact of open notes and patient-centered care plans will be a pathway into the ideas and assumptions of the new approach as long as skeptics are required to use them once they are implemented. In the meetings, the value of finding strengths and creating attributions should be maintained, even if not all are offering ideas and suggestions.

Perhaps the role with the most impact on the success of skill development for progress on the T.E.A.M. Way is the facilitator. Team members use their regularly scheduled meetings (as opposed to the patient/family/team meetings above) to work together to address issues of patient care, to refine work flows, to discuss the instances of mutual observation and feedback, and to practice skills like reframing, solution-focused questioning, creating attributions, and improving patient-centered care plans. As the team addresses these difficult challenges, someone needs to be watching the process rather than the content. In most teams, the facilitator will be one of the team members, though this is not required. On some teams it will be a role that is passed to different members in different situations or for different tasks the team needs to take on. The facilitator may be a doctor, who is also thought of as the leader of the team, or a behavioral health clinician who has experience and training in facilitating groups, or another team member who is particularly good at organizing meetings so that they keep to an agenda. It should be someone who understands the multiple purposes of the meetings. Over time, team meetings will inevitably develop patterns that are expected by team members. The facilitator should have an eye on the patterns that are being developed and how they serve the learning and transformation of the team.

An example of a pattern of interaction that a team might develop over time for a specific function could be the organization of the discussion of patients. It will be a type of conversation that will be very frequent in team meetings. This type of conversation might have common elements that become regular parts of most patient discussions. Perhaps the person who raised the name of the patient for discussion might be expected to say what made them want to discuss this patient today and what outcome would lead them to believe the time was well spent. There could be a moment to seek input from other team members who had very different experiences with the patient. They can briefly share the story of how their interaction has been different from the member who wants new ideas for helping the patient. The team could try to find ways that these differences could fit into one consistent picture. Is there a reframing that might allow the patient and team members to talk about the concerning situation or behavior more easily? Team members could look for examples of strengths or past solutions from their knowledge of the patient and talk about what questions might elicit the patient's story of these strengths or unique outcomes. The team could talk about what attributions about the patient might be useful to help activate the patient to be more comfortable and active as part of their own team. Finally, they might discuss whether there are questions that they might ask the patient, or similar patients, about how the team can improve care for them. Over time, it would help to make a template for discussion among team members. The template could be used as a guide, though not a required format. The facilitator would have their eye on building templates and using them to guide the team generally in processes that have been found to work best for them. Team meetings are taking precious time, so someone should have the job of helping them stay on topic, rather than letting things ramble.

The facilitator can also be sure that an appreciative inquiry approach to assessing the team's processes is followed [16]. Appreciative inquiry [17] is an organizational approach that can be very helpful in building the culture of a team. It is a way of studying what works in an organization, of focusing on what people do well. It tends to both elevate and activate team members. When people are "caught in the act" of doing well, they tend to become energized to continue to do well. They become more confident, more willing to try to improve.

Frankel and Beyt, authors of the AMA module on the topic, claim that as appreciative inquiry becomes the norm in meetings, people tend to get more efficient. Team members are more engaged and more invested in mutual success. The authors offer ideas such as the "appreciative check-in" at the start of a huddle or team meeting in which one or more team members are asked to briefly describe something that has already gone well today. There is the "appreciative debrief" at the end of a team meeting in which people say briefly something they noticed that went well in the meeting. While there may be some reports from people of their own good experiences, these brief reports are also likely to draw team members' reports on what other team members did well.

A few minutes taken every week or month to have commentary about what is working on the team particularly well, or to recount brief stories of team members' excellent functioning, can be bonding for the team as a whole. It improves the sense of mutuality in the work if everyone is enfranchised to notice another team member doing things well. Effective feedback, because that is what appreciative inquiry is promoting, highlights the specific behavior of the team member and says briefly what about that behavior was particularly useful or supportive in the situation. The team member hearing the report will be most influenced if the description of the behavior was specific, so that they can envision the exact situation being described. This calls for a very brief narrative rather than a description in professional language. This is an experience for the one who is described that is likely to make the person better able to repeat the behavior. The process of team self-observation is an example of the self-assessment that was described by Senge [7] discussed above.

Crabtree et al. [5] refer to this sort of change when they say that patient-centered care requires a change in the "mental models of care." The team becomes a learning organization. Each member at one time or other is a learner and a teacher, passing along learning and experiences the other members of the team did not have. The more the team is focusing on patients with complex health needs, as described in Chap. 4, the smaller the role of medical expertise and the greater the role of behavioral expertise have in the learning of all the team members.

11.3 Retaining an Expert Team

The process of growing an expert team also grows the expertise of each individual team member.

In general, people enjoy their work more as they learn new things and take on new tasks. It is rewarding to a team member who was trained in the "squad" model (Chap. 2) to be recognized as offering leadership in some area of the team's work. A counterforce to this pattern, however, can be the difference in pay on the team. In some settings there is the flexibility to create new pay categories or other competency-based structures to adjust salaries and job titles when new competencies are demonstrated and new duties are taken on. In other settings, HR job categories or union contracts make this much more difficult. Tom Bodenheimer, in his study of 15 cases in which primary care practices developed high-functioning teams [18], mentions a "downside" of teams in that staff members who gain competencies and responsibilities are more prone to leave for higher-paying jobs or for training programs to get additional credentials. A team member who has experienced the development process involved in the T.E.A.M. Way and has operated professionally in the routines and relationships of a mature team will be a valuable catch for another organization. Because the T.E.A.M. Way involves an unusually rich development process and because it is built on the unique culture developed by the team, the loss of any team member means the loss of an important element of team culture. A plan for retaining team members is almost as important as the plan for growing the team.

The team can be used to grow its next generation of members, but this is only workable in the long run if continuity of team members and of the relationship of those members to the team's panel of patients is the rule. In residency training practices, the turnover of doctors is inevitable. In those settings the consistency of contact with other team members can be what creates the experience for patients of having an ongoing healthcare team. As one patient in a residency practice put it:

> Even though there have been two or three doctors, I still had the same nurses or medical assistants, seeing the same ones. I usually see the same two, and I feel comfortable around both to them. I feel as though I have a healthcare team. (Morse et al. [19])

As the team becomes settled into regular patterns in its meetings, patterns such as the structure of conversations about patients, practicing the skills of the T.E.A.M. Way, using quality improvement steps such as PDSA (see Chap. 12) on its workflows, and the occasional patient/family/team meetings, its meetings become an excellent ongoing training environment for growing trainees who could become its future members. By shadowing team members, trainees can get hours of time observing and practicing the skills that experienced team members use in providing care. The team becomes a nexus of expertise and of different mental models of care. Trainees who experience the team in its day-to-day functioning will develop much more quickly than the original team members who built the team when there was no model to observe.

There is likely to be a significant demand for the team to create a formal, efficient training model. The team will probably want to use some of the time of one of the members as the training officer to manage the administrative details of choosing, orienting, and monitoring trainees. Training will impact the work of every team member and take time. Working to have efficient training routines, with a minimum of didactic time, will help to maintain the efficiency of team functioning. The team might want to invite a representative group of patients to participate in the training process, especially teaching trainees the life experience of coping with complex health needs and offering observations on attitudes and behaviors by team members that have been especially helpful.

The creation of a training function means that each member of the team will be adding expertise as a trainer to the list of new skills they are building. Members who are successfully involved in innovative ways of practicing constitute valuable human capitol in an organization. Some team members of the early T.E.A.M. Way teams in an organization will show themselves to be particularly good trainers. In a large organization, these people can become part of the training and onboarding process across the organization. The organization will need trainers for different roles, for different sites, and for the organization as a whole. Trainers of each role will be needed for people in that role. Trainers from any role can be part of the training of new team members within the same site. Trainers in leadership roles can provide orientation to new sites as they start up.

In the development of the T.E.A.M. Way, the value of the additional time given to growing the team can be returned manyfold through lower costs for the care of high-utilizing patients provided by the continuity in team relationships with these patients. In order to retain these employees, they need a way to continue to develop their skills and responsibilities. They also need to look forward to increases in salary that match their increases in expertise. One way of accomplishing this without losing the continuity of relationship in the team is to implement a career ladder of steadily increasing responsibility and increased salary within the team. Such a career ladder facilitates team members acquiring additional training and even new credentials and new licensure without having to leave their work and their paycheck.

The New Hampshire Primary Care Behavioral Health Workforce Initiative (www.NHPCBHWorkforce.org) is a project funded by the Endowment for Health in New Hampshire. The Initiative began by assessing the behavioral health workforce needs, current and projected, in the federally qualified health centers and rural health centers in New Hampshire. The project found a broad array of roles on primary care teams. This multiplicity is important in planning for the future of a workforce. Equally important is the pattern in the USA that when a BH clinician with their new expertise is added to a primary care practice for the first time, the integration of behavioral health changes the practice of all the health professionals in the setting [20]. New screening procedures are initiated. Behavioral health needs are more broadly identified. All professionals become more involved in behavioral healthcare to some degree, though they are not doing counseling or psychotherapy. New staff roles are likely to be added such as care managers, community health workers, navigators, health coaches, and so forth which the NHPCBHWI called "care enhancers" [21]. The work of care enhancers is highly behavioral in nature.

The Initiative website (Resources) offers a career ladder that outlines a path for team members in entry roles to advance into care enhancer roles that have more patient care responsibility and higher salaries and ultimately to positions as licensed behavioral health clinicians.

The authors of the Workforce Assessment reviewed training programs that could help someone who entered primary care in one of the entry roles to become competent to fill one of the care enhancer roles. They looked for online training programs that could prepare a staff member to function as a care manager, care coordinator, navigator, patient advocate, or health coach. In many cases some elements of these roles were already part of the duties of the entry-level roles, but the additional training can improve their skills and offer a credential for a change of job title and an increase in pay. The Initiative also found online programs that could provide the training and credentials so that someone in a care enhancer role could become a licensed BHC. They were looking for Masters programs that would allow a worker to continue in their current employment without having to leave for training. This is advisable so the worker doesn't have to give up their salary for a period of time and because for a team member in the T.E.A.M. Way, it would be very difficult to create an experience as appropriate as continuing on their current team to prepare them for additional responsibilities.

The career ladder can be an ongoing method to improve the diversity in the workforce of an organization. Healthcare organizations have a much easier time finding medical assistants, community health workers, and medical interpreters from diverse backgrounds that represent important populations in their communities, rather than trying to find the same diversity in masters or doctoral-level professionals. If the entry-level workers who can enhance ethnic, racial, and language diversity, over time become the new professionals on the team, the diversity of the workforce is spread and maintained.

In a setting committed to partnership, the role of orienting new trainees can be greatly enhanced by giving formal roles in the training to selected patients. Patients can tell the story about successful coping with chronic illnesses and psychological and social challenges. Experiencing the T.E.A.M. Way from the patient role can be an effective learning experience that these patients can offer to new trainees with stories of what kind of behavior by their team members were most engaging and useful to them. Going to patients for crucial learning is a lesson in itself for trainees in the place of partnership in the organization.

In some cases, patients who have had a role in teaching new trainees about coping with multiple health and life challenges may ultimately decide to get training to be a community health worker, medical assistant, or medical interpreter. The presence on the team of a former patient of the T.E.A.M. Way would offer similar benefits to the ones documented by the use of "peers" in mental health settings [22]. Someone with life experience of similar illnesses can build an engagement with some patients that is very difficult for team members who do not have that experience. The evidence of the perceived impact of asymmetries of power and social status in the primary care visit to preventing engagement by many patients with low incomes, trauma histories, and complex health needs was discussed at length in Chap. 5.

Encountering a team member who has successfully traveled the same road can help build an engagement for some patients who are especially troubled by these differences in status.

11.4 Summary

The literature on learning organizations helps in describing the process of growing a team that can learn to use the elements of the T.E.A.M. Way, to engage, empower, and activate patients with complex healthcare needs. The process uses regular routines of team interaction on behalf of its patients rather than an extensive training program to build skills, develop new understanding, and, ultimately, transform mental models of care. The continuity over time of team members working together on behalf of a panel of patients contributes to building relationships that empower both patients and team members.

The skills and relationships built through this process become valuable capitol for the practice and its larger organizational context. The T.E.A.M. Way sets an environment for learning and skill development for both patients and team members. Both can develop into training resources for the organization. The development of a career ladder creates a way of targeting and documenting growth in knowledge and skills to facilitate increases in responsibility and salary for team members. It gives the organization a chance to retain the capital that these team members represent.

Appendix

Patient/Family/Team Meeting

A patient/family/team meeting provides a way to improve the engagement between the patient and the team and a means to solve problems that affect the health of the patient in his or her social network. Situations in which adding the patient to the team meeting can make an important difference can be as follows: a patient who is at odds with the team or one member of the team, when the patient is not successfully managing their illness and the usual approaches are not helping, times when the patient disagrees with their family about their care plan (whether the patient supports the plan and the family disagrees or vice versa), or when there is conflict in the family or between the patient and another agency that creates stress that impedes the patient's self-management.

The idea of the meeting can be intimidating to some team members, to patients, and to family members. For team members, framing the meeting an opportunity for them to practice the skills of the T.E.A.M. Way is one possible way to reduce their uneasiness. Another possibility is to make participation by team members voluntary. A third approach that can also lower patient or family reluctance is to include only team members who have a relationship with the patient to make the process less imposing. Family members or agency members invited to the meeting have to be selected by the patient. Often the likely candidates are already listed in the patient's care plan as the people who are trusted to receive information about the patient's illness and healthcare. Defining the meeting as an assembly of the extended team involved in helping and supporting the patient's progress can be a way of starting an engagement between team and family. This definition makes patients and other members of the network feel that they reasonably have a place in the meeting.

One person should facilitate the meeting. The facilitator may or may not have a role in the patient's care. Often teams will ask the behavioral health clinician to facilitate the meeting. A meeting that is actively structured by the facilitator will tend to reduce uneasiness in people who have not previously been a part.

The Stages of the Meeting

Welcome and Introduction

The facilitator makes a brief introduction in the beginning of the meeting. She/he makes sure people know where the bathrooms are and that everyone has coffee, tea, or water, if those are available. The introduction explains the purpose of the meeting and the steps that they will follow to achieve the purpose. The purpose given is general enough to allow room for individual goals on the part of meeting attendees. It is defined as helping the team learn to be better informed about what the patient and his family face in trying to help him cope with his illnesses. The outcome sought is that the team is wiser about how to be helpful and that patient, team, and relevant family or agency members can work together more effectively. Each member is asked to introduce themselves and to say a couple of words about their role in relation to the patient.

Current Situation

The facilitator then introduces the process of the meeting. She says that in meetings like this, the team has found it helpful to start by getting a brief description from each member who is willing to speak about what is currently going well or is working in the patient's healthcare and what their one or possibly two top concerns are for the patient's care. She is clear that whatever is currently working is part of the foundation on which the group is building. (The foundation metaphor tends to settle people, make them for comfortable, and create a period at the start of the meeting that is less stressful than they worried it might be.) She says that after the group has identified the foundation, what is working, she will ask the group to help identify the next step in building toward better care, something that is doable by the people in this room with leadership from the patient. Then the group will take a minute to identify resources that might be needed and attempt to leave with a brief but clear plan for taking the next step.

The facilitator confirms briefly that this plan sounds acceptable to the patient and people attending the meeting. In most cases the patient and other meeting members are happy to have the meeting led and to follow what to the team seems to be a familiar set of steps. They tend to agree quickly. If a family member raises a concern or a complaint at this point, the facilitator makes clear that the person is raising just the sort of concern that we hope for as part of the "current situation" portion of the meeting. In all likelihood addressing that concern will be part of the plan.

After the crucial step of asking the patient and family for permission for the team to start the descriptions of the present situation, she asks the doctor to go first. The doctor delivers a brief "sign out" of the patient's medical situation with some attention to the challenges that attend any person's attempt to adequately manage such a medical picture. The doctor uses the mindset of the Minimally Disruptive Medicine approach [23], to describe the "footprint" of care and self-management for the patient. This makes for an easier time finding what the patient is doing right in their relationship with the team and in their own care. It is a patient-centered view introduced at the start of the meeting. Having the doctor at the beginning prevents a problem that can arise later if the patient or a family member should make a comment about the patient's health that is medically uninformed. Their embarrassment when they need to be corrected can set back the cooperation which had built to that point in the meeting. After the medical summary, doctor adds something complementary about the patient. This may require a bit of the reframing that has been part of the transparency training for the T.E.A.M. Way. Finally, she suggests one or two concerns about the patient's health or healthcare briefly, building off the foundations of what is working that they listed earlier, if possible.

The next to be recognized is likely to be the team member who spends the most time with the patient or who knows the patient the best from the past. This is the person who, more than likely, can do a robust job of pointing out the aspects of the patient's behavior and of their relationship to the team that are working best. Their top concern is listed as a follow-up to the descriptions of what is working or has worked in the past. Because of their time with the patient, any brief mention of solutions that have been identified or of attributions that have been part of the patient's activation can be good to mention. Then other team members in turn speak very briefly in the same pattern descriptions of what is working and what their top concern or two for the patient are.

By the time the team members have finished, there have been multiple descriptions that could be reframes of previous behavior, solutions that have been gleaned, and attributions that increase the patient and family members' experience of the team work that has gone well and the patient's role in supporting that team work. A patient who has been argumentative might have been called "always willing to share what is on his mind" or "doesn't try to hide from the team the parts of his life that make his self-management very difficult." A patient who never argues but who rarely takes her medicine and has not cut back on her drinking may have been described as "protecting us from things that keep her plan from working so that we can both enjoy our visits together" or "a considerate member of her family who seems to try to keep us from asking about her home life so that the privacy of her family members is protected."

By the time the three or four team members have finished their brief contributions, patients and family members are likely to be a bit more relaxed. The meeting is shaping up to be less blaming and more supportive than they expected. They have also been exposed to a way of working that sets a tone for the meeting. As the process continues with the patient and the family or agency members, the facilitator actively moves the conversation from person to person, making the transitions by reflecting the contribution of each person. This makes each person experience themselves as heard. A bit of pressure toward brevity is maintained by the facilitator by the reminder that we are looking for only one or two concerns that can help us identify the next step toward better health. If there is overt blaming, a reminder that we are all here to help the patient with his journey to better health can help to defuse it.

The reframing skills of the facilitator can be very useful when the family members disagree as they are having their turns to talk.

Example of the "what is working discussion" and reframing

Patient: Since I got my own place, I get to be in charge of myself and my own medication.

Parent: I think he is not taking his meds as regularly as when we got to see what he was taking and when. I am not sure this is a step forward.

Facilitator: So, it sounds like your family has made real progress because Marvin is managing a lot more in his life, but there is no less caring on the part of his parents. They worry like most parents when they can't know as many details about his life. Does that sound right?

Identifying the Next Step

When all of the people in the meeting who want to speak about what is working and what their top one or two concerns are have finished, the facilitator tries to make a summary statement, reiterating the general picture of what is working well and repeating a very brief synthesis of the main concerns that have been offered. She asks the assembled participants what would be the next step on the way for more effective healthcare for the patient. She reiterates the charge that we are looking for one step that is doable by the patient and people in this room, one that will be noticeable when it works. At this point, she leaves a silence. It is hoped that the first suggestion comes from the patient or family members. If it needs to come from one of the team members, a great deal of checking back to confirm support from the patient, agency representatives, and family members will be part of vetting the idea. The facilitator my want to check to see if there are other ideas, saying that the more choices we have, the greater the chance that we will pick an idea that is a good choice and the more choices we have to fall back on if the first one is not helpful. When an idea is settled upon (e.g., the patient will begin walking three times a week and three designated family members will each take one day to walk with him), the facilitator checks with the patient about what others can do to help. Sometimes family or team members are perceived as helpful if they check on how the plan is going and sometimes the patient thinks it is more helpful not to check. Whichever way the patient requests, the people who are requested too respond a certain way are asked it that would be possible, at least as a trial. If they don't agree, they can be asked how they think they can best support the step that was identified.

The roles of the healthcare team are also detailed. Sometimes the doctor or the team member who spends the most time with the patient can ask to do their own check. The doctor says that often additional exercise will contribute to some health metric (e.g., lowering of HbA1c). She will monitor that number for the patient to see if he is getting a benefit in addition to feeling better from the exercise. The care manager may say that it has sometimes been hard in the past for the patient to keep exercising. If this time the patient keeps going beyond 2 weeks, she would like to ask him what he is doing to keep things working this time and to share what they learn with the other family members who were at the meeting. That way they will all learn more about what works for the patient. If possible, the actions of the team are defined as fitting into the plan of the patient and family. If that definition doesn't fit, the team is described as supporting the plan in trying to do their part to help the patient stay healthy.

At this point, the meeting has taken 20 minutes to ¾ of an hour. A brief arrangement is made for follow-up. Usually the follow-up can be the summary at the patient's next visit with the team. It is shared with the people who came to the meeting and worked on behalf of the patient, assuming the patient doesn't want to limit the distribution in some way. The meeting is not reassembled unless there is a reason that is clear to both the team and the patient. The hope is that after the meeting, the team and patient are doing better at working together for the patient's health. If the patient customarily comes to visits with family members, those people would be likely to continue coming unless the patient is functioning more autonomously than before. When the other family members continue to come, it is still possible to continue to notice or to stress what the patient is accomplishing with their support, rather than what they should do to guide or care for the patient.

References

1. Osborn J, Raetz J, Huntington J, Overstreet F, Ross V, Charles C, Maukshc L. A curriculum on care for complex patients: resident perspectives. Fam Med. 2016;48:35–43.
2. Peek CJ, Baird MA, Coleman E. Primary care for patient complexity, not only disease. Fam Syst Health. 2009;27:287–302.
3. Pratt R, Hibberd C, Cameron IM, Maxwell M. The Patient Centered Assessment Method (PCAM): integrating social dimensions of health into primary care. J Comorb. 2015;5:110–9.
4. Mauksch LB, Dugdale DC, Dodson S, Epstein R. Relationship, communication, and efficiency in the medical encounter: creating a clinical model from a literature review. Arch Intern Med. 2008;168:1387–95.

5. Crabtree B, Nutting P, Miller W, Stange K, Stewart E, Jae'n C. Summary of the National Demonstration Project and recommendation for the patient-centered medical home. Ann Fam Med. 2010;8(Supplement 1):S80–90.
6. Berwick D. Developing and testing changes in delivery of care. Ann Intern Med. 1998;128:651–6.
7. Senge PM. The fifth discipline: the art and practice of the learning organization. New York: Currency; 1990.
8. Infed.org. Peter Senge and the learning organization. 2018. Downloaded 17 Sept 18.
9. American Psychiatric Association & Academy of Psychosomatic Medicine. Dissemination of integrate care within adult primary care settings: the collaborative care model. 2016. https://www.psychiatry.org/File%20Library/Psychiatrists/Practice/Professional-Topics/Integrated-Care/APA-APM-Dissemination-Integrated-Care-Report.pdf
10. Dixon A, Hibbard J, Tusler M. How do people with different levels of activation self-manage their chronic conditions? Patient. 2009;2:257–68.
11. Kreiman G, Koch C, Fried I. Imagery neurons in the human brain. Nature. 2000;408:357–61.
12. O'Craven KM, Kanwisher N. Mental imagery of faces and places activates corresponding stimulus-specific brain regions. J Cogn Neurosci. 2000;12:1023–34.
13. Cappas NM, Andres-Hyman R, Davidson L. What psychotherapists can begin to learn from neuroscience: seven principles of brain-based psychotherapy. Psychother Theory Res Pract Train. 2005;42:374–83.
14. Seys D, Wu AW, Van Gerven E, et al. Health care professionals as second victims after adverse events: a systematic review. Eval Health Prof. 2012;36:135–62.
15. Schutzbank A. Personal communication, 9/29/18. 2018.
16. Frankel R, Beyt G. Appreciative inquiry: fostering positive culture. Steps forward. American Medical Association. 2017. https://www.stepsforward.org/modules/appreciative-inquiry
17. Cooperrider DL, Whitney D. A positive revolution in change: appreciative inquiry. Oakland: Berrett-Koehler Publishers; 2005. https://www.goodreads.com/book/show/221785.Appreciative_Inquiry
18. Bodenheimer T. Building teams in primary care: 15 case studies. San Francisco: California Healthcare Foundation; 2007.
19. Morse J, Valeras A, Geffken D, Eubank D, Orzano AJ, Dreffer D, DeCook A, Valeras AB. Using a team approach to address avoidable emergency department utilization and rehospitalizations as symptoms of complexity through quality improvement methodology. In: Sturmberg JP, editor. The value of systems and complexity science in healthcare. New York: Springer; 2016.
20. Hall J, Cohen DJ, Davis M, et al. Preparing the workforce for behavioral health and primary care integration. J Am Board Fam Med. 2015;28(Supplement 1):S41–51.
21. Blount A, Fauth J, Nordstrom A, Pearson S. Who will provide integrated care?: assessing the workforce for the integration of behavioral health and primary care in New Hampshire. Center for Behavioral Health Innovation, Antioch University New England, Keene. 2016. https://bit.ly/2LdzQqd
22. Davidson L, Chinman M, Sells D, Rowe M. Peer support among adults with serious mental illness: a report from the field. Schizophr Bull. 2006;32:443–50.
23. Leppin AL, Montori VM, Gionfriddo MR. Minimally disruptive medicine: a pragmatically comprehensive model for delivering care to patients with multiple chronic conditions. Healthcare. 2015;3:50–63.

Resources

Tools for Mutual Observation and Feedback

Patient Centered Observation Form: MA/Nurse https://bit.ly/2VcCzUJ.
Patient Centered Observation Form- Clinician version http://www.pcof.us/.
Online training in using both forms of the PCOF – http://www.pcof.us/

A Tool for Assessing Patient Complexity

Training in using the Patient Centered Assessment of Complexity – www.pcamonline.org.

Building a Workforce for Team-Based Care

New Hampshire Primary Care Behavioral Health Workforce Initiative – Website www. NHPCBHWorkforce.org.

Chapter 12
Quality Improvement, Data, and Partnership

12.1 Improving Quality for Patient-Centered Care

We have been gradually building a model of interaction between health professionals and patients in which the patient is a fully enfranchised partner, fulfilling a unique role, and the final judge of what treatments, that are supported by the health professionals, will be followed. Using data to improve quality is part of the definition of patient-centered care. The commitment to being patient-centered requires that healthcare teams be constantly trying to improve care for the particular patients they are serving. This entails keeping data about their patients' health and the patterns of service they are given and using the data as feedback for improving quality. Unfortunately for patient-centeredness, the people who decide what data will be collected and what will be done with the data are usually in a powerful role that is distinct from the people about whom the data is collected. In other areas of patient-centered care, the challenge has been to move from taking the wishes and preferences of patients into account when health professionals are designing care, to achieving partnership with patients in designing their courses of treatment. In the effort to use data to improve care, there have been relatively few examples of partnering with patients in deciding what data they would like to have collected, what information that data could supply, and what actions or improvements could be possible because of having that data.

First, we should discuss current practice in designing quality improvement processes, and then we will discuss the role of patients in designating data to be collected. Donald Berwick was one of the leaders of the Institute of Medicine's endeavor to create a blueprint for a new healthcare in the USA that is detailed in the Quality Chasm report [1]. He was also the founder and CEO of the Institute for Healthcare Improvement in Boston, MA. It is hard to overstate his influence in the area of improving healthcare for patients. He pushed for quality improvement approaches that are clear, specific in what they are designed to accomplish, focused on the needs of patients rather than the needs of the organization, designed to change

© Springer Nature Switzerland AG 2019
A. Blount, *Patient-Centered Primary Care*,
https://doi.org/10.1007/978-3-030-17645-7_12

systems rather than to make change within systems, constantly making small improvements rather than holding out for the "best possible" change, and constantly measured so that innovations can be kept, changed, or rejected based on their usefulness for patients [2]. To accomplish these changes, Berwick recommends the Plan, Do, Study, Act approach or "PDSA cycle."

The PDSA cycle approach gives an alternative to the cumbersome quality improvement processes that are sometimes attempted in health organizations. These often involve outside quality improvement professionals, extensive study of current patterns, design of complicated changes in protocols, and long implementation and evaluation periods. Such quality improvement efforts take up so much time and attention that they have to "get it right" the first time to justify their cost. This is not usually possible. The PDSA process is designed to make the quality improvement process shorter, less formal, and more adaptable. The Plan stage of the process can be as brief as a conversation with one patient to identify or consider a possible improvement. The Do stage can be a trial of a change as small as discussing an issue differently with one patient or sampling the reactions of patients who come on a given day or week. This can be enough to give data for the Study stage which can provide information from which patterns can be observed and hypotheses about meanings can be drawn. The Act stage is the implementation of the action suggested by the hypotheses that have been developed through the previous stages. At that point, the cycle often repeats since getting a good solution is not possible every time.

The example below is a trio of PDSA worksheets from a practice that wanted to get patients to fill out a feedback form about the care they were receiving [3].

Cycle One

- **Tool**: Patient feedback
- **Step**: Dissemination of surveys
- **Cycle**: 1st try

Plan

- **I plan to**: test a process of giving out satisfaction surveys and getting them filled out and back to us.
- **I hope this produces**: at least 25 completed surveys per week during this campaign.

Steps to execute:

1. We will display the surveys at the checkout desk.
2. The checkout attendant will encourage the patient to fill out a survey and put it in the box next to the surveys.
3. We will try this for 1 week.

Do

What did you observe?

- We noticed that patients often had other things to attend to at this time, like making an appointment or paying for services, and did not feel they could take on another task at this time.

- The checkout area can get busy and backed up at times.
- The checkout attendant often remembered to ask the patient if they would like to fill out a survey.

Study

What did you learn? Did you meet your measurement goal?

- We only had eight surveys returned at the end of the week. This process did not work well.

Act

What did you conclude from this cycle?

1. Patients did not want to stay to fill out the survey once their visit was over. We need to give patients a way to fill out the survey when they have time.
2. We will encourage them to fill it out when they get home and offer a stamped envelope to mail the survey back to us.

Cycle Two

- **Tool**: Patient feedback
- **Step**: Dissemination of surveys
- **Cycle**: 2nd try

Plan

- **I plan to**: test a process of giving out satisfaction surveys and getting them filled out and back to us.
- **I hope this produces**: at least 25 completed surveys per week during this campaign.

Steps to execute:

1. We will display the surveys at the checkout desk.
2. The checkout attendant will encourage the patient to take a survey and an envelope. They will be asked to fill the survey out at home and mail it back to us.
3. We will try this for 2 weeks.

Do

What did you observe?

- The checkout attendant successfully worked the request of the survey into the checkout procedure.
- We noticed that the patient had other papers to manage at this time as well.
- Per checkout attendant only about 30% actually took a survey and envelope.

Study

What did you learn? Did you meet your measurement goal?

- We only had three surveys returned at the end of 2 weeks. This process did not work well.

Act

What did you conclude from this cycle?

1. Some patients did not want to be bothered at this point in the visit; they were more interested in getting checked out and on their way.
2. Once the patient steps out of the building, they will likely not remember to do the survey.
3. We need to approach them at a different point in their visit when they are still with us – maybe at a point where they are waiting for the doctor and have nothing to do.

Cycle Three

- **Tool**: Patient feedback
- **Step**: Dissemination of surveys
- **Cycle**: 3rd try

Plan

- **I plan to**: test a process of giving out satisfaction surveys and getting them filled out and back to us.
- **I hope this produces**: at least 25 completed surveys per week during this campaign.

Steps to execute:

1. We will leave the surveys in the exam room next to a survey box with pens/pencils.
2. We will ask the nurse to point the surveys out/hand them out after vitals and suggest that while they are waiting they could fill out our survey and put it in box.
3. We will see after 1 week how many surveys we collected.

Do

What did you observe?

- Upon self-report, most nurses reported they were good with pointing out or handing the patient the survey.
- Some patients may need help reading the survey, but nurses are too busy to help.
- On a few occasions, the doctor came in while patient was filling out the survey, so the survey was not complete.

Study

What did you learn? Did you meet your measurement goal?

- We had 24 surveys in the boxes at the end of 1 week. This process worked better.

Act

What did you conclude from this cycle?

1. Approaching patients while they are still in the clinic was more successful.
2. Most patients had time while waiting for the doctor to fill out the survey.
3. We need to figure out how to help people who may need help reading the survey.

The PDSA cycle is repeated and refined by the information gained in the previous cycles. In the example above, there were meetings of a core group working to accomplish the task in order to create a process that produced adequate numbers of patient feedback forms. Once a method of collecting the expected number of forms was created, those forms could be used to inform other targeted QI improvements, probably involving another core group using the PDSA approach.

12.2 Patients as Partners in Quality Improvement

In Chap. 4, we discussed the evolution of the IOM's definition of patient-centered care from "conscientious, explicit, and judicious use of current best evidence and knowledge of patient values" (IOM [1], p. 76) to "care planned, delivered, managed, and continuously improved in active partnership with patients and their families … to ensure integration of their health and health care goals, preferences and values" (Frampton [4]). The shift from understanding the preferences and needs of patients in designing care to making patients partners in the design of their own care is not trivial. The process of designing and collecting data about care is particularly challenging because of the complexity of possible data collection and analysis systems. The amount of training and expertise potentially required is daunting to most health professionals, much less to most patients. At this point, however, we should remind ourselves of our earlier discussions of how daunting the effort to make patients partners in their own healthcare can be, when the training and expertise of physicians and other health professionals seem so far above that of most patients, particularly multiply-disadvantaged patients. In that discussion we came to see that partnership in their healthcare, especially in the case of multiply-disadvantaged patients, is the best approach to achieving good outcomes for their complex needs.

Mutter and his colleagues [5] make the point that the burden of data to be collected in primary care is already unsustainable because so many stakeholders expect primary care to supply data needed for their purposes. They advocate for a standard set of measures of healthcare delivery that is specific to primary care. They assert that many quality improvement approaches have failed in primary care because they were not guided by the core principles of primary care. They want to see data collection schemes that are focused on "optimizing holistic patient and population health, harnessing the Quadruple Aim as a dynamic whole, applying measurements as tools of quality, not outcomes of quality, and prioritizing therapeutic relationships" (Mutter et al. [5], p. 931). First, data collection for quality needs to support wholistic assessments of patients, not just a set of measurements of their body functions. Measurement needs to be an intervention toward quality, not just a check on the quality of other interventions, and it needs to be built on the assessment of relationships between health professionals and patients.

Getting to those goals may be enhanced by adding the additional element of patients' participation in the design of their own individual data tracking. It can also be enhanced by having patients be part of the practice-wide data design. So, what might a program that was designed to partner with patients in quality improvement look like?

Morse et al. have documented such a process in a primary care health center with a residency training program that is attached to a regional hospital. The hospital at the time had the highest rate of emergency department (ED) use in the state. Half the use of the ED by the patients of the health center was made by the population as a whole, and the other half of the use was made by a small group of "high utilizers." In looking for a way to partner with these patients to address their high utilization of the ED, Morse and the team defined "high-utilizing" patients as people who used the ED four or more times in the previous year. Instead of designing a program to try to impact these patients and then trying the program out to see if it was a fit for them, the team (which was one of three healthcare teams in the practice) decided to ask the high-utilizing patients to join them in the QI effort. All 127 patients in the practice who met the criteria of "high utilizers" were invited to become part of a Patient Advisory Committee (PAC) for the team.

This was a very innovative approach and might seem risky to many health professionals. Usually when a practice forms a PAC, they invite the most articulate and invested patients to join. This tends to produce a group of middle- or upper-income patients who are comparatively healthy. Asking the patients who have experience with the difficult problem that the practice wants to address seems obvious, but it is not very common. In this case, of the 127 patients invited, 6 joined the group.

The PAC met monthly for 1.5 hours over a period of 6 months. The meetings were recorded (with the patients' permission) and transcribed as part of the effort. A member of the team facilitated but did not lead the meetings.[1] The healthcare team met weekly for 20 minutes to discuss the emerging themes from the PAC and how to use them in refining care for high-utilizing patients. Over 6 months, the PAC offered ways that the practice could improve its delivery of urgent care in the areas of patient perception, communication, and relationship with the healthcare team. Problems that the PAC identified included patients not understanding what triage was or what the range of urgent care services in the practice was. They pointed out

---

[1] Facilitating a group of patients without being the expert in the room who gives information and directs the process is a skill that many health professionals do not possess. The process is described in detail in Doherty and Mendenhall's "citizen healthcare" method [7].

a pattern in the responses of nurses answering triage calls that contributed to high utilization. Triage nurses usually advised patients who called with urgent problems to go to the ED if inserting them into the schedule at the time of the call might impact the smooth flow of care during the day.

After only 3 months, members of the PAC began to ask if the clinicians and staff in the health center knew who was on the committee. They said they noticed their interaction with the health professionals in the practice was improved, smoother, and more pleasant. The answer was that the doctors and other team members, outside of the two people who recruited the PAC, had not been told who was on the committee. The patients were detecting a change that was based on the feedback and discussions the project had generated up to that point.

Ultimately, working together the PAC and the team created an addition to the patient-centered care plan, an urgent plan of care (UPOC). The UPOC outlined the common sequence of events and symptoms on the part of the patient that had led to ED utilization in the past. It identified who on their care team or from an outside agency the patient felt understood their needs best and who had been most helpful in urgent situations in the past. Finally, it asked specifically what patients wanted to have done when they were experiencing urgent need and how best to follow up on whatever urgent care was provided.

Team members, from their perspective, reported a general shift in the attitude of their colleagues from "no" to "yes" when patients called with urgent needs. One person noted that their own thinking had shifted from a program-protecting to a problem-solving attitude, seeing calls as problems to be solved rather than as potential inconveniences for the team. At the same time, team members were noticing a change in patients' responses to the way care was offered. The "new day" was noticed and appreciated by both patients and the teams.

Ultimately, there was a significant reduction in ED utilization among the 127 identified high utilizers even though only 6 took part in the PAC. The patients of the healthcare team that was conducting the project had the greatest percentage of reduction, but the patients in the group of 127 who were cared for by the other two teams also showed statistically significant reductions as well.

Members of the team conducting the quality improvement project were very aware of the project's impact on their own knowledge and ideas, not just those of the patients.

> Eliciting direct patient input from high utilizers allows the healthcare team to understand their patients' decision-making processes in regards to choosing the place of care for their urgent care needs, highlighting both individual and system contributions. This feedback served as the impetus for the transformational learning amongst the team that eventually changed their patient interactions. ([6], p. 234)

This project involved a number of PDSA cycles in making the progress that it did, each with the addition of an active partnership with patients in generating information that was crucial for informing both the evaluation of previous efforts and in the design of subsequent steps in the overall endeavor. Might we call this pattern a PPDSA approach (Partnering, Plan, Do, Study, Act)?

12.3 Reconsidering Data from a Partnership Prospective

In a chapter on information that supports partnership, it is appropriate to say a bit about the difference between information and data. Having a clear distinction in one's mind is important for navigating the complexities of data and information in the understanding and assessing of healthcare. There is no dearth of attempts available to clarify this distinction. One that I like is the "DIKW pyramid" [8]. The metaphor of a pyramid is used because each "level" is thought of as built upon the foundation of the levels below. The pyramid, from the bottom to the top, is data, information, knowledge, and wisdom. The example Doyle gives is:

- **Data**: I have one item. (*The data collection displays a 1 and not a 0.*)
- **Information**: It is a tomato. (*Now we understand the item and its characteristics.*)
- **Knowledge**: A tomato is a fruit. (*We can identify patterns in the information and apply them to the item.*)
- **Wisdom**: Tomato is never added to a fruit salad. (*There is an underlying commonly understood principle that governs the item's purpose or use.*)

I find this example useful, but it could be misleading in that it is a-contextual. Unless the reader is careful, she/he can get the impression that this is the only hierarchy of ways of knowing a tomato. For example, in many contexts a tomato is a fruit, i.e., the knowledge that is relevant. In other contexts, however, the knowledge could be very different, without defining the first example as incorrect. In an Elizabethan theater in sixteenth-century England, such as the Globe in which Shakespeare's plays were presented, the gentry sat in seats in balconies, and the poorer folks, the "rabble," stood on the ground in front of the stage. To the unlucky actor or playwright whose work was judged as low quality by the rabble, a tomato was a projectile to be avoided. While the question of whether a tomato is a fruit or a projectile is a tongue-in-cheek example, the point is not trivial. We can leave to the philosophers the question of whether facts are facts no matter who is the observer or are facts dependent on who is distinguishing what to observe and what those observations mean. When we talk about making partnership with individuals of a certain population, the perspectives of the members of that population on their health and their healthcare have to be a determining factor when we design our approach. This includes the need to have the patients' experience and perspective reflected in the data we decide to collect and in how we conceptualize what to make of that data.

In healthcare, a four-level pyramid modifying the example above can be defined and an additional layer added to invite an understanding of context into the conversation. My hierarchy is data, information, pattern, meaning, and action.

- **Data**: The number of items.
- **Information**: The characteristics of those items.
- **Pattern**: The patterns that can be noticed in the numbers and characteristics of items observed.

- **Meaning**: The meanings we infer about the domain of the data from the patterns we identify.
- **Action**: The actions that seem logical based on the meanings we have derived and the purposes for collecting the data.

As an example, consider the two perspectives in the relationship of a health professional or team on one hand and a multiply-disadvantaged patient on the other. Remember that such patients, particularly those who are at low levels of activation as measured by the Patient Activation Measure [9], tend to believe that the role of the patient is not to achieve self-management but to do what the doctor tells them to do [10], though in many cases they also experience interactions with their doctors as potentially coercive and demeaning (see Chap. 5). There is little experience of partnership on either side. Below are the two perspectives involved in the care of a person with complex healthcare needs and their doctor on the data from the patient's lab work for their diabetes (Table 12.1). The hemoglobin A1c reading is a measure of the average level of sugar in the patient's blood over the preceding 3 months. A good reading is 5.6% or below. Above 7% is concerning.

In this case, the same data represents different information to the HP and the patient, leading to different perceived patterns, different meanings, and different sorts of actions. They are different largely because there has been no discussion or agreement about what data to collect, what information is wanted, and to what purpose. In this case, the decisions about what data to collect are made unilaterally by the team (as required by the health system or the regulators and payers who influence the health system). The patient above has a low level of activation and low engagement in the process. He expects to be told to follow directions and to be measured on how well he does what he is told. When there is little partnership and shared purpose between the patient and his health team, then the process of collecting this data, the information it provides to the team, the pattern that is observed, and the actions taken by the team tend to support the patient's unstated assumption

Table 12.1 Healthcare information hierarchy

Case #	Perspective	Data	Information	Pattern	Meaning	Action
1	Health professional	HbA1c = 8.5	Pt is at risk for many bad outcomes	Over the last few months, pt. is not making progress. Risk is increasing	Pt must not understand the seriousness of the risks	Spend more time talking about importance of diet, exercise, and med adherence
1	Patient	HbA1c = 8.5	My Dr. will think my HbA1c is a bad number	Every time she thinks that, I get a lecture	She doesn't like me; I let her down and waste her time	"Forget" to go for HbA1c blood draw or to attend next visit

that doctors have a lot of power, that he has no say, and that the only way of having some impact on his healthcare is to decide when to cooperate and when not to.

This example shows the common difference between health professionals' assumption that data is "objective" and the experience of some patients that data is political, reinforcing the asymmetry of power in the doctor-patient relationship.

I have also experienced patients using data collection as a way of communicating with health professionals that the system does not expect. In many years of practice as a psychologist in primary care, almost every patient I saw for a scheduled appointment had filled out a PHQ-9 screening form for depression. The PHQ-9 asks about nine possible symptoms of depression. For each symptom, the response is numerical, from 0 to 3, with 3 being the most serious. The possible scores a patient can have on the form range from 0 to 27. A score below 10 is considered not concerning, 10–14 suggests mild depression, 15–19 indicates moderate, and 20 and over represent severe and very concerning depression [11]. In my many years of seeing the PHQ-9 scores of my patients, I almost never saw a score in the 23–26 range. If I did, I responded with the appropriate level of concern and action for the serious situation I took the score to represent. On the other hand, it was not terribly uncommon to see a score of 27, usually with each 3 circled in an emphatic way. I rarely had to address the most serious possible level of depression in those visits. I learned to take a score of 27 to mean "I am as miserable as I can possibly be. There can be no score that indicates more misery than I have. What are you going to do about it?" My patients were using the form of information that doctors pay attention to, data, as a means of communicating the intensity of their feelings about their care. Even data that we want to interpret as "objective" and "only about the patient, not a relationship" is about the relationship to some degree.

The high levels of life stress faced by some patients should be a consideration when determining what outcome measures are going to be chosen by a health system. The logic that was important in minimally disruptive medicine, trying to keep the footprint of treatment in the patient's life as small as possible, applies as well to these same patients when the data for evaluation is being considered. It is important to keep the footprint of data collection on the patients' care as small as possible, as little intrusive as possible. These are patients whose engagement may be tenuous. Assessing them can make them feel judged if they have no role in deciding what will be assessed. If patients experience partnership in relation to the data that was collected about them, they are more likely to try to cooperate in their interactions with our data collecting tools, just like partnership influences the way they make decisions about whether or not they follow the suggestions of their doctors.

Evaluating programs that serve multiply-disadvantaged patients requires consideration of the experiences and needs of the population. Patients with complex needs and complex treatment plans require longer evaluation times than are typical in healthcare. It may take several months to successfully house a patient for whom that step is the most important intervention and months after that for the benefits of the predictability of lower life stress that being housed provides to impact the person's health status [12]. Efforts to improve the lives of these patients are more complex and involve more types of services. The outcomes become harder to define. This is complicated by the heterogeneity of the population. Housing may be the key need of one patient, while transportation to a day treatment program may be the most important added service for another. The addition of a service somewhere outside the health system can be the change that, over time, makes the most difference in outcomes that are measured by the health system and for which the health system may be held accountable by payers. Raven, Romm, and Ajayi [12] stress principles for evaluating treatment for complex patients (1) allow adequate time to evaluate impact of a new element in a treatment plan, (2) look beyond dollars using validated tools to measure quality of life and use generally accepted values to measure the quality of the end of life, and (3) link existing data sets to discover more comprehensive program effects. While it is challenging to identify patterns that cross data sets from different services in a community, those patterns that can be identified will be particularly valuable in promoting collaboration among services. The launching of a medication-assisted treatment program for opioid use disorder in a primary care practice might lead to a reduction in recidivism in the local criminal justice system. It will take some forum for sharing efforts and results for a community to be able to identify these patterns.

12.4 Making Data Collection Support Partnership

In the context of partnership between a patient and the team, there would be some explanation, discussion, and (hopefully) agreement on what data to collect before a protocol for collecting information is set up. The conversation would address what information the data could provide, what types of patterns the team (including the patient) might see, and what the meanings of those possible patterns could be. The information would be experienced as facilitating the work of the whole team, which includes the patient, in the effort of keeping the patient healthy so that she/he can do the things they want to do in life.

Building partnership using data from the domain of the single patient can be done in at least two ways. The first is by considering the understanding and preferences of the patient in designating the information that is drawn from the data, and the second is by using data collected by the patient as a crucial part of the care the team provides.

A good example of changing the information drawn from data by considering the patient's understanding and preferences can be found in the routine practice of weighing patients at every visit. For many heavy patients, it is a moment of shame and perceived stigma. Patients commonly presume that the information collected and the pattern that their doctor observes are that they are too heavy and not losing weight. Doctors write the word "obese" in the record to indicate a specific range of BMI measures. Most patients read the word "obese" to mean "really fat." The only meaning many of these patients can imagine their health professionals are assigning to the pattern is that the patient continues to be personally weak and out of control of their lives. Some patients spend much of their visit distracted, waiting for their doctor to mention their weight. They don't feel less judged when the doctor makes no mention of it. They just assume the doctor is being polite about such an obvious personal flaw.

Yet there are multiple reasons for weighing patients beyond just to see if they are still heavy. How different might it be if the information shared when the patient was weighed went more like this:

MA taking the weight:	"Good, your weight is relatively stable. That is a good sign." Patient: "I'm still 5'4 and 180 lbs. How in the world is that a good sign?"
MA:	"If someone loses or gains a lot of weight between visits, it can mean many different things, good and bad. If they lose weight and don't mean to, it could mean that they have a cancer or some other serious condition that needs attention. So, knowing that your weight is stable helps the doctor rule out something serious going on that we don't know about."

The data is the same, but the information changes from "obese" to "stable" which changes the pattern the patient is likely to infer, from "really fat" to "still at the same weight." This might change the meaning of the patient from "my doctor thinks I am a failure" to "my doctor is watching out for changes in my health."

In the new world of patient portals and available test results, health professionals are sharing the data, but they often don't explain to the patient what information the health team is drawing from their data nor discuss the patterns HPs are looking for or what meanings they make of those patterns. Patients with low levels of activation are not likely to ask. If we want actions toward partnership from patients and from health providers, we have to create a shared understanding of the information that they observe in the patients' data and the patterns and meanings it supplies to them. Assertively soliciting or coaching patients to ask questions can gradually educate them about their health data and what it means [13]. In this way they become partners in receiving information and identifying patterns in their test results. Because the patient is the only member of their team who continuously observes their own life, stresses, and health behavior, they can observe patterns between their actions and the test results, patterns that are not available to the health professionals. Partnership with the patient improves the possibility of refining the patterns and the meanings that the healthcare team uses in their part of designing the patient's treatment.

An example of using data collected by the patient as a crucial part of the care that the team provides is the use of patient's tracking of their own health indicators. This can be a logical extension of the information taken in a patient's visit as they present the complaint that brought them. Imagine that the doctor asks how often the patient has the headaches that she came to talk about today. The patient reports that she is not sure, but she guesses it is about three or four times a week. The doctor then asks how intense the pain usually is on a scale of 1–10 and what sort of pain characterizes them, burning, stabbing, throbbing, or dull and where on the head she feels the pain. By this point many patients are not sure what to say. They weren't watching for all these aspects of a headache. At this point, the doctor might suggest that the patient get a pad of paper and keep track of her headaches for some number of days and bring the information to the next visit. She should note when she takes her medication, the number of her headaches, the time of day, the intensity, the character of the pain, the part of her head involved, and any other symptoms that occur with it. The *data* that the patient brings to the next visit provides *information* to the doctor, so he can find a *pattern*, allowing him to narrow down the possible headache type (*meaning*) and helping to make the decision about what *action* to take toward diagnosis or treatment. The patient becomes a partner in the process of her care by collecting data that only she has access to.

The T.E.A.M. Way of using tracking is not unique in the way it helps patients and clinicians gather data, but the way that data is used to create information and patterns is unusual if not unique. The T.E.A.M. Way looks for specific patterns in the patient's data, times when the patient succeeded or did not have as intense a loss of functioning as might have been expected. This approach to interpreting the data helps to give patients and other team members access to new information. In Chap. 8 we talked about empowering multiply-disadvantaged patients by focusing on their strengths or successes as a means to foster their engagement with their care team and vice versa. Tracking enables a patient to put their experience into data in a fashion that is easily understandable and offers access to patterns in their life and their health that will be meaningful to the patient and their team. Having data that the patient generated and understands allows the team and the patient to identify instances of successes or solutions, however nascent, by the way in which they approach the data. When the patient brings the tracking form to a visit, instead of studying the day those things were worst by looking at all the problem patterns surrounding that day, it is part of the empowering of the T.E.A.M. Way to study the day when things went best. If the patient was happiest on Tuesday, the team member should start there to understand what the patient did or thought that helped to create the best day. Another version of the same approach is to look at times when it would be natural to expect things to go poorly and they did not. Suppose the patient's energy level was the same on most days, but on 1 day their pain level went from 5 to 8. The team member might ask how the patient managed to keep their energy up even when faced with increased pain. Tracking allows for a patient to experience their own self-management successes and perhaps to accept activating attributions about their commitment to their health (see Chaps. 8 and 9).

While the data in one patient's tracking form cannot be aggregated with other patients' data (when one person says his happiness was a 5 out of 10, it is not possible to assume that the number represents the same experience as another person who reported the same score), the data is valid for the team and the patient who made the ratings. This is the type of data, in its collection and its interpretation, that builds partnership and opens new avenues for effective clinical conversation (see the Appendix for details on designing, using, and interpreting patient tracking using the approaches of the T.E.A.M. Way).

And in the future, we will see the continuing spread of health systems trying to support partnership by giving patients access to their medical record, a pattern coming to be reflected in the architecture of health data systems. The idea has moved from the patient having access to their test results and to communication with their doctor through a patient portal, to the patient having the ability to see their clinicians' notes (OpenNotes), to the idea that patients should "own" their individual record in some way and should have decision power over which professionals can access their health record. The patient's record would be separate from the EHR of any health setting. At this point, this is primarily a proposal that is being worked on by some data professionals in concert with a few medical professionals.

The concept of the patient file being separate from the electronic health record will make intuitive sense to some and will take others a while to fit into their understanding of software. Most computer users understand the difference between a file and a program. I can have a file that is a spreadsheet, for example, with the data that is the income and expenditures of my business for a year. Imagine that for the sake of security, I keep this spreadsheet on a detachable hard drive. It sits there and nowhere else. I want to assure myself that I am the only one who can access it. The file can be opened by a few different kinds of programs made by a few different software companies. I can open it in Excel, Google Sheets, and others. Each one can let me manipulate the data, find totals, add data, or graph monthly patterns. When the spreadsheet is saved again, it is changed in whatever way I have manipulated it, but it is the only place that my business information is kept. I don't need to keep it with my Excel or Google Sheets programs.

Peter Elias [14] is proposing a patient-centered health record in which the relationship of the patient file to the EHR that can manipulate the date in the file is analogous to the relationship of my spreadsheet and the programs (Excel, Google Sheets) that can manipulate its data. The patient-centered health record is an approach that embodies the ideal of a system in which the patient has full access to their health information and all records while controlling who else, professional or personal contact, can have access. The idea is that each person's health record would reside in "the cloud" and be available at all times to anyone to whom the patient gave access. When a professional in a health organization was given access, the professional could access the record through their EHR, modify the record to document the treatment of the patient, and then store it again in the patient's file back in the cloud. The information that was added would be added to the patient's health record, and the patient would have their usual access, and the health organization would continue to have access unless the patient withdrew it. When a patient sought care in a health setting, they would be required to give permission to the setting to access their record, which would have all previous health and care information about the patient. If the patient sought care with another clinician in another health organization, they would simply give permission for the second clinician's EMR to access their health record in the new organization's EMR. The new clinician would encounter a fully up-to-date record, and their additions would be ready for access by the patient or the next clinician involved. Within each organization, the data in the patient's record could be part of any manipulations the organization wished to make concerning its patients' data without compromising the organization's proprietary software. While this idea will take some standardization of the record format and interface between the file and EHRs, work to accomplish this is currently in progress in multiple venues.

Mark Byers [15] stresses the fundamental redefinition of electronic health record that occurs when it ceases to be solely a mode of retaining data and communicating that data between health professionals and administrators and becomes a mode of communication between health professionals and patients. The challenge for smooth movement of information is no less important in communicating with patients, but the additional functions of engaging and educating patients are added to data exchange. The addition of the patient as consumer of information in the EMR can facilitate the addition of the patient as provider of information. The patient is the best source to clear up a lack of clarity or redundancy of information.

But patient control is not partnership. It does not guarantee understanding by the patient, nor does it guarantee the confidence or willingness to participate. Early implementations of patient-centered data architectures have produced fairly low rates of acceptance and participation by both providers and patients [16]. The T.E.A.M. Way, with its focus on the skills needed by health professionals to craft a patient-centered care plan, teaches the development of partnership to take advantage of the opportunities provided by the newest data structures. One of the challenges in previous implementations of patient-centered care plans was the lack of the presentation of the care plan when new clinicians accessed the patient's record in the EMR in which it resided. When each patient's record is the only source of information about the patient for any healthcare service, the ability to design the presentation of the information, including the patient's self-description as elicited for the PCCP (see Chap. 10), makes the question of acceptance by patients and providers seem much more likely. The health goals identified in a patient-centered care plan provide an opportunity for patient-level outcomes to be measured across an organization without requiring that all patients be measured by the same outcomes.

The broad field of healthcare data is so large, so complex, and so fast moving that it is unrealistic to make specific suggestions meant to be useful for any reasonable time into the future, particularly in a book that is not constantly updated. It is easy to see how the constant innovation in how data can be collected, manipulated, interpreted, and communicated can make attention to the elegance of data systems much more compelling than focusing on the complexity and messiness of some patients' lives. My hope is that the discussion of partnership with patients in the creation and use of data will be an interesting challenge for many of the people who will be a part of the field's exciting future.

Appendix

Tracking Patient Data to Improve Partnership and Foster Clinical Improvement

Asking patients to keep track of some aspect(s) of their experience (symptoms, health behaviors, environmental challenges) is a common practice in medical care. The results of a patient's tracking can be used by the health professional and the patient for encouraging the patient or for problem-solving. The person who goes significantly off their diet on weekends or the smoker who lights up 30% more times on Mondays or the person with diabetes who has blood sugar readings that are significantly elevated on the mornings after days when he works late at the office; in each of these cases, there is an opportunity to discover the factors or barriers that effect the patient's self-management program. Finding out that the obese patient can't pass up the extra sweets when the family gets together on weekends, that the smoker drinks extra coffee to get going on Mondays and smokes with each cup, or that the person with diabetes has doughnuts to keep up their energy when they work late at the office each can help the patient and clinician focus on very particular skills that can help with the patient's self-management. In each case, the tracking results can augment the memory of the patient so that the problems are easier to define.

Tracking using the T.E.A.M. Way is particularly useful for working with patients with complex biological, psychological, and social health situations. It can be used by the doctor, the behavioral health clinician, or a care enhancer on the team. The elements of the patient's experience to be tracked are suggested by the clinician on the basis of the patient's narrative and have to be accepted as representing possibly useful information by the patient. The process supports partnership by giving an opportunity to validate the patient's concerns by having tangible follow-up on what the patient has identified and adding additional data on other elements of the patient's life experience that can contextualize and illuminate patterns in the patient's life that neither the clinician nor the patient currently know about. The tracking form is highly structured and yet gives a great deal of latitude in how it can be used (Table 12.2).

Each column allows a patient to track one element of their experience. Each row holds the rating on a simple scale (0–10 is most common) of the element or a total of the number of times that an element occurred. A small number of examples of events that might be counted are headaches, drinks, panic attacks, cigarettes, minutes of joy, minutes of enjoying child or spouse's company, minutes of exercise, ounces of sugared soda, washing of hands, rushed trips to the bathroom, and on and

Table 12.2 Blank tracking form

		Tracking form				
Name: _____				**Date:** _____		
	I am tracking	**I am tracking**	**I am tracking**	**I am tracking**	**I am tracking**	**I am tracking**
	_____	_____	_____	_____	_____	_____
	_____	_____	_____	_____	_____	_____
Date:	**How:**_____	**How:**_____	**How:**_____	**How:**_____	**How:**_____	**How:**_____
25-Sep						
26-Sep						
27-Sep						
28-Sep						
29-Sep						
30-Sep						
1-Oct						

on. A small number of examples of things that can be rated are pain, happiness, hope, productivity, stress of work, stress with family, relationship with some person, fear, confidence, and on and on. When possible, I find it useful to make 10 the desired end of the scale, though some elements, like pain, are so commonly structured with 10 as the most undesired end that changing would confuse the patient. Occasionally the tracking will be a yes or no answer each day when it monitors the occurrence or nonoccurrence of some event. The patient is always told to fill out the sheet at the same time of day and to estimate, not to take up time in the day with counting or rating. It is important to keep the process from intruding in the day any more than necessary.

When choosing elements to be tracked, the symptoms or occurrences that are most concerning to the patient should be in the first column(s). The next columns can track events or actions that could be related to the occurrence of the chief concerns, other events or actions that might offer alternative theories about what leads to the symptoms, and events or actions that can be examples of successful coping or relating or improvements on the part of the patient.

The choices made in defining the elements to be observed can open opportunities for collecting new patterns from the patient's life, often impacting their experience and their behavior. Keep in mind that any aspect of a person's experience that becomes their focus is likely to become more prominent in their assessment of themselves or the people around them. For example, observing the number of minutes that a parent enjoys having their child around can set a different tone and a new perception of the child as opposed to a rating of how bad the child's behavior was on the same day. A parent who begins to notice enjoying a child's company will be likely to give different cues to the child about how their behavior is being experienced, eliciting somewhat different behavior from the child. In the repetitive sequences of interaction between people, a change at any point in the sequence can lead to subsequent changes on both sides as the sequence progresses.

When going over a tracking sheet with a patient, the clinician focuses on the day that went best, not the one that was worst.

Example

Clinician: "Wow, you had some very difficult times this week. I am struck by what happened on Tuesday. That was the day you rated highest for happiness, even though you were at your usual level of pain. What was it that happened on Tuesday that made it the happiest day?"

Patient: "I guess it was the time I got to spend with my granddaughter. She always cheers me up."

Clinician: "What is it about being with her that you enjoy so much."

Patient: "I guess it is because I am helping my daughter and doing something fun at the same time. My granddaughter just wants me to read and play games. She doesn't ask me about my pain all the time."

Clinician: "I notice that your pain was a little higher the next day. Did you expect that?"

Patient: "Oh, yes, I knew it was coming, but it was worth it."

Clinician: "Sounds like you are willing to take on extra pain if it benefits the ones
               you love. Is that typical of you that you sacrifice for others?"
Patient: "Yup. I have always been like that."
Clinician: "How about if we add a new column for the number to times you did
               something to help somebody else on each day? Then we can look for
               times when you could be helpful and not increase your pain because of
               it."

Tracking offers the possibility of using data collected by the patient to create
patterns of information that are new to both the clinician and the patient, patterns
which can be highlighted by the clinician to support the meanings that are particularly useful in the T.E.A.M. Way.[2] The tracking result gave the clinician the opportunity to identify an incident of strength in that the patient helps even when she was
in her usual level of pain (empowerment). From that event, the clinician could make
an attribution that the patient accepted (activation) using types of data suggested by
the clinician and kept by the patient (mutual). These new types of attributions
become part of the conception of the patient's character and life situation that are
reflected in the clinician's notes to which the patient has access (transparency).

Many health professionals reading this account have already said to themselves
that however great this tracking can be, it is not likely that most patients, especially
multiply-disadvantaged patients, will do it or if they do it, they will forget to bring
it in. This happens, but much less commonly if tracking is introduced as a "no-fail"
exercise. Usually patients are interested in the process of choosing the elements to
be tracked and in the explanation of how the tracking is done. At the point that it is
time to give the fully constructed form to the patient, the clinician stops the process,
while they are still holding the form. The clinician instructs the patient that if filling
out the form might add any stress to their already very stressful life, the patient is
not to do it at all. If filling it out on a particular day is inconvenient for any reason,
even if they just don't feel like it, they are not to do it that day. They can start filling
it out again on another day. Any data is helpful, but only if it is not making things
worse for the patient. Noting that the patient already has enough stress in their life
will get agreement from almost anyone. In essence, the clinician is trying to fore-
close the possibility that the patient feels the tracking is something they were told to
do. It is something they were told not to do if they didn't feel like doing it. This
tends to greatly increase the number who bring it back.

If the patient does not bring back the form, the clinician thanks them. Most
patients will be curious at this response, though it is a sincere appreciation. The
clinician notes that she/he had asked the patient not to do the tracking form if it was
not a fit for them and their lives. They have done just what the clinician suggested.
The partnership is affirmed. In many cases, the patient, seeing that the clinician
appreciates what they have done, will offer to try again to fill it out or to remember
to bring it to the visit. At the second visit with no tracking results, it makes sense for

---

[2] See Blount and Adler (2008) for a detailed example of the use of tracking in a successful team-
based brief treatment of a young man with somatization disorder.

the clinician to live up to their instructions about not doing what is stressful or inconvenient and stop the process. The partnership will have been shown to be the most important goal. Even when it is successful, the process of tracking should be continually assessed for its contribution to the ongoing partnership and to the treatment. When it stops generating new patterns of information from which new and useful meanings can be drawn, it should be discontinued.

Case Example

A 48-year-old man named Jim Roberts comes for a review of his hypertension medication. In addition to hypertension, he has a BMI of 32, chronic knee pain, and a distant history of alcohol abuse. His BP is 150/90, better than it was in the past, but not at target. The visit is uneventful. Toward the end, the doctor offers him congratulations that he has a better BP, but he replies, "To tell you the truth, Doc, I don't care as much as I used to. I haven't been sleeping that good. When I'm not at work, I don't have the energy to do much of anything. I haven't been to a choir practice at church in a long time. My wife and the kids go out and do things, but I just don't feel like going. I am mostly just sitting around the house eating and gaining weight. I don't know what's wrong with me."

The doctor is quietly dismayed. This was supposed to be one of the less complex visits of the day. He has known Mr. Roberts for a while. Jim is not a complainer. The visit had a clear focus, and the doctor had expected it to go quickly. Now he is looking at a need to follow up on sleep, fatigue, weight, and probably on depression. The patient already listed four symptoms of depression (doesn't care or anhedonia, loss of energy, weight change, poor sleep) before he was asked any questions about it. Rather than trying to follow up on several discrete issues, or telling Mr. Roberts that he doesn't have time for all the issues he named, the doctor decides to use tracking and an early next visit to see if Jim's many complaints can be related and might generate a pattern. It takes about 5 minutes to set up the tracking form and give him the necessary instructions about not letting the process add stress. In this case, the doctor suggested items for Jim to track based on his concerns, the doctor's concerns for Jim, and the doctor's experience that when people find they spend more enjoyable time with their family, they tend to be less depressed, with less background stress and easier BP control. The choice of the wording for the assessment of depression was to track something that the HP and the patient would like to see more of, since in general when you start watching some element that was unnoticed before, it tends to occur more often. Jim Roberts leaves happy, in that he feels his doctor took him seriously. He is also interested in what keeping track of these aspects of his life might discover (Table 12.3).

One might think that the focus would be on Wednesday when the tracking form was discussed. It was clearly the worst day. The T.E.A.M. Way would suggest that this set of patient-collected data is an opportunity for finding strengths and solutions that can build an engagement, increase the patient's feeling of self-efficacy, and provide the data for reframing the patient's situation. In this approach, the first question would be more likely to be something like:

Table 12.3 Jim Roberts' tracking form

		Tracking form				
Name:	**Jim Roberts**			**Date: Sept 24**		
	I am tracking	I am tracking	I am tracking	I am tracking	I am tracking	I am tracking
	I am happy and energetic	**# hrs sleep in last 24**	**I ate right today**	**Enjoyed time with family**	**BP at bed time**	**drinks in last 24 hrs**
Date:	How: **1–10**	How: **#**	How: **1–10**	How: **# mins**	How: **homecuff**	How: **#**
Tu-9/25	3	6	3	20	156/92	4
W-9/26	2	5	4	0	160/90	2
Th-9/27	6	5	5	45	153/88	1
F-9/28	6	6	5	35	150/85	1
Sa-9/29	5	6	4	60	150/84	0
Su-9/30	6	7	6	45	147/80	1
M-10/1	7	7	7	40	145/80	0

It looks like Wednesday was your lowest day in terms of your happiness and energy, and yet you came roaring back on Thursday. Even though you didn't get a lot of sleep the night before, you drank less, you spent a lot of enjoyable time with your family, and even your eating pattern was a little better. Is there anything that you did or that someone else did that helped you make those improvements on that day?

Notice that you don't expect every element to go up or down together. You pick the patterns that seem to support the empowerment and activation aspects of the T.E.A.M. Way while still being open to data that counters the meanings you are looking for. If someone's data takes a terrible dive at some point in the tracking period, you would ask about the events that surrounded the plunge, but once you knew that the events did not seem to be the beginning of a new and concerning pattern, you would spend much more attention on whatever process the patient showed in getting back on track.

Tracking can lose its impact over time as the data starts to show consistency in improved or not improved patterns in the data. At that point, it can be dropped, and the conversation between the patient and the health practitioner shifts toward the ways that the patient is keeping their life and health on track for the improved patterns. Often this is at about the third to fifth iteration. If there are elements that have showed no improvement and are concerning, a new approach can be tried for impacting those elements, with new types of tracking used if appropriate. When this happens it can also be appropriate to go to another approach than tracking. And at any time that the patient seems less interested or committed, the process should be discontinued.

References

1. Institute of Medicine. Crossing the quality chasm: a new health system for the 21st century. Washington, DC: National Academies Press; 2001.
2. Berwick DM. A primer on leading the improvement of systems. BMJ. 1996;312:619–22.
3. Agency for Healthcare Research and Quality. https://www.ahrq.gov/professionals/quality-patient-safety/quality-resources/tools/literacy-toolkit/healthlittoolkit2-tool2b.html. Downloaded 25 Oct 2018.
4. Frampton S, Guastello S, Hoy L, Naylor M, Sheridan S, Johnston-Fleece M. Harnessing evidence and experience to change culture: a guiding framework for patient and family engaged care. National Institute of Medicine. 2017. https://nam.edu/harnessing-evidence-and-experience-to-change-culture-a-guiding-framework-for-patient-and-family-engaged-care/
5. Mutter JB, Liaw W, Moore MA, Etz RS, Howe A, Bazemore A. Core principles to improve primary care quality management. J Am Board Fam Med. 2018;31:931–40.
6. Morse J, Valeras AS, Geffken D, et al. Using a team approach to address avoidable emergency department utilization and re-hospitalizations as symptoms of complexity through quality improvement methodology. In: Sturmberg JP, editor. The value of systems and complexity sciences in healthcare. New York: Springer; 2006. p. 231–8.
7. Doherty WJ, Mendenhall TJ. Citizen health care: a model for engaging patients, families, and communities as coproducers of health. Fam Syst Health. 2006;24(3):251–63.
8. Doyle M. What is the difference between data and information? DQ Global Blog. 2014. https://www.dqglobal.com
9. Hibbard JH, Stockard J, Mahoney ER, Tusler M. Development of the Patient Activation Measure (PAM): conceptualizing and measuring activation in patients and consumers. Health Serv Res. 2004;39:1005–26.
10. Dixon A, Hibbard J, Tusler M. How do people with different levels of activation self-manage their chronic conditions? Patient. 2009;2:257–68.
11. Kroenke K, Spitzer RL, Williams J. The PHQ-9: validity of a brief depression severity measure. J Gen Intern Med. 2001;16:606–13.
12. Raven MC, Romm IK, Ajayi T. Evaluating complex care programs: is it a zero-sum game? NEJM Catalyst. May 15, 2017.
13. Kaplan SH, Greenfield S, Ware JE. Assessing the effects of physician-patient interactions on the outcomes of chronic disease. Med Care. 1989;27:S110–27.
14. Elias P. The patient-centered health record. 2016. http://thehealthcareblog.com/
15. Byers M. EHR integration: keeping patients at the center. July 24, 2015. http://HealthcareItNews.com.
16. Krist AH, Woolf SH, Bello GA, et al. Fam Med. 2014;12:418–26.

Resources

Data Synthesizers

I2I
Innovacer

PDSA Cycle

Agency for Healthcare Research and Quality
Institute for Health Improvement
AMA – Steps Forward

Patients and Families in QI

https://www.nichq.org/resource/family-engagement-guide-role-family-health-partners-quality-
improvement-within-pediatric
Patient-Reported Outcomes Measurement Information System - short form. (Promis Global 10)
https://www.codetechnology.com/promis-global-10/

Chapter 13
Articulating the Model

In the USA and around the world, the more robust a nation's primary care service, the better are the health markers seen in the population, and the lower the comparative cost of healthcare. In the USA, primary care has been under stress for some time, under-supported financially with too small physician workforce and overtaxed by demands to impact the population as a whole. The Institute of Medicine (IOM) and other leaders have attempted to remedy the quality problems of the healthcare system by calling for a reorganization of primary care into a medical home that is patient-centered, evidence-based, offering improved access, better ongoing contact, and coordination of care [1]. In a medical home, care would be delivered by a team, taking pressure off the physician who was leading the team and adding resources for increased patient engagement and support. A medical home would be self-improving through the use of relevant data on its own functioning and its effectiveness with its patients. It would be supported through payment systems that reward the maintenance of health rather than the delivery of service.

The IOM's ten rules for the redesign of healthcare include some that are focused on systems change in the delivery of care and others that are focused on change in the relationships of doctors (and other health professionals) with their patients. The systems change rules have been easier to implement. These have been associated with improved health markers and lower cost of care for many patients. The improvements associated with the change of the relationship of the physician and healthcare team to the patient have not been nearly as impressive, and some have said that to fully achieve these changes requires a change in the "mental models of care". It is in this area that the next steps in patient-centered care can be achieved, especially for patients with complex health needs. Therefore, it is in this area that the next steps to a more equitable delivery of healthcare must take place.

The transition to team-based care within primary care is a foundational step in building an environment that promotes the sort of relationship between patients and clinicians that is truly patient-centered. Changing from an individual provider with staff support to a team is the first step in the change in "mental models of care" called for by the evaluators of the National Demonstration Program [2]. The change

© Springer Nature Switzerland AG 2019
A. Blount, *Patient-Centered Primary Care*,
https://doi.org/10.1007/978-3-030-17645-7_13

can be characterized as a change from a squad to a team. It is a transition from a small group that is hierarchical with an unchanging leader to a group with greater participation among team members and flexibility in leadership. This change gives greater flexibility in the delivery of the services that make a difference to patients. It has been shown to lead to improvement in group cohesion, improved patient satisfaction, improved quality of services, and lower burnout for both clinicians and support staff. Many general descriptions of a well-functioning team are available in the literature, but there is comparatively little guidance concerning the steps that should be taken to develop a team that meets these descriptions. One requirement that seems to be emerging is the dedication of time for team meetings, both daily and weekly, that is commensurate with the importance of the team's successful functioning to the successful delivery of care. Others are steps such as the same team members consistently working together, daily preparation for care using huddles, regular conversations about mission, mutual participation in the review of quality data, and iterative innovations aimed at improvements are a start in overcoming the legacy of the squad organization.

For practices that are attempting to develop patient-centered team-based care, the addition of a behavioral health clinician (BHC) is a logical step along the way. When done well, adding a behavioral health clinician enhances the fit of the expertise of the team to the needs of many of its patients. Behavioral healthcare within the primary care practice greatly increases access for patients by being a better fit to their understanding of their needs and therefore increasing its acceptability. The patterns of communication among team members that make for successful team-based care are the same ones that make for successful integration of a behavioral health clinician. The expertise that is added to the team by a behavioral health clinician can help to foster the change in "mental models of care" that has been discussed as underlying the transition to both patient-centered and team-based primary care. In addition, for patients with significant challenges in the area of the "social determinants of health," a team member who is able to enhance the care provided by the team, sometimes called a navigator, care manager, or health coach (i.e., a "care enhancer") [3], is also a crucial part of an effective team.

Over time, the IOM's call for patients to be the source of control in their care has been represented differently from the original ideas presented in the Quality Chasm report. The definition of "the patient as the source of control" has evolved from the clinician's taking the patient's preferences and values into account in designing care to a partnership between the clinician and the patient in making the choices necessary to plan care. This is a particularly challenging standard because both health professionals and many of their patients have been socialized to the model of the doctor leading the care. Even when both the doctor and the patient would endorse the idea of partnership, their difference in knowledge and in their perspective on the patient's illness makes partnership difficult. One group of authors termed the pattern of communication created by the difference in approach to the illness between the doctor's knowledge, training, and protocols on one hand and the patient's experience of their illness and the demands that it places on their life, on the other, "parallel play" [4]. This makes partnership challenging, even if the difference in levels of knowledge about the patient's illness is reduced by patient teaching based on the patient's health literacy.

A number of programmatic approaches to improving doctor-patient communication been offered in the hopes of improving patients' participation in their treatment and in making themselves healthier. Motivational interviewing, shared decision-making, minimally disruptive medicine, addressing health literacy, relationship-centered care, and coaching patients to be more assertive in relating to their physician, each of these approaches can be an important contribution, and each one demands extra attention and time to be effectively taught and implemented. In all these approaches, in as much as they call for a change in the feelings or thoughts about the patient on the part of health professionals, there is the risk of the "be spontaneous" paradox, an expectation that the professionals deliver, when instructed to do so, reactions toward the patient that are inherently spontaneous, and not possible to be produced on demand. Successful transition of health professionals' understanding of their complex patients is likely to be based on new routines of practice that lead to new ways of experiencing these patients and subsequently to new feelings or thoughts about them.

For an important group of patients, the divide created by their differences in knowledge and perspective from their doctors and their health teams is a chasm. These patients are variously identified in different parts of the literature, as "complex" (either because they utilize so much care or because they bring multiple chronic illnesses plus behavioral health diagnoses), as "deprived" because they are coping with challenges of low income and struggles with the "social determinants of health," or as "trauma victims" because they report high levels of adverse childhood experiences and exhibit the high levels of chronic illness, mental health problems, and substance abuse issues associated with these experiences. In the literature on the doctor-patient relationship, they are sometimes called "heartsink" patients [5] because their expectations of their doctors and their doctors' expectations of how patients should behave are so wildly at odds.

Doctors and other health professionals commonly make assumptions about the ability of these patients to be active parts of the development of their treatment plans. Even doctors and health professionals who are interested in partnership are likely to adjust their approaches to their care, using behaviors that are less patient-centered rather than more so. For their part, these patients are less likely to trust their relationship with the members of their healthcare team and to be less confident in their own ability to improve their health states. For many such patients, their likelihood of adhering to a medical regimen is correlated with their experience of the caring and support coming from their healthcare providers. Their relationship with their doctor can become a reciprocal interactive process, featuring negative generalizations about the other which underlie the failure of partnership. The best of team-based patient-centered care is required to develop a different interaction pattern in the care of these patients. Trauma-informed care (TIC) can provide guideposts needed to develop a pathway to partnership and healing for these patients and their healthcare teams. There is no generally used term that reflects the complexity of these patient's challenges with life and with the healthcare system. As we go forward in outlining a method for engaging these patients in patient-centered care, the term "multiply-disadvantaged" patients will be the most common term we will use, though from time to time, we will use terms such as "complex patients" depending on the context and the literature being reviewed.

To engage multiply-disadvantaged patients in self-management, the relationship between the patient, the doctor, and other members of the team is the first consideration. A robust approach combines what is known about caring for these patients in multiple literatures, combining the care management and team approach of the "complex" patient literature with the respect and cultural competence of the low-income patient literature and the support and refusal to be directive and re-traumatizing of the trauma-informed care (TIC) literature. The delivery of integrated primary care, including behavioral health clinicians and care enhancers, is particularly crucial in the success of patient-centered care for these patients. In addition, using skills learned from primary care behavioral health practice can help promote a culture in the team that generates the new mental models of care and the corresponding routines of practice needed for developing true partnership with these challenging patients. These new routines of practice can be characterized by the mnemonic, T.E.A.M., for Transparent, Empowering, Activating, and Mutual.

The relationship of multiply-disadvantaged patients with their health professionals is often characterized by a lack of transparency on both sides. In order to allow the kind of communication that builds trust, increases patient adherence, lowers healthcare costs, and improves the care experience and the health of the patient, increasing transparency is important. Transparency in doctor-patient relationships generally has taken a big step forward with the wide implementation of "OpenNotes," a software that allows patients to read their doctors' notes about their care. Open notes, as a concept, is appreciated by patients more readily than doctors; however, doctors have generally come to like it in practice. For multiply-disadvantaged patients with complex illnesses, low SES, or who are members of minority groups, i.e., patients for whom trust and adherence have tended to be more difficult, open notes have been particularly effective and appreciated. When notes are available to patients, researchers in the field suggest that doctors should adjust their language a bit to make the notes more engaging. It is important, however, that the notes' usefulness as communication with other professionals or with monitors of quality care not be compromised. The adjustments in language, while not extensive, can make the notes a positive clinical tool. Guidance on "reframing" from behavioral health literature can be useful to the team's learning to be comfortable with these changes. These same adjustments can be used to allow clinical conversations between team members about patients to occur in the presence of the patient, enabling much more meaningful patient participation in their care. The practice of speaking about the patient in the patient's presence can allow a much more effective transfer of positive relationship with the patient from one team member to other members of the team. This improves the ability of the whole team to treat the patient efficiently and makes the process more rewarding for the team members and the patient.

Empowerment of patients is a critical element in primary care that improves clinical outcomes and lowers costs. Patients who experience themselves as partners with their doctors are generally more active in caring for their own health. For multiply-disadvantages patients, the steps to partnership have to include both building trust in their health professionals and developing the experience of self-efficacy in relation to their lives and their health. For these patients the definition of empowerment that is used in trauma-informed care, that care is built on enhancing strengths rather than highlighting deficits, offers a place to start. The methodology of solution-focused interviewing provides a pathway to achieving this sort of empowerment. Solution-focused approaches to communication have an empowering effect for both patients and professionals. These methods can be adapted smoothly to the communication with patients of doctors, behavioral health clinicians, care managers, and other team members. Approaching treatment with multiply-disadvantaged patients by building on patients' strengths in self-care and their histories of coping in their lives can be the step to empowerment that is the foundation for the shared decision-making called for by the IOM. The enhancement of self-confidence and self-efficacy of patients and their healthcare team members based on evidence from the fields of neuroscience and memory makes sensible the use of interviewing techniques that otherwise might be counterintuitive to many health professionals.

The concept of patient activation is one of an array of concepts designed to help health professionals encourage patients, particularly patients with chronic illnesses, to be active in caring for themselves. These concepts began to be developed by researchers when the evidence became overwhelming that simply instructing patients on how to care for themselves was inadequate to produce the required health behaviors, especially for patients with complex biological, psychological, and social challenges. The Patient Activation Measure has proved to do an excellent job at distinguishing which patients are most likely to be successful at self-care. While the PAM can identify a group of patients as having low activation, professionals gain options when they consider these patients in terms other than their low level of activation. In general, these are the same patients designated as complex and as needing care management, as disadvantaged and as needing information targeted to their health literacy, and as patients with a high likelihood with traumatic experiences as measured on the ACEs screen and needing trauma-informed care. They tend to be multiply-disadvantaged patients. We have described previously the way in which a solution-focused approach can be adapted to fostering patient empowerment. If we consider the evidence of the impact of changing expectations between helper and client from Rosenthal's work on the Pygmalion effect, we find support for an approach that uses explicit attributions about patients to change the expectation of the patients' success at self-management on the part of both health professionals and the patients themselves. Attributions of activated intent or behavior that are believable to patients about themselves, when delivered by health professionals, can have an activating impact on patients toward better self-management.

Transparency, empowerment, and activation can be supported by institutionalizing the mutual creation of the treatment plan that guides patients' care in their primary care and in the health system more generally. A care plan is a brief distillation of the information that is needed to inform a successful treatment. It includes an assessment of a patient's needs, the medical and social history necessary to understand those needs, and the general steps planned to address them. The desire of patients to participate in creating the documentation of their care that emerged in the pilot of OpenNotes can be addressed and made central to the design of their care through a process called a patient-centered care plan. A patient-centered care plan elicits a patient's self-description, values, and preferences needed to help health professionals work together with multiply-disadvantaged patients successfully. For patients who are likely to have a history of difficult experiences in the healthcare system, the patients' view of the ways that their health teams should relate to them in difficult moments can be part of keeping partnership intact through difficult or upsetting times. When done well, multiple members of the team, including the patient, are involved in creating a document that reflects the patients' ideas and values on which a successful relationship would be built.

Growing an expert team is more a matter of building a culture than implementing a model. Enacting the T.E.A.M. Way of working with multiply-disadvantaged patients requires learning new behaviors on the part of every team member. Rather than a primary focus on the training of individuals and the implementation of new routines, the success of the endeavor is built on a process of team learning through mutual experience. Team learning develops over time through mutual observation and feedback, sharing narratives of individual experience, mutual practice of new skills, and problem-solving meetings with patients and their families. As the team proceeds, some of the basic assumptions team members hold about patients and their care evolve, just as is called for by the IOM in the Quality Chasm report. This learning creates value for the practice and for the individuals involved.

Professionals who learn to use transparent notes, to engage in transparent clinical conversations, who use solution-focused interviewing in their exchanges with patients, who are able to use targeted attributions to support patient activation for health, and who are able to combine these skills to create a patient-centered care plan will have opportunities in other settings and will not be easy to replace. Without a plan to maintain the team, each departing member takes with them an important piece of team culture. One approach to maintaining the expert team is to help each member take on a training role for future professionals. New professionals provide a reserve workforce to maintain the knowledge and functioning of the team as a whole, and learning to train new professionals solidifies the gains in skills of current team members. A second approach is to build a career ladder within the organization so that the increase in expertise of team members can be reflected in increases in salary and responsibility. When an increase in responsibility must be supported by additional credentials, the option to obtain those credentials while keeping their employment and salary can make the difference in retaining or losing a valuable team member. An example of a way of creating such a career ladder has been created by the New Hampshire Primary Care Behavioral Health Initiative.

In order for the team, including the patient, to refine and improve the care plan, they need regularly collected, up to date, actionable information about their own functioning in relation to the goals of the plan. The current requirements on primary care in relation to information that is collected and that can be delivered to larger health systems, regulators, and payers are daunting. Adding additional information to be collected is likely to be acceptable to team members only if it can be done with little increase in time spent and then only if it immediately useful in improving care. The personalizing of information to be collected, based on the goals in the PCCP, can contribute to the activation of the patient in the role of data source on their own functioning for review with the team, either face to face or through asynchronous communication at a distance. In this way the care plan continues to provide guidance and structure to the team as it evolves to reflect the refinements contributed by team members including the patient. Rather than specify what information should be collected for all patients, this approach allows the team and the patient to identify easily obtainable information that is most meaningful in assessing the progress of the team in carrying out the treatment plan. In the long run, changes in the architecture of EHRs and the addition of new add-on software, such as the addition of OpenNotes or population health management packages, have facilitated advances in patient-centered care. Continued changes on the horizon can be even more effective in developing agency for patients and their partnership with health professionals.

Each element of the T.E.A.M. Way is based on evidence though its diverse elements require a synthesis of elements from several domains. Team-based patient-centered primary care as a general effort has moved forward with an iterative approach adding one targeted innovation to another to try to engage the most complex patients. The T.E.A.M. Way synthesizes these varied steps into an approach which could be called a "meta-integration" of behavioral health in primary care. Rather than being built solely on the integration of behavioral health clinicians, the T.E.A.M. Way leverages the work of every team member, without changing their role, to forward a behaviorally enhanced pathway to partnership with multiply-disadvantaged patients. This makes it truly possible to offer patient-centered care, in the form of partnership between patients and their health team, to everyone.

References

1. Institute of Medicine. Crossing the quality chasm: a new health system for the 21st century. Washington, DC: National Academy Press; 2001.
2. Crabtree B, Nutting P, Miller W, Stange K, Stewart E, Jaén C. Summary of the National Demonstration Project and recommendation for the patient-centered medical home. Ann Fam Med. 2010;8., Supplement 1:S80–90.
3. Blount A, Fauth J, Nordstrom A, Pearson S. Who will provide integrated care: assessing the workforce for the integration of behavioral health and primary care in New Hampshire. Concord: Endowment for Health; 2017.
4. Kruse RL, Olsberg JE, Shigaki CL, Oliver D, Vetter-Smith M, Day T, LeMaster J. Communication during patient-provider encounters regarding diabetes self-management. Fam Med. 2013;45:475–83.
5. O'Dowd TC. Five years of 'heartsink' patients in general practice. BMJ. 1988;297:528–30.

Index

© Springer Nature Switzerland AG 2019
A. Blount, *Patient-Centered Primary Care*,
https://doi.org/10.1007/978-3-030-17645-7

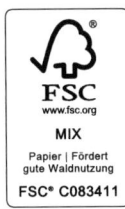

Zeitfracht Medien GmbH
Ferdinand-Jühlke-Straße 7
99095 Erfurt, Deutschland
produktsicherheit@kolibri360.de